MEDICAL PROCEDURES FOR REFERRAL

MEDICAL PROCEDURES FOR REFERRAL

Practical Information for Physicians

RICHARD SADOVSKY, M.D.
author and editor

DAVID H. GORDON
RICHARD M. STILLMAN

MEDICAL ECONOMICS BOOKS
ORADELL, NEW JERSEY 07649

Library of Congress Cataloging-in-Publication Data
Sadovsky, Richard.
  Medical procedures for referral: practical information for
  physicians/Richard Sadovsky, David H. Gordon, Richard M. Stillman.
  Includes bibliographies and index.
  ISBN 0-87489-498-0
  1. Medical protocols. 2. Medical consultation. 3. Family
medicine. 4. Patient education. I. Gordon, David H.
II. Stillman, Richard M., 1947- . III. Title.
[DNLM: 1. Diagnosis—methods. 2. Referral and Consultation. WB
141 S126m]
RC64.S23   1989
616.07'5—dc20
DNLM/DLC
for Library of Congress   89-3287
                                                                          CIP

ISBN 0-87489-498-0

Medical Economics Company Inc.
Oradell, New Jersey 07649

Printed in the United States of America

The authors and publisher have exerted every effort to ensure that drug selection,
dosage, and therapeutic modalities set forth in this text are in accord with current
recommendations and practice at the time of publication. However, in view of ongoing research, changes in government regulations, and the constant flow of information relating to drug therapy, and drug reactions, the reader is urged to check the
package insert for each drug for any change in indications and dosage and for added
warnings and precautions. This is particularly important when the recommended
agent is a new or infrequently employed drug.

To Tom for his ideas and Paul for his encouragement

R.S.

Contents

Authors

Richard Sadovsky M.D.
Associate Professor and Associate Chairman
Department of Family Practice
SUNY Health Science Center at Brooklyn

David H. Gordon M.D.
Professor of Radiology
SUNY Health Science Center
at Brooklyn

Richard M. Stillman M.D.
Attending Surgeon
Northwest Regional Hospital
Margate, Florida
West Boca Raton Medical
Center
Boca Raton, Florida

Contributing Authors

Michael J. H. Akerman M.D.
Assistant Professor of Medicine
SUNY Health Science Center at
Brooklyn

Howell R. Goldfarb M.D.
Clinical Assistant Instructor of
Anesthesiology
SUNY Health Science Center at
Brooklyn

Roger W. Kula M.D.
Associate Professor of
Neurology
SUNY Health Science Center at
Brooklyn

Matthew Lefkowitz M.D.
Assistant Professor of
Anesthesiology
SUNY Health Science Center at
Brooklyn

Justin McKendry M.D.
Clinical Assistant Instructor of
Anesthesiology
SUNY Health Science Center at
Brooklyn

Jeffrey Schwartz M.D.
Postdoctoral Fellow in
Anesthesiology
Columbia-Presbyterian Hospital

Peter R. Smith M.D.
Assistant Professor of Medicine
SUNY Health Science Center at
Brooklyn

Arnold M. Strashun M.D.
Associate Professor of
Radiology
SUNY Health Science Center at
Brooklyn

Joel Mann Yarmush M.D.
Clinical Assistant Instructor of
Anesthesiology
SUNY Health Science Center at
Brooklyn

Foreword

There was no need for a book of this kind when I graduated from medical school in 1950. Sending a patient for a urinalysis, CBC, chest x-ray, or upper GI hardly produced white knuckles or an acute anxiety attack. Today, the primary-care physician has access to a multitude of complicated technological procedures, both for diagnosis and for management, that may indeed cause anxiety among patients and their families.

The caring physician wants to prepare the patient for the trials and tribulations of progress through a complicated series of examinations, as well as have each patient share in health decision making. The primary-care physician may be well versed in analyzing the *results* of such technological powerhouses as CT scans, procedures in nuclear medicine, cardiac catheterization and others, but he or she may have never witnessed these procedures or become fully aware of the preparation, discomfort, or risk that the patient goes through while submitting to such examinations.

Time has marched past some of us, and the tests that are constantly being developed and the procedures that accompany them may tax our knowledge of their complexity and risks. Being of an "older" generation, I now have the dubious distinction of not only being a physician but also a patient. I have recognized that my colleagues, either because they do not wish to acknowledge that my physician's fund of knowledge may have eroded somewhat or because they themselves may be unable to discuss the complexities of the various technological procedures that I have to experience, have left me completely in the dark. I have been acutely aware of the potential anxiety of "not knowing," and I find that I am a less cooperative and less manageable patient under these circumstances.

With this background, I had hoped that someone would develop a book of the kind that you will soon be using as a reference when discussing potential diagnostic procedures and complicated management scenarios with your patients and asking them to help with their own health decision making. I believe that the authors of this book have accomplished the task to my satisfaction. It is not possible to review every procedure, but it is possible to take those most common procedures that may indeed produce some anxiety and put them together in a compendium of the kind that the authors of this book have designed. I believe that the primary-care physician will feel much more comfortable in dealing with the patient who has an impending examination by being able to pick up this book from the corner of the desk and saying to the patient, "Please sit down and I will review for you what to expect when you have your test."

Thomas L. Stern, M.D.

Preface

The primary-care physician uses both medical and educational skills in recommending medical procedures for diagnostic and therapeutic purposes. Decisions are made about the procedure's likelihood to provide the desired information or results without undesirable after effects. Once these decisions are made, the primary care provider's work has just begun.

Patients want to be informed about the procedures being planned. Full information exchange is required for medicolegal reasons about all potentially hazardous procedures, but the need for patient/physician rapport and understanding underscores this information exchange. The physician who simply tells a patient about a medical procedure without any explanation or communication violates the law and jeopardizes future efforts to improve the patient's health. Patients want to know more, and they have a right to know more.

The primary care physician's obligation does not end with the planning of the procedure and appropriate referral along with explanation of the procedure. Additional questions may arise prior to the date set for the procedure from the patient or other family members. The physician must be prepared and willing to respond to these questions, and this, in itself, is not only an obligation but a gratifying aspect of communication between patient and trusted care giver. After the procedure has been performed, the referring physician again becomes the interpreter and further manager of the results. This involves resolving short-term problems, complications, or questions that arise following the procedure.

For the primary-care physician to provide appropriate referrals, educate the patient about a procedure, use the procedure results in ongoing care decisions, and manage any long- and short-term complications of the procedure, some intimacy is required with modern diagnostic and therapeutic procedural techniques. This book is written to help the physician review many of the procedures now in common use. Written specifically for the primary-care provider, the book contains short but comprehensive reviews of indications, contraindications, patient education information, and potential complications of a number of procedures for which primary-care physicians routinely refer patients. An additional section accompanying each procedure description clearly discusses the questions and concerns most often held by patients about specific procedures. The goal is to have the patient understand:

- The reason for the procedure or test
- How it will be performed
- Potential risks and benefits
- Alternative ways of obtaining the needed information or obtaining the desired results
- References if desired for further information.

The referring physician is obligated to be knowledgeable about the complications of procedures. Patients are often unwilling or unable to reach the physician or operator who performed the procedure. To provide follow-up care, an understanding of postprocedure instructions and potential problems with accompanying consequences is required. These are described here for each of the procedures discussed.

It would be impossible to include all the procedures known to medicine in a book of this size. This volume is limited to those procedures for which primary-care physicians commonly refer patients. Most of the procedures are diagnostic ones, although some have therapeutic or combined diagnostic and therapeutic value. The procedures are listed by name and arranged according to organ system or modality being used to perform the procedure.

This book is not meant to be a comprehensive index of all medical procedures. Neither is it meant to dictate when certain procedures are indicated. All procedure indications require individualization to the patient who is involved. Neither is this book meant to be a comprehensive reference work for the described tests and procedures. The determination of when to do a specific procedure and which one to do depends on resources available, as well as clinical indications, potential risks, and anticipated benefits.

This book is not meant to provide all the information required for obtaining informed consent. Patients should be given maximal information about a procedure, depending on their desire to know and their intellectual ability to comprehend the information. Close relatives and friends are entitled to the information as well, as long as the patient does not request otherwise. Informed consent should be obtained with maximal information exchange.

Many primary-care physicians may perform some of the described procedures in their offices. The inclusion of a procedure in this book is not meant to imply that it cannot or should not be performed in the office of the primary-care practitioner. Our purpose is to enhance information exchange and the proper use of procedures.

Used as a reference and refresher, this book provides primary-care practitioners with:

1. Updated and informative summaries of the status of commonly performed procedures and tests;

2. Illustrations intended to educate the health care professional and the patient;
3. Guidance in providing postprocedure care; and
4. Questions commonly asked by the patient.

Written by a family practitioner with the help of specialists in other medical areas, the book concentrates on patient education rather than on the procedure itself. The illustrations and photographs are intended to convey to the patient general information about how the procedure is performed. Patient questions were obtained from the practice of primary-care providers as well as those of other specialists who perform the procedures on a regular basis. The answers are not intended to be medicolegally complete but are designed to educate the patient and to allay fears. Each procedure section was reviewed by a physician or operator who performs the procedure regularly.

We suggest that this book be used to make medical procedures less mysterious for both patients and primary-care practitioners and we hope that this will lead to better communication, improved patient compliance with well-thought-out medical advice, and, most important, healthier and happier patients.

I
Cardiovascular System Procedures

1

Ambulatory ECG Monitoring (Holter Monitoring)

RICHARD SADOVSKY

Ambulatory electrocardiogram (ECG) or Holter monitoring is a diagnostic technique that involves recording the patient's heart rate and rhythm for 24 hours on a magnetic tape that is then analyzed for evidence of arrhythmias or abnormal electrical waves. The patient wears a tape recorder connected to electrodes placed on the chest and follows a normal day's activity during the evaluation. The tapes are generally read by a computer permitting correlation of cardiac variations with the patient's activities and symptoms.

INDICATIONS

Ambulatory ECG monitoring is indicated for diagnostic purposes in the presence of symptoms of syncope and dizziness, evaluation of therapy, or identification of asymptomatic patients with a high risk of sudden death. Patients with cardiovascular symptoms such as palpitations, dizziness, or syncope, and those with suspected arrhythmias may reveal the cause of their symptoms on the 24 hour tracing. Patients with coronary artery disease may demonstrate typical ST segment changes while arrhythmias may demonstrate conduction defects or myocardial irritability.

When evaluating therapies such as the effectiveness of antiarrhythmic medications, the efficacy of pacemaker function, or any other treatment of arrhythmia, the tracing is valuable to demonstrate an adequate period of ECG activity to permit accurate determinations. Asymptomatic patients with high risk of sudden death can be identified with ECG changes representative of myocardial infarction or cardiomyopathy.

The cardiologist reviews the 24 hour tracing with the patient's diary. Holter monitor recordings can demonstrate the relationship of symptoms, such as syncope, shortness of breath, and chest pain, to an arrhythmia or episode of ischemia. Ambulatory monitoring is mandatory in the diagnosis of Prinzmetal's angina because exercise testing is usually normal and many episodes of ST segment depression are clinically silent. Patients with nocturnal ischemia or ischemic episodes at rest may demonstrate transient ECG changes. Quantification of these changes is possible in a way that cannot be done by any other practical technique in ambulatory patients. The silent episodes may be caused by coronary vasospasm or by borderline occlusive disease that intermittently obstructs myocardial perfusion.

Real time ambulatory ECG systems record the number of events rather than the entire ECG. Although monitoring occurs in a continuous manner, recording is noncontinuous because of the limitations of memory. All that is retained are noncontinuous excerpted electrocardiographic examples. This is appealing to cardiologists because of the automaticity but there is little technician interaction with the actual tracing. Another type of recording that has a patient activated monitor can be worn for 5 to 7 days allowing the patient to manually begin the recording when symptoms are experienced. These techniques do not permit review of the actual tracing but often demonstrate the presence or absence of significant pathology.

ALTERNATIVES

Clinicians have been slow in adopting ambulatory ECG monitoring as a method for diagnosing ischemia. In the practice of medicine currently, exercise treadmill tests and coronary angiography are the primary means for diagnosing coronary artery disease. Ambulatory ECG recordings have achieved use primarily in the subset of patients with suspected Prinzmetal's angina, but even in this condition, patients are generally hospitalized and the disease documented by 12 lead electrocardiography performed during pain or by ergonovine provocation of coronary arterial spasm during coronary arteriography.

The graded exercise stress test has the advantage of revealing immediately whether exercise will induce arrhythmias; but in Holter monitoring, the arrhythmias are detected only in retrospect. Holter monitoring, however, is more sensitive in detecting arrhythmias and has also been found to detect a greater complexity of arrhythmias than the graded exercise stress test.

It is possible that 24 hours of tracing may be insufficient to make the diagnosis if the patient did not have the symptom on that particular day. Transtelephonic ECG monitoring employing small FM transmitting devices, which send the ECG over telephone lines, can be used during a symptomatic episode. These devices have recently been modified to provide 20 to 40 seconds of memory so that a recording can be done even if the patient cannot get to a phone. The disadvantage here is not recording the onset of the arrhythmia.

POSSIBILITY OF FAILURE

If the cardiac abnormality being evaluated does not occur during the period during which the monitor is recording, this procedure will fail to recognize the problem. Occasionally, the physician will ask the patient to perform slightly more strenuous activities during the day of recording or ask the patient to perform activities that have brought about symptoms previously. If the recording shows no abnormality, then clinical judgment will be needed to determine the likelihood of disease and the need to perform additional cardiac tests.

CONTRAINDICATIONS

There are no contraindications to ambulatory electrocardiographic recording.

PREPROCEDURE PREPARATION

There is no specific preprocedure preparation.

PATIENT EDUCATION

The patient must be informed about what the procedure is and told that the test may or may not pinpoint the cause of the symptoms being experienced. The test requires the patient to wear a small tape recorder that weighs about two pounds for 24 hours. A strap or belt will be provided so that the recorder can be attached to the body in a comfortable and convenient manner. Once the equipment is in place with the positioning of the leads, there is no alteration in daily activities for the patient. A sponge bath should be done if bathing is necessary during the period of cardiac monitoring. Magnets, metal detectors, electric blankets, and high voltage areas should be avoided but will probably not affect the recording.

PROCEDURE

The procedure is begun either in the physician's office, the ECG laboratory, or the patient's hospital room (figure 1–1). The number of electrodes vary from three (for a single channel monitor) to four or five (for a dual-channel monitor). The patient is also asked to keep a diary of activities and symptoms. Chest hair may need to be shaved to assure electrode stability.

Virtually all systems currently in use utilize two bipolar leads. The electrodes are taped into place, and the monitor is turned on, and placed in a case that is strapped to the patient's waist by means of a belt. The patient returns to the doctor's office or laboratory 24 hours later, and the monitor is removed.

POSTPROCEDURE INFORMATION

There is no specific postprocedure information.

COMPLICATIONS

There are no reported complications associated with ambulatory ECG monitoring.

PATIENT QUESTIONS

Is this test likely to discover my cardiac rhythm or myocardial perfusion abnormality?

In major studies, only half of patients with appropriate symptoms experience these symptoms during the monitor recording. The use of the ambulatory recording to evaluate chest discomfort is limited. Exercise testing or radionuclide studies are more sensitive and specific. Frequent episodes of spasm, however, may be detectable with proficient monitoring. Ventricular premature beats in patients with known coronary artery disease or in patients with dilated or hypertrophic cardiomyopathy are associated with higher risk. The role of ambulatory monitoring in the diagnosis of silent ischemia has not been clearly defined, and the significance of this observation has not yet been clarified.

Why must I record the timing of my symptoms?

It is essential to document the temporal relationship between the symptom and a specific rhythm abnormality. If there is no correlation between the two, then any arrhythmia noted cannot be assumed to be the cause of the symptoms. Most

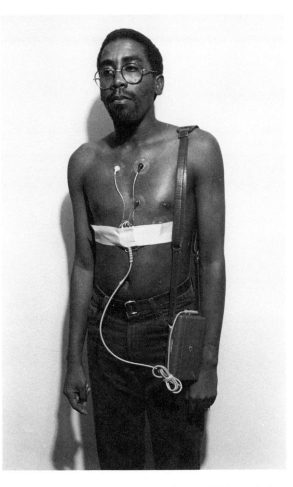

Figure 1–1. Patient prepared for ambulatory electrocardiogram (ECG) monitoring.

arrhythmias found in patients who report palpitations, chest pain, or lightheadedness produce no symptoms. A clear correlation between symptoms and arrhythmia should be established before therapy is initiated.

Will ambulatory ECG monitoring be affected by proximity to microwave ovens, pacemakers, or other electronic equipment?

The monitor is adequately shielded to prevent interference from any external electrical source. In addition, the presence of the monitor and recorder will not cause any other electrical source to malfunction.

CONSENT

Informed consent is not needed for ambulatory electrocardiographic monitoring.

SELECTED BIBLIOGRAPHY

Berman DS, Rozanski A, Knoebel SB: The detection of silent ischemia: cautions and precautions. *Circulation* 1987;75:101.

Johansson BW: Evaluation of alteration in consciousness and palpitations. In Wenger NK, Mock MB, Rinquist I, eds: *Ambulatory Electrocardiographic Recording.* Chicago: Year Book Medical 1981:321.

Kennedy HL, Wiens RD: Ambulatory (Holter) electrocardiography using real-time analysis. *Am J Cardiol* 1987;May 1:59:12:1190.

Pepine CJ: Detection of transient ischemic episodes by ambulatory ECG recordings. *Cardiol Clin* 1984;Aug:2(3):441.

Schmidhofer M: Indications for holter monitoring. *Fam Pract Recert* 1988;Feb:10:2:93.

2

Arteriography and Digital Subtraction Angiography

DAVID H. GORDON

Arteriography is the study of the arterial vascular system and the organs supplied by arteries. Arteriograms can be obtained by direct puncture of an artery and injection of a contrast material into the vessel. Digital subtraction angiography uses a computer to convert the images into an array of numbers that allows "subtraction" of the images of the vessels without contrast material from the images of those that contain contrast medium. This removes the nonvascular background densities and allows clearer visualization of the vasculature. The use of subtraction techniques has greatly enhanced the field of arteriography.

INDICATIONS

Arteriography is performed to (1) demonstrate abnormalities of blood vessels, (2) demonstrate extrinsic pressure effects on the vessels from mass lesions, (3) evaluate the presence or absence of vascularity in an already identified mass, and (4) identify vascular anatomy for the surgeon.

The most common type of arteriography is called peripheral angiography. It involves the study of the aorta and vessels of the leg for peripheral ischemic vascular disease and for evaluation of vascular structures prior to recommending surgery. The patient may present with pain, paresthesia, and coolness of the extremity. Intermittent claudication is another frequent symptom of arterial insufficiency. In addition, arteriograms are used to evaluate cerebral, abdominal, renal, pulmonary, and coronary circulation.

Cerebral arteriography may be used in patients with symptoms of carotid occlusion, transient ischemic attacks, aneurysms causing sensory motor changes, facial numbness, headaches, or confusion. Abdominal arteriography is employed to visualize the aorta and its major arteries and is used to evaluate symptoms of aortic aneurysms, gastrointestinal bleeding, renal artery problems (hypertension and stenosis), and suspected vascular malformations (figure 2–1.). Pulmonary arteriography is performed in cases of suspected pulmonary embolism and in patients with congenital heart disease. Arteriography is required before the performance of angioplasty. Viewing a patient's blood vessels allows the identification of stenosis, aneurysms, and arteriovenous fistulas. Arteriography is also performed to view the vasculature within an organ.

Digital subtraction angiography is less invasive, has fewer risks when done intravenously, and is less costly than conventional arteriography. This test can be done on out-patients and uses a much smaller volume of contrast material intraarterially, permitting the use of smaller catheters and decreasing the risk of embolization and other complications. Intraarterial subtraction angiography may produce satisfactory studies of the carotid and coronary arteries without selective catheterization. It is becoming the preferred technique over intravenous digital subtraction arteriography. Some researchers, however, are finding a slight increase in complications with digital subtraction angiography over conventional arteriographic techniques. Comparisons of complications of intraarterial subtraction angiography and conventional arteriography are in progress, and studies seem to show a lower percentage of complications with the newer technique.

ALTERNATIVES

The information obtained by arteriography and digital subtraction venous angiography can be obtained by other procedures such as Doppler studies, radionuclide imaging, and computerized tomography (CT) scanning.

Angiography is an invasive procedure requiring injection of a quantity of contrast material directly into the artery to be studied.

Problems with digital subtraction angiography include small image intensifiers, allowing only a limited viewing field. Therefore, a greater number of injections are needed. The major disadvantage is the poor spatial resolution caused by noise in the electronic imaging system, which yields inadequate results in small vessels and fine details. For example, intracranial aneurysms may be discovered, but the detail is insufficient for detailed preoperative evaluation. In addi-

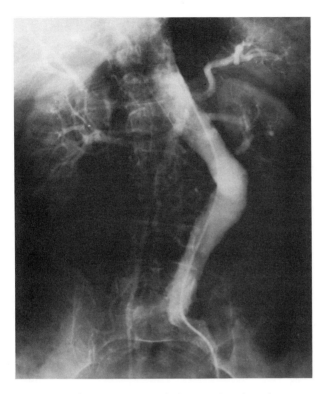

Figure 2–1. Arteriogram demonstrating the abdominal aorta and renal arteries.

tion, most studies are nonselective and vessel overlap may obscure pathologic features. Patients who are uncooperative or who have low cardiac output cannot be studied in this manner.

Doppler studies and plethysmography are acceptable screening tests but do not identify specific pathologies and generally do not allow for therapeutic decisions. The combination of digital subtraction angiography and ultrasound has been found to be helpful in carotid bifurcation evaluations.

Radionuclide studies have been used to study vasculature in areas such as the lung; scanning should precede angiography if embolism is suspected. If the scan is negative, then embolism is highly unlikely, and the pulmonary arteriogram is not needed.

Computerized axial tomography is helpful especially when performed with contrast in evaluating a space-occupying lesion. In addition, a CT scan is often better than angiography for tumor staging by evaluating more fully extension and metastases. The CT scan does not, however, clearly identify the blood supply of masses and angiography becomes essential.

Most mass lesions of the pelvis are now identifiable with CT or with ultrasound without angiography.

POSSIBILITY OF FAILURE

Clearly, arteriography is the best way to view vascular structures and their patency. A high-quality examination will be very informative. There are, however, situations in which another test may reveal additional information. An example is the ability of computerized tomography to define the limits of an aneurysm that may have looked smaller than its true size on arteriography because of the filling of the lumen with thrombus.

CONTRAINDICATIONS

Contraindications for arteriography include allergic reactions to contrast, renal failure or insufficiency, congestive heart failure, uncontrolled or severe hypertension, various arrhythmias (particularly bradyarrhythmias), recent myocardial infarction, and various coagulation abnormalities including use of coumarin or heparin. All these complications are relative rather than absolute and must be balanced against the need for the arteriographic study. These contraindications can be managed, at least on a temporary basis, allowing performance of a much needed arteriogram.

Allergic reactions are difficult to predict unless the patient has a history of reaction during a prior contrast study. The common minor reactions can be dealt with by reassurance and the administration of diphenhydramine or a steroid preprocedure when needed. Steroids can be used for three days prior to the procedure if the patient has a history of severe contrast reactions and the arteriography is strongly indicated. In these patients, an anesthesiologist should be available on standby to treat a serious anaphylactic reaction. Recent data suggest that administration of prednisolone 12 and 2 hours prior to the procedure may be as effective as the use of nonionic contrast material in diminishing allergic reactions. Nonionic contrast material is less likely to cause allergic responses, but is more than 20 times as expensive as ionic contrast materials.

In patients who have severe underlying renal disease or are diabetic with compromised renal function, the renal toxic effects of contrast material can be minimized by hydrating the patient well prior to the procedure. The injection of mannitol at the conclusion of the procedure will cause an osmotic diuresis, removing contrast material from the body and enhancing continued renal output.

Heart failure can be treated with digitalis and diuretics. Hypertension can be brought under control by aggressive medical therapy such as intravenous diazoxide or nitroprusside, lowering the diastolic pressure to below 120 mm Hg, which is the absolute maximum pressure at which arteriography should be attempted.

Arrhythmias are managed in an appropriate manner to minimize complications. The angiographer should be familiar with the use of cardiac stimulants and atropine if problems arise. Arteriography should be postponed 6 to 10 weeks after myocardial infarction because of the risk of a severe vagal reaction, although there is now work demonstrating the value, in specific patients, of coronary angiography in the hyperacute phase of myocardial infarction.

Coagulation defects are treated by halting the cause if it is medically indicated. This may require time to allow the blood-thinning medication to be cleared from the circulation. If arteriography is urgently needed, the coagulopathy is reversed by the administration of fresh-frozen plasma and vitamin K parenterally. Other coagulation abnormalities must be appropriately investigated and, generally, arteriography should not be attempted if the prothrombin time or the partial thromboplastin time is more than 50% above normal. It may be necessary to perform a bleeding time to evaluate platelet function if there is any reason to expect it to be poor, such as chronic renal insufficiency or leukemia.

PREPROCEDURE PREPARATION

The patient should anticipate shaving the right and left groin with the understanding that, if the right femoral artery is unacceptable for any reason or if the catheter cannot be advanced through the vessel, the left femoral artery will be used. The axillary vessels are used much more rarely. The patient is given parenteral sedation on call to the arteriography laboratory to reduce anxiety and to lower the pain level. The patient is kept well-hydrated and is not permitted to eat solid foods after the midnight prior to the procedure. If the procedure is being done late in the day, the patient should take nothing by mouth for 6 to 8 hours before the procedure. The bowel may need to be evacuated if an abdominal study is being done. The patient will require an intravenous line throughout the procedure in case of allergic reaction.

Routine blood tests include renal function tests, coagulation studies (including platelets), and a complete blood count.

PATIENT EDUCATION

The patient should be well informed about the procedure and the possible risks. In addition, the patient should be aware that, if any unexpected complications such as embolization occur that require urgent care such as embolectomy, the appropriate measures will be taken immediately. Reassurance that all will be done to prevent complications is important to the patient.

It is anticipated that the patient will have some pain. If the pain is severe, the angiographer should be informed immediately as excessive pain could mean improper passage of the catheter with resulting intimal irritation or tear. Complications may be avoided by the patient's cooperation in reporting pain. The patient should know that he or she is under constant electrocardiographic monitoring.

PROCEDURE

For angiography, the patient is placed supine on an x-ray table with an intravenous infusion maintaining hydration and permitting the emergency administration of medications, if needed. Scout films are done first, and the puncture site is prepared in a sterile manner.

Arteriography is usually approached from the right femoral area, although the left femoral or axillary regions may be the site of the initial puncture.

The right femoral approach involves anesthetizing the groin with lidocaine, after which a small incision is made in the skin to allow passage of the catheter. Deep anesthesia is also given. The patient can expect a sensation of pain with the initial puncture. A flexible guide wire is inserted once it is certain that the needle is in an intra-arterial position as determined by a free backflow of blood. The patient should be aware that a warm feeling may occur when the initial spurt of blood hits the leg or the drape.

The guide wire is then advanced up into the aorta and into the desired position. The patient must be encouraged to inform the angiographer about any pain because this may hint of subintimal passage of the wire. A catheter is then inserted over the wire to the desired level. In the case of a peripheral runoff study after the catheter is placed, an injection is made to visualize the aorta from below the renal arteries to well below the knees and even to the ankles if an in situ saphenous vein bypass is indicated. The patient may experience back pain and a feeling of increased intraabdominal pressure similar to that felt during defecation when the injection is given and the contrast enters the pelvic arteries and vessels supplying the bowel. In addition, a warm sensation will occur in the lower extremities. As the contrast material circulates, the patient may feel a metallic taste in the mouth and a wave of nausea. The painful sensation of the first injection lasts about 5 seconds and can be diminished by the concurrent injection of lidocaine with the contrast material. Doses of lidocaine must be measured carefully to avoid lidocaine toxicity. If the patient has a seizure disorder or a hypersensitive nervous system, lidocaine should not be administered.

Translumbar arteriography for evaluation of the peripheral runoff involves placing the patient in a prone position. A needle is inserted directly into the aorta from a translumbar approach. A lumbar puncture is made at a level between L-1 and L-3 and about 8 to 10 centimeters to the left of the midline. Once the puncture of the aorta has been accomplished, the needle is flushed with a heparin and saline solution and contrast is injected. No selective studies can be done from the translumbar approach in which dye is injected directly into the abdominal aorta. Only a peripheral runoff study is obtained. In most centers this test is being replaced by the femoral approach, but it is still useful if groin pulses are not palpable.

Nonionic contrast material can be used to reduce pain, but it is too expensive to use on a regular basis.

After the injection, radiographic filming is done with the table moving to allow filming at appropriate levels. After the films are developed and reviewed by the angiographer for completeness of study, more views are obtained if needed. When the needed views are completed, the catheter is removed, and compression is done at the puncture site for at least 15 minutes.

The patient is returned to the hospital room with instructions to report any bleeding occurring at the puncture site to the nurse or physician. Circulation to the extremity distal to the site of injection should be assessed. The patient should remain in bed for all activities for 6 to 8 hours. Most complications will show themselves within 1 hour of the procedure. Hematomas can be avoided by appropriate bed rest.

With the recent increase in arteriography on an outpatient basis, it is important that the patient be accompanied by a responsible family member or friend. Under these circumstances, the patient is held in the recovery area for 4 to 6 hours after the procedure and should go home by car rather than public vehicle, which might require standing and waiting. No other special precautions are required.

Selective arteriography into specific branches involves the same procedure. Localized warmth and pain can be expected in the area being injected. This pain should decrease quickly as the blood washes the contrast away.

Digital subtraction angiography involves the precontrast injection storage in the computer of a "mask" of background structures. This mask can then be automatically subtracted from the views obtained postcontrast. This technique eliminates bone and soft tissue images and highlights the contrast material. Antecubital venous injection of contrast material may be acceptable for pulmonary or aortic arch subtraction angiography, but central injections are needed for most examinations.

POSTPROCEDURE INFORMATION

If the procedure is done on an inpatient, then hospital personnel will provide the medical support needed. If the test is done on an outpatient, a close friend or family member should accompany the patient to the test to help him or her get home. Since most complications occur during the first hour following arteriography, generally the patient is monitored at the testing site for this period. When the patient gets home, the friend should help the patient to rest for several hours in a position that avoids movement of the puncture site, and to help the patient to watch for bleeding. Optimally, if the friend can test the pulses on the punctured extremity regularly for the first 12 hours following the arteriogram, continued patency of arterial blood flow will be assured.

COMPLICATIONS

Arteriographic procedures should not be done when the risk to the patient is excessive and when the results will not alter the treatment plan. Many of the potential complications are related to the pathophysiologic effect of the iodinated contrast material. These include red-cell hemolysis with accompanying sludging in patients with sickle cell anemia, cardiac arrhythmias including vasovagal bradycardia with resulting hypotension, neurotoxicity including seizures and cortical blindness, and renal toxicity.

Hypersensitivity may cause major responses such as cardiac arrest, hypotension, pulmonary edema, convulsions, laryngeal edema, and bronchospasm. More minor, self-limited reactions to contrast occur more frequently and include nausea, vomiting, itching, and transient urticaria.

Angiographic complications from catheter effects include thrombosis, bleeding, embolism, and vessel-wall injury. Puncture-site bleeding is the most common complication.

Digital subtraction angiography is also accompanied by the complication of hypersensitivity to the contrast preparations. Although embolic phenomena do not occur since a catheter is not placed in the artery, embolism-like symptoms have occurred such as transient vision loss and progression of hemiparesis. These rare episodes are probably caused by hemodynamic changes rather than embolic events. The rapid injection of high volumes of hypertonic contrast media and the resultant hemodynamic and cardiac effects can cause problems in the elderly or in patients with known cardiac disease.

PATIENT QUESTIONS

Does the procedure involve pain?

The patient should be informed that the procedure does involve mild pain occurring mostly at the time of the initial incision to access the artery. Pain during the remainder of the test should be minimal. Pressure may be experienced as the catheter is inserted. Any pain noted during the procedure, especially during movement of the catheter and guide wire, should be reported to the angiographer as it may mean subintimal invasion. Mild pain will also be felt when the contrast material is injected. If it appears that concern about pain makes a patient unwilling to have the procedure, use of the more expensive nonionic contrast material can be offered.

What type of anesthesia will I have?

Angiography may be performed under a local or general anesthetic. General anesthesia is advantageous for patients undergoing cerebral angiography for optimal patient comfort and immobility. The disadvantages of general anesthesia include inability to use the state of consciousness for neurological evaluation and the risk of increased intracranial pressure. It is used very selectively. Local anesthesia is widely preferred for all noncerebral angiography. Digital subtraction angiography never requires general anesthesia.

How long does the test take?

The patient will be asked to remain still on a hard, flat x-ray table for 30 minutes to 3 hours depending on the complexity of the test and the number of vessels that are being studied. The patient should be warned that he may have some temporary stiffness following the examination.

What happens when the test is over?

The patient is returned to the room and put in a comfortable position in the bed. Generally, the patient lies flat on his back or on the side of the procedure for the initial few hours. Flexion of the limb where the puncture was made should be avoided. Any blood on the dressing or feeling of dampness should be reported to the nurse immediately. These instructions should be followed even if the test is done as an outpatient.

Can anything go wrong?

The patient should be made aware of all the potential risks and complications that may have a significant impact on his specific situation. The cue should be taken from the patient about how much he wishes to know, but the angiographer must obtain detailed, informed consent prior to the arteriogram. The patient's anxiety can be best handled by explaining the management of complications and by emphasizing the therapeutic necessity and value of obtaining the results of an arteriogram. The patient will be closely monitored during the procedure, and every effort will be made to detect potential complications before they become serious.

CONSENT

Informed consent is clearly required prior to arteriography with complete documentation that the patient has been informed of the major and most common side effects and complications.

SELECTED BIBLIOGRAPHY

Ball JB, Lukin RR, Tomsick TA: Complications of intravenous digital subtraction angiography. *Arch Neurol* 1985;42:969.

Carmody RF, Yang PJ, Seeger JF, Capp MP: Digital subtraction angiography update. *Investigative Radiology* 1986;December:21:12:899.

Gonzalez CF, Doan HT, Han SS, DeFilipp GJ: Extracranial vascular angiography. *Radiol Clin North Am* 1986;Sept:24:3:419.

Massey JA: Diagnostic testing for peripheral vascular disease. *Nurs Clin North Am* 1986;Jun:21(2):207.

Rossi P, Pavone P, Tempesta P, Ambrogi C Castrucci M, Rossi M: Present and future prospects for angiographic techniques. *Radiol Med* 1986;June:72(Supp. 1):51.

Wilbur AC, Spigos, DG: Angiography. In Bernard Sigel, ed: *Diagnostic Patient Studies in Surgery,* Phiadelphia: Lea and Febiger, 1986;153–186.

3

Cardiac Catheterization and Coronary Angiography

RICHARD SADOVSKY

Cardiac catheterization involves passing one or more long catheters to the heart from a peripheral vein or artery. The catheter is moved to the chosen position in the heart where pressure can be recorded or contrast material introduced, allowing radiographic imaging on film. This procedure is generally performed by a team of trained personnel.

INDICATIONS

The main indication is the need to establish the presence and extent of organic heart disease in a symptomatic patient. Presenting symptoms may include chest pain, dyspnea, cough, peripheral edema, hepatic congestion, syncope, or palpitations.

Specific indications for catheterization vary widely between patients, but catheterization is usually done when the patient's life style is significantly altered by symptoms related to the heart. The procedure then determines the precise nature of the organic disease or the absence of disease when no abnormality is present. The anatomic and physiologic status of the heart can be determined.

This knowledge about the heart is valuable to make an accurate diagnosis, determine a proper intervention, assess the results of the intervention, reassess surgical results when symptoms recur, and it is being done more recently to follow up patients with myocardial infarction. This latter indication is to determine "other vessel disease" that may require bypass surgery and to evaluate left ventricular function. Improved survival has been proved to occur in patients receiving bypass surgery for triple vessel disease or with critical narrowing of the left main-stem coronary artery. These lesions are found in over 40% of postmyocardial infarction patients. It has been suggested that bypass surgery or postinfarction angioplasty for these lesions would improve survival, and, since catheterization appears to be a safe procedure if done 3 to 4 weeks after myocardial infarction, there may be value in identifying surviving patients with these particular coronary artery lesions.

Occasionally catheterization is undertaken to determine the extent of an asymptomatic lesion, especially in the case of suspected congenital lesions such as atrial septal defect, ventricular septal defect, or patent ductus arteriosus. In infants, catheterization is a different project. Conditions indicating the need for catheterization in the very young are generally life threatening.

In most cases, cardiac catheterization follows other ancillary tests including electrocardiogram, exercise stress test, cardiac fluoroscopy, ambulatory electrocardiogram recording (Holter monitoring), and possibly, radionuclide studies.

Depending on whether the catheter is inserted into a vein or an artery, the catheterization evaluates the right or the left side of the heart. The coronary arteries originate in the aorta just above the aortic valve. To examine them, the catheter is advanced to the opening of each artery, and the contrast medium is injected.

Pressure measurements can be performed by advancing the catheter to the area of interest. The other end of the catheter is attached to a pressure transducer and converts the pressure reading into an electrical signal that can be viewed on an oscilloscope or recorded on paper. On the right side of the heart, pressures are recorded from the right atrium, right ventricle, and pulmonary artery. If the catheter is advanced until it can go no farther, it wedges in a small pulmonary artery and records a pulmonary wedge pressure, which is, in effect, the left atrial pressure. Pressures in the aorta and the left ventricle can also be recorded.

Abnormalities in pressures can indicate obstruction of flow caused by mitral or aortic stenosis. The wave formation of the recorded pressures is valuable also in evaluating valve regurgitation or opposition to atrial emptying.

Blood sampling can be done for analysis of oxygen content and is helpful in evaluating a patient with a suspected intracardiac shunt. This can help distinguish a septal defect or tetralogy of Fallot.

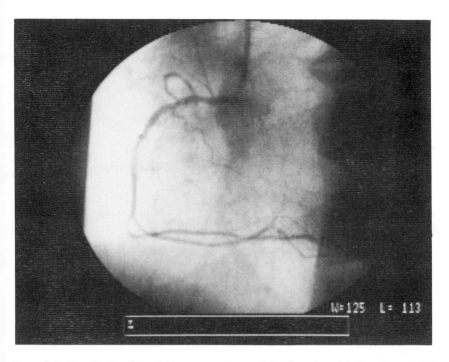

Figure 3–1. Visualization of the right coronary artery and its bifurcation with the catheter visible coming down from the top.

Cardiac output measurement can be done by a variety of techniques including the Fick method, indicator dilution method, thermodilution method, and the angiographic method. This allows an accurate estimation of cardiac function at the time of catheterization.

Coronary angiography refers to the injection of a radiopaque substance into the region and the recording of the image on film (figure 3-1). The recording may be made either on cinematic film (cineangiography) or as one or more independent radiographic films (cut film angiography).

A high-power syringe injects a bolus of the contrast material through the catheter to look at the large chambers of the heart. Opacification of the coronary arteries can be done by hand injection. Oblique pictures are generally taken to allow a true three-dimensional view of any lesion or narrowing of a vessel. With coronary catheterization, it is possible not only to determine the presence of disease but also to quantitate its severity. These findings have important influence on patient management. Often, catheterization is the deciding factor when choosing between medical and surgical management of cardiac and coronary vessel disease.

ALTERNATIVES

No other diagnostic tests provide the quantity of information about the heart as is offered by cardiac catheterization. Catheterization remains the standard by which other tests are measured. Exercise stress testing can be used to divide patients into high-risk "ischemic" and low-risk "ischemic" groups. If angina develops during stress testing or an ST depression of greater than 1 mm occurs, there is a greater probability of significant coronary artery disease.

Left ventricular dysfunction can be assessed by radionuclide angiography or two-dimensional echocardiography. In addition, most structural lesions such as ventricular septal defect, severe mitral regurgitation, or a large, left-ventricular aneurysm can be detected by the combination of clinical findings and the same noninvasive techniques. Thus, cardiac catheterization is not necessary to define gross structural lesions of the heart causing poor, left-ventricular function. If surgery is contemplated, then the catheterization data and pictures become necessary.

^{201}Thallium myocardial scintigraphy is being used to detect the presence of jeopardized myocardium or area of inducible ischemia.

Cardiac digital angiography is a new technique based on the premise that a digital format would facilitate the extraction of quantitative parameters from images and thus improve diagnostic accuracy and reduce subjective variability. With digital angiography, images can be added or subtracted, enhanced and filtered, giving a clear picture of structures and cardiac events. Cardiac digital subtraction angiography using intravenous contrast injections injected into the vena cava or right atrium allows high quality left ventriculograms with good spatial resolution. This allows assessment of left ventricular function and is beginning to offer information about coronary artery flow reserve. Motion artifacts still cause problems with this technique, and the patient is required to hold his breath. Advantages of digital ventriculography include reproducibility, rapidity, less contrast-material dosage, and serial assessment of left-ventricular function during catheterization. Some cardiologists feel that, when fully automatic processing and adequate storage and retrieval are available, this method will replace film in the cardiac catheterization laboratory.

POSSIBILITY OF FAILURE

The major weakness of conventional cardiac catheterization and coronary angiography is that subjective interpretation of coronary stenosis severity is neither accurate nor reproducible. This makes the procedure ideally suitable for resolution by automated computer imaging.

Cardiac catheterization is currently considered the most accurate measurement of cardiac disease, chamber dysfunction, and coronary artery lesions.

CONTRAINDICATIONS

The relative risk of the procedure varies considerably depending on the patient's clinical status. A patient having frequent episodes of chest pain at rest even when on optimal medical therapy is at significantly greater risk than the patient with stable, exertional chest pain. Similarly, the patient who is hemodynamically unstable is at greater risk during the procedure.

The safety of cardiac catheterization has improved greatly in recent years. Acute myocardial infarction, cardiogenic shock, recurrent ventricular tachycardia, and congestive heart failure are no longer considered absolute contraindications. Some feel that the only absolute contraindication is the refusal of the competent individual to consent to the procedure.

Relative contraindications include recurrent ventricular arrhythmias, severe hypertension, left ventricular failure in which acute pulmonary edema can result from administration of the dye, fever (during which hemodynamic responses may be exaggerated and infections may spread), severe anemia, digitalis toxicity, hypokalemia, renal failure, acute myocardial infarction, and abnormal coagulation profiles secondary to disease or to administration of anticoagulant therapy.

PREPROCEDURE PREPARATION

It is important to know whether the patient has previously had angiography performed and whether any adverse reactions occurred. If the patient is taking anticoagulants, aspirin, or any other medication that affects platelet aggregation, the drug is stopped 1 to 2 weeks prior to the procedure.

Precatheterization orders typically include laboratory tests such as complete blood count, prothrombin and partial thromboplastin time, urea, creatinine, and electrolyte studies. Some physicians order blood for type and hold because of the potential need for transfusion. A chest roentgenogram and ECG are usually performed.

The patient is often given a sleeping medication the night before the procedure. Premedication may consist of a minor tranquilizer by mouth or intramuscularly when the patient is called for the catheterization.

The patient's vital signs are recorded and reviewed prior to the procedure, and the patient generally goes to the catheterization by stretcher.

Children are more anxious than adults and may require more sedation and reassurance.

PATIENT EDUCATION

The nature of the procedure and its risks and benefits should be carefully explained to the patient. Many institutions use a portable audiovisual tape recorder to give patients and relatives a clearer picture of what is involved in the catheterization procedure. The patient's exposure to audiovisual information prior to catheterization has been demonstrated to have beneficial effects by decreasing anxiety and concomitant psychophysiologic arousal, which, in turn, results in lower blood pressures and heart rates during the procedure. There is, of course, a small subset of patients whose apprehension is increased by detailed description of possible risks, so this is not always in the patient's best interest.

Specific patient instructions should include the advice to continue all cardiac medications and to void just prior to the catheterization. The patient should also fast for 6 to 8 hours prior to the procedure because of the risk of nausea and vomiting during catheterization. The patient should also be told to remain in bed for 12 to 24 hours after catheterization.

PROCEDURE

Cardiac catheterization is a sterile procedure performed by trained personnel. The amount of time required for the procedure is approximately 20 minutes to several hours, with the large majority being performed as inpatient procedures. Some centers are beginning to do cardiac catheterizations as outpatient procedures and are having good results. The patient is placed on the catheterization table, the site of entry (usually the right antecubital fossa or right groin) is exposed and cleaned, and the patient is covered with sterile drapes. In adults, percutaneous catheterization of the femoral artery and vein or cutdown into the brachial artery and vein, under local anesthesia is generally the preferred route. In children, cutdown on the axillary vessels, femoral artery or long saphenous vein, or cannulation of the umbilical vessels is occasionally needed.

The site of entry is then anesthetized with an injectable anesthetic, skin incisions are made, and the catheterization is performed. The direct brachial approach may have advantages in patients with coarctation of the aorta or with peripheral vascular disease involving the abdominal aorta or the iliac or femoral arteries. The direct brachial approach may have advantages also in the obese patient because of technical ease. The percutaneous femoral approach has the advantages of not requiring arterial repair and of a lower incidence of infection at the site of catheterization. This is done either percutaneously or by direct visualization of the vein using an incision through the skin. The catheter is a hollow tube with a proximal end that can be attached to a syringe or a pressure transducer and a distal end that has one or more openings for blood sampling, pressure recording, or injection of contrast material. Depending on the indications, a right heart catheterization, a left heart catheterization, or both may be performed.

When the catheterization has been completed, the catheters are removed from the blood vessels. Hemostasis is obtained by pressure on the puncture site followed by a period of strict bed rest. If a cutdown is performed, the artery is usually repaired with fine sutures; the vein is usually ligated.

Aftercare includes observation for signs of bleeding or loss of pulses. Additionally, the contrast material, having a high density, promotes a brisk diuresis that may cause dehydration if not corrected. Patient must be on strict intakeoutput recording and drinking fluids should be encouraged. Vital signs should be observed closely for a minimum of 24 hours.

POSTPROCEDURE INFORMATION

When cardiac catheterization carries a high risk of complication, the problem should be discussed with close family members. The bandage over the incision site can be removed either the evening of the day of the procedure or the next day. An adhesive bandage is needed over the puncture site for one more day. The gauze should be changed if it becomes soiled or wet. The sutures, if any, are removed approximately 5 days after the procedure.

COMPLICATIONS

Minor complications include arrhythmias during catheterization, difficulty with hemostasis after the procedure, or loss of pulse caused by local vascular thrombosis, vasospasm, embolization, or improper vessel repair. These complications occur in less than 2% to 3% of patients and may require surgical intervention. In addition, the hyperosmolarity of the contrast material may cause dehydration and hypotension. The patient must be adequately hydrated both before and after the procedure. About 10% to 15% of patients develop nausea and/or vomiting during the injection of contrast material, and about the same number develop an urticarial rash. A true anaphylactic reaction to the dye can occur, but this is rare.

Major complications include myocardial infarction, cerebrovascular accidents, and/or death within 24 hours of the procedure. The incidence of actual cardiac tissue death is below 0.5% and the incidence of death is below 0.25% for adults in a safe laboratory. The incidence of death in infants and adults over 60 years of age has been found to be slightly higher. Women of advanced age appear to be at especially high risk for this procedure. Disease of the left main coronary artery does appear to correlate with catheter mortality. Most studies report a somewhat higher risk in patients studied by the brachial artery technique although the skill of the angiography team is probably the most important variable. There is also a higher risk of death in patients with left main coronary artery disease and in patients with a left ventricular ejection fraction of less than 30%.

The risks of outpatient cardiac catheterization appear to be about the same as inpatient procedures. Admission is required postprocedure for patients who have severe disease, transient hypotension, severe bleeding at the site of catheter insertion, vasovagal reactions, allergic reactions, and, occasionally, for social reasons.

PATIENT QUESTIONS

Will I be awake during the procedure?

It is necessary for the patient to remain awake during the procedure so that he or she can be of assistance by taking deep breaths, coughing, or turning to the side. A mild sedative will relax the patient; additional sedation can be given before or during the procedure. Patients can also ask questions and tell the technician what they are experiencing during the procedure.

Where should the catheterization be performed, and by whom will it be done?

Cardiac catheterization should be performed by a trained team with a cardiologist present. An inverse relationship between the number of procedures done and the incidence of complications has been reported. This relationship is especially important in transseptal catheterization. A laboratory with a mortality rate greater than 0.3% should terminate coronary angioplasty altogether. Patients should be referred to laboratories having the lowest mortality rate and the highest number of procedures performed within an acceptable geographic area.

Will I have a reaction to the dye?

Some type of reaction to the contrast material is seen in 50% of patients. Reactions range from flushing and mild nausea to severe anaphylaxis and death, which occurs in approximately 1 patient in 40,000. Since the dye is composed primarily of iodide salts, the patient should be asked if he or she has any allergies to iodine, seafood, or the contrast media used during any previous dye contrast study. Pretreatment with steroids and antihistamines is advocated for prophylaxis in patients with previous allergic reactions. Nephropathy can also be caused by the contrast material and is rare in healthy patients and more common in patients with diabetes. This can be avoided by maintaining good hydration or by infusion of mannitol in some patients.

CONSENT

Informed consent is clearly required for this invasive procedure and should be obtained by the team performing the examination.

SELECTED BIBLIOGRAPHY

Cohn HE, Freed MD, Hellenbrand WF, Fyler DC: Complications and mortality associated with cardiac catheterization in infants under one year. *Pediatr Cardiol* 1985;6:3:123.

Fellows KE: Therapeutic catheter procedures in congenital heart disease: current status and future prospects. *Cardiovasc Intervent Radiol* 1984;7:3–4:170.

Katz NM: Discussing coronary artery surgery with the patient. *Am Fam Phys* 1984;Jan 29:1:123.

Klinke WP: Is outpatient cardiac catheterization safe? *Pract Cardiol* 1988;May:14:6:29.

Lloyd-Jones H: Complications of cardiac catheterization. *Radiography* 1986;Jul–Aug:52:604:210.

Stack RS, Carlson EB, Hinohara T, Phillips HR: Interventional cardiac catheterization. *Invest Radiol* 1985;Jul:20:4:333.

4

Cardiac Electrophysiologic Testing

RICHARD SADOVSKY

Clinical cardiac electrophysiology is commonly thought to have originated in the late 1960s when it was observed that programmed electrical stimulation of the human heart was safe and yielded valuable information. It was noted also that the HIS bundle electrogram could be recorded by catheter technique allowing measurement of cardiac electrical activity that could not be detected on the body surface. Clinical electrophysiologic techniques have evolved for the assessment of sinus node, atrioventricular (AV) node, and HIS-Purkinje system function. This use of programmed electrical stimulation to initiate and terminate arrhythmias in a controlled situation has become useful in the study of tachyarrhythmias.

INDICATIONS

Clinical indications for electrophysiologic study (EPS) include bradyarrhythmias, tachyarrhythmias, complex premature ventricular beats, and presumed, but unsubstantiated, arrhythmias. Clinical symptoms accompanying these indications can be syncope of unknown origin, dizziness in a patient with Wolff-

Parkinson-White syndrome, recurrent palpitations, or unexpected cardiac arrest. There is no clinical role for EPS in patients with previously documented sinus node dysfunction or in asymptomatic patients with evidence of sinus node dysfunction that has been previously detected. Asymptomatic patients with AV and intraventricular dysfunction should only rarely require this evaluation. The extent of the study may vary depending on the clinical circumstances in the particular patient.

The indication of bradyarrhythmias may result from dysfunction of the sinus node and includes clinical diagnoses such as sinus bradycardia, sinus pauses and sinus arrest, sinoatrial exit block, and bradycardiatachycardia syndrome. Clinical manifestations may range from none to syncope. Ambulatory monitoring often is the most useful study in these patients, and generally electrophysiologic study is not needed. However, electrophysiologic study may reveal associated tachyarrhythmias or conducting system disease. The indirect measurements used to evaluate the function of the sinus node are sinus node recovery time, sinoatrial conduction time, sinus node effective refractory period, and the intrinsic heart rate. Direct measurement of sinus node activity is generally not done. Testing may be helpful in patients with episodic symptoms, in patients with asymptomatic disease who require drugs that may exacerbate sinus node dysfunction (such as beta-adrenergic blockers, calcium channel blockers, or antiarrhythmic agents), or in patients with recurrent syncope of unknown origin.

Bradycardia may be caused by conduction system dysfunction. Bifascicular block and congenital complete heart block may be evaluated using electrophysiologic testing. The goal is to predict the likelihood of progression to a more serious cardiac problem and to clarify the relation of symptoms to the arrhythmia. The site of block in congenital heart block often has prognostic significance.

Tachyarrhythmias are an indication for electrophysiologic study because of its ability to identify the mechanism of the tachycardia. Clinical symptoms may include syncope or palpitations. ECG findings of Wolff-Parkinson-White syndrome or asymptomatic tachycardia in patients with known structural cardiac disease are also indications for analysis. Studies may not be necessary in all cases when careful study of the surface electrocardiogram yields sufficient information to initiate treatment. The indication for invasive studies is supraventricular tachycardia associated with pronounced symptoms and a ventricular rate of over 200 beats per minute, which is refractory to conventional therapies. Accessory atrioventricular pathways can be identified and thus facilitate subsequent surgical ablation. An assessment can also be made about risk of sudden death.

Prevention of clinical tachycardia can be done by using the electrophysiology laboratory to determine which drug is effective in preventing the induction of a clinical tachycardia. If no drug is efficacious, antitachycardia pacing can been performed. Electrophysiologically guided surgical procedure for the treatment of patients with tachycardia is now a well established technique with a high rate of success. This does require open heart surgery.

Complex, premature ventricular beats (defined as multiform, repetitive, paired, or short runs of nonsustained ventricular tachycardia) are an independent risk factor for sudden cardiac death in patients with a recent myocardial infarction, chronic ischemic heart disease, or cardiomyopathy. Programmed electrical stimulation can help to identify those patients who are specifically at high risk for sudden death, although it is unclear that treatment of the arrhythmia will alter the likelihood of sudden death. The role of electrophysiologic studies in this area is evolving.

For patients who have survived an out-of-hospital myocardial infarction, the identification of an effective antiarrhythmic drug that prevents induction of ventricular tachycardia helps the patient to have decreased mortality and to be free of arrhythmia 18 months after the electrophysiologic study. If no arrhythmia can be induced, then the underlying cardiac disease is treated.

Electrophysiologic testing should be performed in patients with recurrent near syncope or syncope or other profound symptoms that suggest a disturbance in cardiac rhythm as their cause. Those patients with symptomatic, unsubstantiated arrhythmias can be tested in an effort to reproduce the arrhythmia in combination with the symptom. In various studies, rhythm abnormalities have been found in up to 60% of patients with syncope. Abnormalities are the most common in patients with structural heart disease. Ventricular tachycardia was the most frequent abnormality found. Treatment to prevent recurrence was successful in up to 85% of these patients.

Measurements that can currently be made include sinus node recovery time as an index of sinus node function, patterns of atrioventricular block as an index to localize conduction disturbances to specific portions of the AV conducting system, initiation and termination of supraventricular tachycardia demonstrating the site of entry of the abnormality, and premature depolarization demonstrating preexcitation syndromes. This procedure allows activation mapping via catheter electrodes.

The predictive value of electrophysiologic studies allows determination of post myocardial infarction patients who are at risk of developing malignant ventricular arrhythmias. This remains controversial at present.

Therapeutic uses of cardiac electrophysiologic techniques now include ablation of the AV junction. This is useful in patients with incessant or refractory supraventricular arrhythmias but it requires refinement as to the amount of electrical stimulation needed.

Electrophysiologic studies can also be used to identify prospective antiarrhythmic regimens that could prevent spontaneous recurrences of supraventricular

Electrophysiologic studies can also be used to identify prospective antiarrhythmic regimens that could prevent spontaneous recurrences of supraventricular tachycardia. This is based on the hypothesis that medical regimens that prevent the initiation of ventricular tachycardia in a patient in whom the tachycardia could be initiated prior to the drug therapy were effective in preventing recurrent ventricular tachycardia during follow up. This has been substantiated in many studies.

Alternatives

Alternatives to cardiac electrophysiologic studies do exist. Highly regimented, ambient electrocardiographic monitoring and exercise testing has been used to assess antiarrhythmic regimens. Signal averaging promises to be a fairly accurate noninvasive technique for recording His bundle activity and identifying late potentials in patients with prior myocardial infarction and ventricular tachycardia. Esophageal recording and pacing is another somewhat invasive technique that is useful to delineate atrial activity to diagnose complex supraventricular tachycardias and ventricular tachycardias.

Potential for Failure

Electrophysiologic testing appears to have several well-defined limitations. The sensitivity of programmed stimulation is the probability of inducing a tachycardia with stimulation in patients with spontaneous tachycardia. The sensitivity of two extrastimuli appears to be 70% to 80%. With three stimuli, the sensitivity appears to increase to 90%. Specificity, the probability of a negative response to programmed electrical stimulation in a patient who has not had or will not have ventricular tachycardia, is estimated to exceed 95% when two stimuli are used. When three or more extrastimuli are used, specificity appears to be much lower, around 50% to 70%.

Reproducibility should probably not signify a specific clinical response. An artifact is likely to be reproducible.

Definitions are also causing problems in this new diagnostic technique. Definitions of sustained tachycardia vary because of a paucity of data on which any definitions can be based.

There is also a lack of uniformity about stimulation protocols. This problem occurs more in the evaluation of ventricular tachyarrhythmias than in sinus node, atrial, and AV conduction system function where more uniformity exists.

The presence of conduction disturbances, which are substantiated by ECG and clearly require permanent pacing including clear sinus node disease, Mobitz II second-degree atrioventricular block or complete heart block, do not require evaluation by electrophysiologic testing.

CONTRAINDICATIONS

Contraindications for electrophysiologic study of the cardiac conduction system are the same as those for cardiac catheterization with the exclusion of the dye reactions noted in the latter procedure. There are no specific contraindications to intracardiac impulse recording and the concurrent use of electrical stimulation.

PREPROCEDURE PREPARATION

The procedure is explained to the patient who should understand that catheterization of the heart will occur. Usually, all antiarrhythmic medications are discontinued for at least four elimination half lives. Light sedation can be given prior to the test. Otherwise, preparation is the same as that for cardiac catheterization.

PATIENT EDUCATION

The patient should be informed that the procedure may require several hours. Many patients take a nap during the procedure, and this should be encouraged. Simple relaxation exercises can be taught prior to the procedure.

PROCEDURE

The performance of clinical cardiac electophysiologic studies requires fluoroscopy and can be done in a procedure room or a cardiac catheterization laboratory.

One to four electrode catheters are positioned in the heart using established catheterization procedures and fluoroscopic guidance (figure 4–1.). The catheter electrodes are positioned high in the right atrium, across the tricuspid valve to record His bundle activity, and in the right ventricular apex. Surface electrocardiograms are recorded simultaneously with the intracardiac recordings in order to time events accurately. Both sets of readings are displayed on an oscilloscope and reproduced on hard copy for later evaluation.

The stimulation protocol continues to evolve as investigations are reported demonstrating improved specificity and sensitivity. Arrhythmias are induced during programmed electrical stimulation and are often terminated by pacing techniques or by spontaneous reversion to sinus rhythm.

The studies generally require 2 to 4 hours of laboratory time. Standardization and the maintenance of rigid timetables is difficult.

Following the procedure, the patient is told to remain at bed rest for 6 to 8 hours with no bending of the joint where the catheterization was performed.

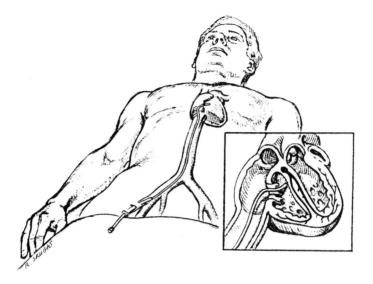

Figure 4–1. Cardiac electrophysiologic study via cardiac catheterization.

POSTPROCEDURE INFORMATION

The patient's family and/or friends should be given the same information as that provided with cardiac catheterization. If a close relative requests, additional information concerning the indications and usefulness of the electrophysiologic study is provided.

COMPLICATIONS

Most clinical reports have indicated that cardiac electrophysiologic studies can be performed safely and with minimal complications. There are little data actually quantifying the actual risks of such studies. The most common serious complication is venous thrombosis and it appears to occur in about 0.2% of studies. This complication is more common in patients of advanced age who have been relatively inactive for long periods or in patients with congestive heart failure.

Death has been reported in 0.06% of studies, occurring almost exclusively in patients undergoing study for evaluation of ventricular tachyarrhythmias. However, deaths have occurred in relatively stable patients with no obvious evidence of mechanical complication. The actual risk of death is probably comparable to that of routine cardiac catheterization and angiography.

Other major complications include cardiac perforation, pulmonary embolism, hemorrhage, and arterial injury. Pneumothorax has been reported when the subclavian vein is used for access. Arrhythmic complications have been reported including abnormal ECG patterns as well as the induction of arrhythmias. Cardioversion may be necessary during electrophysiologic study in many patients with ventricular tachyarrhythmias.

PATIENT QUESTIONS

How much pain will I have?

Patients should be assured that local anesthesia will obviate any severe pain, but they will sense touch and pressure and sometimes be aware of sensations while the catheter is being passed through the veins.

Why should I have this procedure just for dizziness?

If the dizziness reported by the patient is actually episodes of syncope, or a sudden and transient loss of consciousness, the symptom may be caused by decreased cerebral blood flow. The diagnostic workup of the patient with syncope is complex but must be done carefully. The reported one year mortality rate for patients with syncope of cardiovascular origin is approximately 20% and even higher in some studies. The standard ECG or long-term monitoring may be misleading, demonstrating bradycardia that is not the cause of the syncope, or nondiagnostic. Sinus node dysfunction, conduction defects, or tachycardia may be found on the ECG, but the significance of these rhythm disturbances may not be clear. The use of electrophysiologic studies in these patients, after a comprehensive evaluation of the cardiovascular and neurologic systems, is indicated when the syncopal symptoms are recurrent, unpredictable, and disabling. When the EPS study is diagnostic, therapy can be initiated and the patient often remains asymptomatic.

Is there a possibility that my heart will be damaged by this test?

The EPS use of programmed cardiac stimuli can cause the development of arrhythmias such as ventricular tachycardia, and cardioversion may be needed to return the heart rate to normal sinus rhythm. These excitation events, however, do not damage the cardiac tissue and the patient will not be worse off after the examination than before.

Will this test predict the likelihood of a heart attack?

The study of the movement of the electrical stimulation through the conducting system of the heart may allow prediction of the likelihood of sudden cardiac death cause by ventricular arrhythmia. This is one of several causes of cardiac damage and sudden death. Electrophysiologic study does not accurately evaluate all factors involved in cardiac tissue perfusion and cannot be used as a predictor for heart attacks.

CONSENT

Informed consent is required for this invasive procedure.

SELECTED BIBLIOGRAPHY

Horowitz LN: Clinical cardiac electrophysiology: history, rationale, and future. *Cardiol Clin* 1986;Aug:4(3):353.

Michelson EL, Medina RP: Introduction to clinical electrophysiologic studies. *Cardiovasc Clin* 1985;16(1):1.

Rahimtoola SH, Zipes DP, Akhtar M: Consensus statement of the conference on the state of the art of electrophysiologic testing in the diagnosis and treatment of patients with cardiac arrhythmias. *Circulation* 1987;75(suppl 3):III-3.

Tyndall A: A Nursing perspective of the invasive electrophysiologic approach to treatment of ventricular arrhythmias. *Heart-Lung* 1983;Nov:12(6):620.

5

Cardiac Pacing

RICHARD SADOVSKY

A cardiac pacemaker is an electronic stimulator used to send a specified current to the myocardium to control or maintain a minimum heart beat. With modern advances in pacemaker therapy, individualization is possible to match the patient's needs with the most suitable pacing mode and the most appropriate available pacing system. Pacing can be either permanent or temporary.

Pacemakers initiate myocardial depolarization with an electrical impulse generated from the tip of pacing wire delivering electrical energy to the heart. The heart then responds to the impulse with depolarization unless the myocardium has been irreversibly damaged by previous disease.

Pacemaker systems consist of the pulse generator and the lead/electrode system. The pulse generator includes the power source and electronic circuitry responsible for initiating the signal and for sensing cardiac activity. Synchronous, or demand, pacemakers are now the rule. These sense the patient's natural heartbeats and prevent competitive pacemaker firing. Recently, the pacemaker industry has developed a more sophisticated pacemaker that maintains atrioventricular (AV) synchrony. It takes advantage of atrial systole, which contributes approximately 20% to cardiac output. These popular new devices are called "physiologic pacemakers." Asynchronous, or fixed-rate, pacemakers are rarely used today, because they fired at a fixed rate regardless of the patient's heart rate, occasionally causing feelings of palpitations. The most appropriate pacemaker for the patient is determined by the chamber of the heart that needs pacing or sensing. If there is a definite need for the atrial kick to maintain adequate cardiac output, then an AV sequential pacemaker would be the most beneficial. Adequate hemodynamics should be restored when appropriate to help relieve symptoms.

Current lithium pacemakers are very small, with hermetically sealed pulse generator/lead connections. These are used almost exclusively at this time and have an expected life span of 4 to 10 years, depending on the type of battery used. These newer pacemakers can be programmed and allow for telemetry. Nuclear pacemakers are not in use because of the advent of these long-lasting lithium batteries.

The lead/electrode system includes a conductive wire or wires with an electrode(s) at the tip that comes in direct contact with the myocardium. The electrode delivers the impulse to the myocardium and carries information about spontaneous cardiac activity back to the pulse generator. Pacing leads, which are unipolar or bipolar, can be attached to the outside of the heart (epicardially) or the inside of the heart (endocardially). Unipolar leads sense electrical activity in a larger area of the myocardium. However, they can also sense extracardiac signals that may inappropriately inhibit pacemaker activity. Bipolar leads have more specific ability to sense only myocardial information, but can sense only information that arises between the two poles. Lead fixation devices are the special tips of the electrodes that secure contact with the myocardium. Active leads penetrate the myocardium and include screws, barber tips, and metal or nylon barbs. Passive permanent lead tips have wedges or coils that hold the electrode and wire in place.

The heart can be stimulated by the pacemaker in the pacing mode as well as by the interaction of the pacemaker with any underlying rhythm. The three-letter Inter-society Commission on Heart Disease (ICHD) code with two additional letters referring to some of the newer features available on pacemakers is used to classify the different pacing modes. The first letter represents the chamber paced (ventricle, atrium, both), the second letter defines the chamber sensed (ventricle, atrium, dual, or none), the third letter gives the mode of response (inhibited, triggered, dual, no response), the fourth and fifth letters designate programmability (programmable, not programmable, or multiple adjustments) and special features that prevent or stop arrhythmias. Familiarity with this code is helpful in interpreting pacemaker ECGs. Institutions generally use only a few types of pacemakers and maintain reference charts on them.

INDICATIONS

A pacemaker is indicated when the heart's natural pacemaker cells are unable to maintain a reliable rhythm. In addition, sophisticated pacemakers have been developed that have antiarrhythmic properties designed to terminate tachyarrhythmias.

Temporary pacing is used when immediate correction of symptomatic brady-cardia is required. It can be helpful also in uncontrolled tachyarrhythmias in which temporary pacing will override the tachyarrhythmia. Temporary pacing may also be used to ensure a reliable basic heart rate when antiarrhythmics and other drugs have caused the sinus node to slow below an acceptable rate. In addition, temporary pacing is sometimes used as part of a diagnostic procedure such as cardiac catheterization or electrophysiologic studies to evaluate the conduction system and to evaluate the potential for arrhythmias. Frequent use of temporary pacing is made following cardiac surgery.

Permanent pacemakers are usually indicated for symptomatic irreversible bradycardia, bradyarrhythmias due to hypersensitivity of the carotid and refractory tachyarrhythmias, especially when antiarrhythmic medications suppress sinus activity to rates that encourage ectopic rhythms.

There are some controversies about the indications used for pacing of the heart. It is unclear for some indications such as tachyarrhythmias that electrical stimulation will help, and some physicians believe that electrical stimulation will accelerate the arrhythmia to an even more malignant mechanism. Indications for pacemaker insertion must be carefully reviewed and individualized as to the benefit for each patient.

There is no role for physiologic pacemakers in patients with atrial fibrillation.

ALTERNATIVES

There are no satisfactory alternatives to cardiac pacing when the indications are present.

CONTRAINDICATIONS

There are no specific contraindications to cardiac pacing. Relative contraindications to the subclavian, femoral, or jugular approach requiring caution include anticoagulant therapy or uncontrolled bleeding diathesis. In addition, prior surgery or carotid artery disease may be a contraindication to specific approaches.

PREPROCEDURE PREPARATION

There is no specific preparation needed prior to cardiac pacing.

PATIENT EDUCATION

Patients who require temporary pacing want to know about the reason for the procedure but generally have little anxiety because of its transience. Patients who need permanent pacing have a variety of emotional reactions. Those who have experienced some relief with temporary pacing will look forward to the relief offered by the permanent procedure. Patients who are involved in the active resolution of the cause of their arrhythmia face permanent pacing with less emotional disturbance. There are also some patients who maintain steady denial throughout and are disappointed and angry when advised that a permanent pacemaker is indicated.

The amount of information given to the patient before the procedure must be tailored to the needs and desires of each particular patient and family. The reason for the permanent pacemaker installation should be explained with clarification that the "heart block" does not mean that something is obstructing the outflow of the heart. Diagrams of the heart may be helpful in the explanation. The patient should also be given the opportunity to see the pacemaker unit and to ask any questions they might have. Patients who have had temporary pacemakers need to be told that the permanent device is much smaller and is completely hidden beneath the skin.

Preoperative anxiety is expected prior to implantation of the pacemaker. This includes fear that their lives are being taken over by an artificial device and that control is being lost. Effective support should be provided before, during, and after the procedure.

The patient is awake during the entire procedure and a visit to the operating room prior to the procedure is very helpful in reducing patient anxiety. The patient should understand that some local anesthesia will be given and that additional sedation or anesthesia is available throughout the procedure if it is needed.

PROCEDURE

Temporary pacemaker insertion can be done by external pacing through electrodes attached to the patient's chest. With the development of improved surface electrodes, this procedure permits immediate pacing stimuli until a transvenous pacemaker can be inserted. Transthoracic temporary pacing leads can be passed through a cardiac needle inserted in the chest wall into the myocardium. However, capture is not dependable in this method, and there is a risk of cardiac tamponade if the needle ruptures a coronary blood vessel. External and transthoracic pacing is done only during extreme emergent situations such as cardiac arrest. Temporary epicardial pacemakers can be attached to the heart during open heart surgery allowing easy removal several days later. Temporary transvenous pacemaker wires are usually inserted in an x-ray suite. Local anesthesia is administered, and the wire is inserted into the subclavian, jugular, brachial, or femoral vein travelling to the right ventricle where the electrode contacts the myocardium. Continuous ECG monitoring is essential during insertion.

Permanent pacemaker insertion is done by a transvenous/endocardial technique. A small incision is made in the subcutaneous tissue of the upper chest and the lead or leads are inserted through a major vein into the right atrium and then into the right ventricular apex. It is a good practical idea that left handed persons should have the battery generator placed in the right pectoral area and vice versa. Fluoroscopy is used during the lead placement.

The pulse generator is attached to the leads once adequate lead placement is assured by measuring pacing and sensing thresholds. It is then inserted under the skin into a "pocket" in the subcutaneous tissue (figure 5-1.). Absorbable sutures are used to close the incision before the tight, occlusive dressing is applied.

Transthoracic pacemaker insertion requires general anesthesia and the insertion of a chest tube. The leads are sutured directly to the myocardium and fluoroscopy is not needed. The patient should be informed about turning, coughing, and deep breathing exercises after surgery.

POSTPROCEDURE INFORMAITON

Endocardial pacemaker insertion requires a hospital stay of 3 to 4 days. The patient should be told following the procedure that there is no clothing restriction once the soreness disappears and that his or her usual lifestyle can resume 3 to 4 weeks after the procedure. Besides the specific instructions for postimplant patient activities, people living with the patient should recognize that a large percentage of pacemaker recipients feel that they are significantly physically handicapped. This feeling leads to depression and unhappiness. The patient will need repeated ressurance about the pacemaker and the opportunity to ask any questions troubling them. Family members should provide support and comfort, but should urge the patient to seek answers from an appropriate medical person.

The patient may need to be reminded about the necessity for continued monitoring of pacemaker function. Many cardiologists reprogram the thresholds at 3 months after implant to prolong the life of the pacemaker. Frequent checkups are necessary to detect battery exhaustion before it occurs. These are generally done monthly and can be handled by a telephone hookup that relays information about the pacemaker function to the cardiologist's office.

COMPLICATIONS

Complications of temporary pacemakers are rare. Complications of permanent pacemakers can include problems related both to the procedure, to the pace-

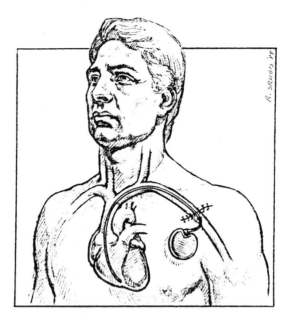

Figure 5□1. Subcutaneous pacemaker with endocardial leads.

maker or to the underlying cardiac disease. The procedure can cause impaired activity secondary to incisional pain, weakness, and drugs. This can be avoided by teaching range of motion (ROM) activities postoperatively and by offering analgesics if they are needed. Bleeding, venous thrombosis, hemorrhage, or infection occur rarely. Hemo and pneumothorax, chest nerve stimulation (diaphragmatic stimulation), and cardiac tamponade are also rare complications of the procedure.

At times, the patient may develop pectoral muscle twitching with pacing. This occurs when the generator of a unipolar pacemaker turns on itself because of a loose pocket, especially in elderly patients with little or loose connective subcutaneous tissue. This usually occurs during sleep when the patient turns from one side to the other. It is easily correctable by manually turning the pacemaker 180 degrees along the short axis using external pressure.

The pacing of the diseased heart may result in congestive heart failure secondary to loss of atrial kick, to the sudden rise in heart rate, tachyarrhythmias, failure to pace secondary to absence of electrical impulse, nonconduction problems, failure to sense, inappropriate sensing, or changes in the pacer rate. In addition, pacemaker runaway can occur. This results from a pacemaker rate of over 120 beats per minute, which can cause fibrillation, congestive heart failure, and even death. These problems are kept to a minimum by appropriately programming the pacemaker.

PATIENT QUESTIONS

What effect will the insertion of a permanent pacemaker have on my lifestyle?

The response to this question depends partly on the surgical approach (endocardial or epicardial) and the patient's preinsertion lifestyle and physical status. The patient can begin ROM exercises immediately following the procedure with strenuous exertion of the affected extremity held off for 3 to 4 weeks. Football, firing a rifle, or any activity that may cause blunt trauma to the area should be avoided. Padding the car seat belt may be necessary to prevent discomfort over the pacemaker implant site. Sexual activity can be resumed as soon as desired, and return to work should be on the advice of the physician. The patient should be reassured that the pulse generator is not damaged by proximity to magnets, high tension wires, or microwaves despite the fact that it might be temporarily confused by them. The currently used pulse generators are well protected against false inhibition by microwave ovens. Even though the current generators are well shielded, it is recommended by some that one avoid using motorized devices such as electric razors and electric tooth brushes. It is also recommended that the patient not work on a motor vehicle engine with the hood up while the motor is running. This may change the pacing mode from demand to fixed, or it may inhibit pacing. Airport screening devices may detect the pulse generator, although no interference will occur. Before boarding an airplane, the patient should request a seat away from the galley, since inflight meals are generally heated in microwave ovens. The patient cannot have a magnetic resonance study done after insertion of the permanent pacemaker. A balanced diet can be resumed unless the doctor feels there is a need for fat or salt restriction.

The patient should be cautioned against feeling and meddling with the pulse generator. Some patients may do this unconsciously, and in some cases, the pulse generator may rotate on its axis, pulling and displacing the electrode from the heart. This is called the "pacemaker twiddler syndrome."

The patient should receive a pacemaker identification card, which should be filled out completely and kept with the patient at all times.

How do I know that the pacemaker is functioning properly?

The patient should be reassured that pacemakers rarely malfunction and that the pacemaker battery can last up to 10 years. If the battery requires replacement, the procedure is easier than the original insertion because the lead to the heart is generally left in place. The patient should be advised to report episodes of palpitation, dizziness, or chest pain to the physician. To ensure proper pacemaker operation, the patient should be taught telephone ECG transmission, should make regular visits to the physician, and should learn how to take his or her own pulse. The physician monitoring the patient should be able to recognize the ECG components of pacemaker activity and should know the type of pacing device being used and its settings.

Will I still need to take medications after the procedure?

Because the pacemaker does not cure the patient's underlying pathology, medications are still an important part of the treatment program. The patient should have a list of his medications, instructions for their use, and a clear understanding of their purpose.

Can I still get a heart attack even with my pacemaker functioning well?

A heart attack is caused by damage to the cardiac muscle resulting from inadequate blood supply. The pacemaker will diminish some of the reasons for coronary insufficiency by regulating the heart rate and rhythm. The pacemaker does not, however, alter the patency of the coronary vessels. If insufficiency is caused by inadequate blood flow secondary to decreased coronary artery diameter, then the patient with a pacemaker may still have a heart attack.

Can my family physician properly monitor the functioning of my new pacemaker?

The family physician can monitor pacemaker function when the proper information is available. This includes the pacemaker registration form and copies of the before and after ECGs. This information is essential when examining the patient for signs and symptoms of pacemaker malfunction. The most common sign of pacemaker malfunction is a drop in pulse. If it is irregular as well as slow, then it is probably a result of heart, as well as pacemaker, malfunction and caused by ectopic beats. Other symptoms to watch for include fatigue, chest pain, lightheadedness, dizziness, fainting, dyspnea, or other signs of congestive heart failure. Every patient should know how to use a telephone monitor to augment his or her own ability to obtain information about the functioning of the pacemaker unit.

CONSENT

Consent should be obtained by the implanting physician prior to the procedure. It must indicate the anticipated risks and complications associated with pacing.

If, in an emergency, the patient's permission cannot be obtained, the family should be contacted and their consent obtained as thoroughly as possible.

SELECTED BIBLIOGRAPHY

Benditt DG, HT Markowitz: Permanent cardiac pacing in the era of peer review. The acceptable indication and the necessary documentation. *Postgrad Med* 1986;Aug:80:2:123.

Guzy PM: Emergency cardiac pacing. *Emerg Med Clin North Am* 1986;Nov:4:4:745.

Parsonnet V, Bernstein AD: Pacing in perspective: concepts and controversies. *Circulation* 1986;June:73:6:1087.

Wirtzfield A, Schmidt G, Himmler FC, Stangl K: Physiological pacing: present status and future developments. *PACE* 1987;Jan:10:1:41.

6

Doppler and Plethysmography

RICHARD M. STILLMAN

Doppler ultrasound flow uses reflected ultrasound waves to detect blood flow. Plethysmography uses cuffs or mercury-in-rubber strain gauges to detect changes in extremity circumference that occur with blood flow. Oculoplethysmography uses pneumatic corneal cups to detect intraocular pressures reflecting extracranial cerebrovascular blood flow. The combination of Doppler flow determinations and plethysmography is a useful adjunct to the diagnosis of peripheral vascular disease. These noninvasive studies are less costly and safer than more invasive vascular imaging studies such as angiography and radionuclide scanning. These tests together have a 95% accuracy rate in detecting vascular occlusive disease that significantly impairs blood flow, that is, hemodynamically significant lesions of 50% or more. However, Doppler and plethysmography may fail in detecting less substantial lesions that nevertheless may be highly significant in the etiology of the patient's problems. These tests are most useful in detecting blood flow in the extremities and the extracranial cerebrovascular system, and Doppler is currently being used in combination with two- dimensional (2-D) echocardiography to measure cardiac blood flow. A number of different manufacturers produce the equipment used for obtaining hard copy of Doppler flow and plethysmographic tracings, and most of these are quite portable, allowing use at the bedside.

INDICATIONS

Indications, procedure, and interpretation are quite different depending on whether the problem is venous disease or arterial disease. Deep vein thrombosis (DVT) may lead to pulmonary embolism, and to long-term disabling problems including leg pain, chronic edema, and venous stasis ulceration. Pulmonary embolism complicates 50% of cases of thigh vein thrombosis and about 10% of cases of calf vein thrombosis. Leg pain or edema typically alerts the clinician to the possibility of DVT, however, in some cases, pulmonary embolism may be the first sign. Because leg findings are variable and physical examination is often unreliable, noninvasive vascular laboratory testing is a useful adjunct to the diagnosis of DVT.

Atherosclerosis is characterized by invasion of a damaged arterial intima by plaque consisting of lipids, necrotic cells, cholesterol crystals, and connective tissue. Although these atherosclerotic plaques are initially asymptomatic, discovered only by diminished pulses or the presence of a bruit on physical examination, progression of disease results in ischemia of the anatomic sites supplied by the atherosclerotic arteries. Physical examination usually is quite reliable in determining the location of arterial occlusive disease, but the noninvasive vascular laboratory test is useful in determining the degree of compromise and is particularly vital in delineating the hemodynamic significance of each component of combined segment disease. Noninvasive evaluation using Doppler and plethysmography allows definition of the likely sites and severity of arterial occlusive disease.

Noninvasive evaluation of the peripheral venous system is indicated for symptoms or signs that suggest the possible presence of venous thromboembolic disease. Such findings include leg edema, leg pain, venous stasis disease (e.g., varicose veins, venous stasis ulcer), and pulmonary embolism. Noninvasive venous testing is also useful as a screening procedure for patients at high risk for venous thromboembolic disease e.g., bedridden, hip-fracture, major orthopedic or vascular surgical, hypercoagulable, or cerebrovascular-accident patients. Because physical examination is only 50% accurate in diagnosing or excluding DVT, objective testing is always required. The addition of Doppler and plethysmography to the history and physical examination increases the accuracy of the diagnosis of DVT to approximately 80%. Serial plethysmography repeated every day or every other day results in a continuous rise in accuracy with each test that is in agreement with the baseline study.

Noninvasive evaluation of the peripheral arterial circulation is indicated for symptoms or signs suggestive of arterial occlusive disease. Such findings include intermittent claudication, ischemic pain at rest, gangrene, palpable aneurysm, audible bruits, diminished distal pulses, suspicion of distal embolization, or vascular trauma. Noninvasive arterial evaluation is also indicated routinely following vascular bypass surgery to monitor graft patency and to detect possible development of new occlusive disease proximal or distal to the bypass graft that might threaten graft patency. Although physical examination by an experienced clinician is highly accurate in detecting or excluding the presence of arterial occlusive disease, noninvasive vascular testing is particularly helpful in patients with combined segment disease, e.g., combined iliac and femoral artery occlusive disease, or combined femoral and infrapopliteal occlusive disease. In these cases, noninvasive testing helps determine the hemodynamic significance of each of the occlusions, which is particularly relevant to determining long-term prognosis and the advisability of surgical intervention. Also, subtle changes in serial plethysmographic tracings and Doppler pressures may be the first indication of improvement or worsening of collateral circulation.

Noninvasive evaluation of extracranial cerebrovascular blood flow is indicated by symptoms or signs suggestive of extracranial arterial occlusive disease (figure 6–1.). Such findings include transient cerebral ischemic attack, reversible ischemic neurologic deficit, cerebrovascular accident, carotid bruit, syncope, dizziness, dementia, or confusion. In the presence of a carotid bruit, noninvasive evaluation of cerebrovascular flow will help to determine the degree of carotid occlusion, and detect the presence of contralateral disease. In the absence of a carotid bruit, noninvasive testing may be the best way to diagnose complete occlusion of the internal carotid artery.

ALTERNATIVES

Contrast radiography is the definitive test in confirming and defining the presence and extent of vascular disease. However, because contrast radiography has several risks, is uncomfortable or painful, and is expensive, noninvasive vascular testing provides, in many cases, a sufficient level of confidence in the diagnosis to supplant contrast radiography.

Radioisotope scanning has also been used to provide a gross image of arterial blood flow and of evolving venous thrombosis; however, it has several limitations that restrict its applicability. Radioisotope scanning of arterial flow provides a poorly resolved image that is inadequate for decisions regarding surgical management. Because radiolabeled fibrinogen is incorporated into only the evolving thrombus, radioisotope scanning for venous thrombosis will be falsely negative if the thrombus is fully formed. Incorporation of enough isotope to provide an image requires about 36 hours. False positives occur in areas of

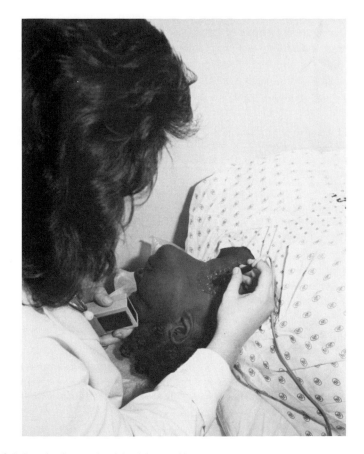

Figure 6–1. Doppler flow study of the right carotid artery.

hematoma, infection, or surgical incisions. Background counts in the pelvis preclude accuracy of diagnosis of pelvic venous thrombosis. Because ^{125}I fibrinogen scanning is such a nonspecific test, it is currently very useful as a research tool.

B-mode venous imaging uses ultrasound to provide images of the deep veins and to demonstrate any thrombi within them. This is a relatively new test and its accuracy has not been thoroughly assessed.

Carotid phonoangiography allows a frequency spectrum analysis of a carotid artery bruit or detection of turbulent carotid arterial flow even in the absence of bruit audible to the physician.

Potential for Failure

In diagnosing DVT, Doppler and plethysmography are approximately 80% accurate. That is, if the test suggests deep vein thrombosis, there is a 20% chance that DVT is not, in fact, present. Conversely, if the test is negative, but if the clinical signs suggest venous thrombosis, there is a 20% chance that the test is wrong and that DVT is indeed present. Serial performance of venous plethysmography every day or every other day results in an increased diagnostic accuracy with each test that agrees with the baseline study. Several factors contribute to the relatively high false-negative and false positive rates of this study. External compression of the major veins by a mass lesion, hematoma, or pregnant uterus will limit venous flow and may lead to a test that suggests venous thrombosis (false positive). Conversely, rapid opening of collateral veins to circumvent a clotted major vein may allow adequate venous flow and give a false-negative result. This is a major limitation of the test because the clotted vein, even though well-collateralized, may still be a source of pulmonary embolism. Therefore, if the clinical suspicion of DVT is strong, and if there is no contraindication, a venogram should be obtained.

In diagnosing arterial occlusive disease, these tests give a general idea as to the degree and location of arterial occlusions. The combination of arterial plethysmography and Doppler are approximately 95% accurate in defining the location of major arterial occlusions. Noninvasive tests, however, cannot distinguish the exact nature or location of occlusive lesions within major arteries. That is, although the noninvasive report may indicate aortoiliac occlusive disease, it cannot determine whether the occlusion is of the aorta, proximal common iliac, or distal external iliac arteries—a distinction particularly important for the vascular surgeon. Noninvasive testing may confirm infrapopliteal occlusive disease, but it cannot specifically determine whether the peroneal artery is open, or at what level the popliteal trifurcation is occluded. In some patients (especially those having diabetes mellitus), heavily calcified arteries may be noncompressible resulting in falsely elevated Doppler pressures. Despite these limitations, in most cases physical examination and noninvasive arterial flow determinations are sufficient to allow nonoperative treatment of peripheral arterial occlusive disease of the extremities. However, if surgery is contemplated, arteriography is usually required to confirm the exact nature of the disease, especially if a vascular operation is contemplated.

In diagnosing cerebrovascular disease, oculoplethysmography is diagnostic only for lesions that limit blood flow (usually these lesions occlude at least 60% of a cross sectional area of the internal carotid artery). Less occlusive carotid artery disease and vertebral artery occlusions are not detected by oculoplethysmography. B-mode ultrasound Duplex scanning of the carotid arteries is somewhat dependent on the skill and experience of the operator, but overall it is approximately 80% to 90% accurate in detecting even small carotid artery plaques. If surgery is not being contemplated, the data provided by history, physical examination, and noninvasive studies provide adequate reliability to avoid invasive testing. However, most surgeons insist on arteriography prior to carotid or vertebral artery surgery.

Interpretation of plethysmographic tracings requires substantial experience. Synthesis of the patient's clinical findings with the information obtained from the noninvasive vascular laboratory tests requires clinical experience and judgment. Legal issues involving noninvasive vascular testing include failure to provide the standard of care in performance of the examination, failure to recognize an abnormality, interpretive errors, and use beyond the physician's skill and knowledge. If venous disease is suspected, an experienced vascular specialist should be asked to evaluate the patient whether the noninvasive study is negative or positive. If arterial disease is suspected, an experienced vascular specialist should be asked to evaluate the patient even if the noninvasive study appears negative. Currently there are no licensing standards for those who perform these examinations.

CONTRAINDICATIONS

There are no contraindications to noninvasive evaluation of the arteries or veins of the extremities. However, to prevent the spread of infection from patient to patient, flow probes and pressure cuffs should not be placed in contact with open, infected or draining wounds. In some cases, this stipulation will limit the completeness of noninvasive examination. Oculoplethysmography should not be performed on patients who have had recent eye surgery or who have eye infections or detached retinas. An ophthalmologist should be consulted prior to considering oculoplethysmography on patients with any other ocular pathology.

PREPROCEDURE PREPARATION

No specific preparation is required for noninvasive testing of the arterial or venous circulation of the extremities. A topical ophthalmologic anesthetic agent is administered 15 minutes prior to performance of oculoplethysmography.

PATIENT EDUCATION

The patient should be informed of the clinical indications for the procedure and what may be learned. The patient should also be advised that this test is not always definitive in diagnosing or excluding the presence of vascular disease. This is particularly important when the purpose of the test is to evaluate a patient for the possibility of deep vein thrombosis, because potential false-negative results may dictate the need for venography. The patient may be reassured that the test is painless and noninvasive and that no drugs will be administered. Clothing must be removed from the area to be examined; therefore, the patient should not wear tight fitting garments that may be difficult to remove. The test takes 30 to 60 minutes.

PROCEDURE

For the Doppler examination, the patient lies supine on the examining table. The Doppler flow probe is placed sequentially over accessible vessels. The patient may be allowed to hear the signals, or the examiner may listen through headphones. The arterial sound is pulsatile; the venous sound is a more continuous "windstorm," varying only with respiration and with compression of the extremity distal to the probe site. Plethysmography involves placing pneumatic cuffs or mercury-in-rubber strain gauge wires snugly around the extremities. Changes in air pressure or in electrical impedance are measured through a transducer and plotted on a strip chart recorder. The primary care physician receives a report of the suspected pathology based on synthesis of the data obtained from the two tests.

The physician or technician evaluates a venous disease noninvasively using the following two techniques.

1. **Venous Doppler examination.** The 8 mHz Doppler instrument allows the physician to hear flow in the deep veins including the posterior tibial, popliteal, and femoral veins. There are three findings that suggest normal flow. First, the "windstorm" sound of venous flow at rest; second, augmentation of this sound by calf compression; third, fluctuation of this sound by deep respiration. The absence of any of these findings suggests deep vein thrombosis. Most important is documentation of a substantial difference between the involved and uninvolved sides.

2. **Venous plethysmography.** Plethysmography provides tracings of segmental limb venous flow. Strain gauge or impedance plethysmographic techniques measure volume changes in the leg before, during, and after proximal thigh occlusion with a cuff to evaluate for venous outflow disorders. This is done by applying a blood pressure cuff to the calf, inflating to 5 to 20 mm Hg and attaching it to a transducer and strip chart recorder. A second blood pressure cuff is applied to the thigh and inflated to 40 to 60 mm Hg. This latter cuff occludes venous outflow. As the calf veins fill, the calf cuff pressure slowly rises, and is reflected as a rise in the amplitude of the tracing. When this amplitude reaches its plateau, the thigh cuff is rapidly deflated. The calf cuff reflects the rapidity of venous outflow. Using a nomogram, the physician plots the maximal amplitude (segmental/venous/capacitance) against the rapidity of decline (maximal venous outflow). In addition, the segmental venous capacitance of the involved side is divided by the segmental venous capacitance of the

contralateral side. This ratio (segmental/venous capacitance ratio) should be approximately 1.0. Deviations from normal of these parameters lend support to the diagnosis of deep vein thrombosis.   The physician or technician evaluates arterial disease noninvasively using the following two techniques.

1. **Arterial Doppler examination.** The Doppler instrument allows the physician to hear blood flow in arteries that may have pressures too low to provide a palpable pulse.   Doppler pressures are obtained by listening to the posterior tibial or dorsalis pedis artery while inflating a blood pressure cuff around the calf. The pressure at which the Doppler signal disappears is recorded. Dividing this ankle pressure by the brachial systolic blood pressure results in the ankle/arm ratio, a useful prognostic indicator. For example, a patient with an ankle pressure of 60 mm Hg and a brachial pressure of 150 mm Hg has an ankle/arm ratio of 0.4, suggestive of a highly occlusive proximal lesion. Especially in diabetic patients, the physician must beware of calcified blood vessels, which may compress poorly and cause a falsely elevated ankle/arm ratio.

2. **Arterial plethysmography.** Plethysmography provides tracings of overall segmental limb flow. Plethysmography is performed by applying blood pressure cuffs to the thighs, legs, ankles, and, sometimes, toes. Cuffs are sequentially inflated to a pressure of 40 to 60 mm Hg and attached to a recorder that measures the small changes in pressure that occur with each heartbeat. Normal circulation provides a wave with known amplitude and form. Abnormal circulation due to proximal arterial disease is reflected by abnormally shaped or blunted waveforms at the level supplied by the diseased artery. In some cases, the patient will be asked to exercise by walking on a slow treadmill and the tracings repeated after this period of exercise. This stress test tends to exaggerate abnormalities in the tracings and in distal arterial pressures by diverting flow through collaterals.

The physician or technician will perform noninvasive evaluation of cerebrovascular arterial disease using **oculoplethysmography**. Oculoplethysmography requires the placement of sterile plastic cups (similar to contact lenses) onto the anesthetized cornea. The cups are attached by fine plastic tubing to the transducer, which measures and plots the intraocular arterial pressure, differences between arrival of the pulse wave at each eye, or (rarely) timing from pulse arrival at the eye versus pulse arrival at the ear with ear plethysmographs.

POSTPROCEDURE INFORMATION

There are no special instructions for family members. The patient may come and go from the noninvasive vascular laboratory without assistance. Outpatients may leave the test area immediately. The physician should be contacted in the rare event of prolonged symptoms following noninvasive vascular testing.

COMPLICATIONS

Some patients, especially those who have undergone treadmill exercise testing immediately before, may have mild muscular pain for several hours after the procedure. Following oculoplethysmography, the topical anesthesia will persist for about one hour, and subsequently there may be some eye redness and pain for up to 24 hours. There are essentially no complications following Doppler ultrasound and plethysmography.

PATIENT QUESTIONS

Is this the same as an angiogram?

No. Angiography is an invasive procedure requiring the injection of a radioopaque contrast material (dye) to allow visualization of arteries or veins on x-ray film. Doppler and plethysmography do not require the use of radioopaque dye nor of roentenograms. There is no needle puncture and no pain.

How accurate is this test?

In the diagnosis of venous occlusive disease, this test is approximately 80% accurate. That is, if the test suggests deep vein thrombosis, there is a 20% chance that you do not have deep vein thrombosis. Conversely, if the test is negative, but if your clinical signs suggest venous thrombosis, there is a 20% chance that the test is wrong and that you do have deep vein thrombosis. If deep vein thrombosis is suspected, and if there is no contraindication, a venogram may be obtained. In the diagnosis of arterial occlusive disease, these two tests give a general idea as to the degree and locations of arterial occlusions. Angiography may be required to confirm the exact nature of the disease.

If the angiogram is so much more accurate, why not just obtain an angiogram?

Although an angiogram may be required, there are several absolute and relative contraindications to angiography. These include history of anaphylactic reaction to radioographic contrast materials, renal insufficiency, and pregnancy. If the physician believes that the benefits of angiography outweigh the risks, angiography may be performed anyway, but only after pharmacologic blocking of the allergic response using an antihistamine or a corticosteroid. If renal insufficiency is present (usually judged by a blood test showing an elevation in serum creatinine and blood urea nitrogen), the injection of radiopaque contrast material may cause a worsening of the renal problem or even permanent kidney failure. In such a case, angiography is best avoided. Nevertheless, if angiography is absolutely necessary, and if the potential benefits outweigh this very major risk, angiography is performed after carefully monitored intravenous fluid administration and with close observation of renal function. If the patient is pregnant, angiography may be contraindicated because of potential effects of the contrast agent on the fetus, or because of the fear of radiation exposure of the fetus. Nevertheless, if angiography is absolutely necessary, the fetus should be shielded from radiation exposure as much as possible.

Will another test be needed before I have surgery?

Yes. In most cases, the surgeon will need a highly detailed road map prior to performing a vascular surgical operation. This degree of detail and accuracy is possible only with angiography.

CONSENT

Written consent is not required.

SELECTED BIBLIOGRAPHY

Atik M: Venous thromboembolic disease. In Moore WS, ed: *Vascular Surgery—A Comprehensive Review.* Orlando, FL: Grune and Stratton, 1983;821.

Bergan JJ, Yao JS eds: *Cerebrovascular Insufficiency.* Orlando, FL: Grune and Stratton, 1983. A comprehensive text about diagnosis and therapy of cerebrovascular disease, with a surgical emphasis.

Greenfield LJ: Pulmonary embolism: diagnosis and management. *Curr Prob Surg* 1976;13:1.

Samson RH, Scher LA, Veith FJ: Combined segment arterial disease. *Surgery* 1985;97(4):385.

7

Echocardiography

RICHARD SADOVSKY

Echocardiography is a noninvasive technique using sound waves to follow movements and measure dimensions of cardiac structures. To accomplish this, an echocardiogram requires three pieces of equipment: an ultrasonic transducer, an echoscope, and a recording device. These allow transmission and reception of ultrasonic impulses, display of the images of cardiac spatial anatomy and function created by the reflected impulses, and a permanent recording of the reflected image.

Recordings of movement of the valve leaflets, ventricular walls, and the interventricular septum are made. Changes in any cardiac chamber during the cardiac cycle can be assessed and abnormal chamber filling can be noted. A time/motion study of the heart (M-mode echocardiography) is possible because the ultrasonic beam follows the motion of various cardiac structures over a period of time. The angle of the ultrasound beam is kept still. This permits position and motion information to be displayed as a function of time.

A second kind of scan is produced in two dimensional echocardiography as the angle is changed within a sector. This technique demonstrates cardiac structures more fully by movement of the sound beam through a given plane resulting in a tomographic image on display.

Contrast echocardiography involves injection of a dye into the cardiac chambers through cardiac catheterization. This is an invasive procedure and is generally used when it is crucial to follow the flow of blood through the heart clarifying valvular insufficiency disease and other abnormalities. It is anticipated that eventually this technique will allow accurate determination of intracardiac pressures using resonant frequency analysis of precision microbubbles. This technique is currently being developed. Work with peripheral contrast injections is under way and may allow for the diagnosis of intracardiac shunts.

Echocardiography combined with Doppler techniques can detect flow disturbances, and when combined with two-dimensional echocardiography, the severity of valvular flow abnormalities can be clearly assessed.

INDICATIONS

Both M-mode and two-dimensional echocardiography show cardiac anatomy and the dynamics of cardiac structures so that the physiology and pathophysiology of the heart can be interpreted in light of other clinical facts known about the patient. M-mode echocardiography is able to evaluate cardiac motion well. Its use in detecting pericardial effusion and guiding needle placement during pericardiocentesis is now routine in the hands of the skilled technician. Two-dimensional echocardiography has been developed more recently giving a good view of overall cardiac anatomy and motion. A multidimensional display of anatomy is possible as is the ability to integrate motion occurring in disparate areas of the heart. This allows segmental assessment of ventricular function and is an asset in diagnosing congenital and coronary artery disease.

A combination of M-mode and two-dimensional echocardiography gives the best analysis of complex heart motion and gives increased access to information about the heart. Details of the interior anatomy of the heart can be examined and may provide sufficient information to avoid more invasive tests.

The test is most often used to investigate suspected aortic or mitral valve disease, idiopathic hypertrophic subaortic stenosis, left ventricular disorders, pericardial effusions, hypertrophy, and subacute bacterial endocarditis. Echocardiography, alone, using calculations made with estimated cardiac chamber volumes at different stages in the cardiac cycle, or in conjunction with newly developing Doppler techniques, can also evaluate cardiac functions such as stroke volume, ejection fraction, and blood flow through the valves. Other uses include assessing a patient before and after cardiac surgery, monitoring the progress of a cardiac disorder, exploring the advisability of cardiac catheterization for suspected operable lesions, and investigating a malfunctioning prosthetic valve.

Exercise echocardiography is a technique that evaluates myocardial response to exertion. Advances in computer technology coupled with Doppler studies are making possible the evaluation of indicators of ischemia such as wall motion and thickening, as well as abnormal blood flows.

Transesophageal echocardiography expands the role of cardiac sonography in patients who are difficult to examine externally, and allows continuous monitoring. This study is somewhat invasive due to the need for placing the transducer in the esophagus in order to visualize the heart from the back. This test does have a level of morbidity.

ALTERNATIVES

Echocardiography is a noninvasive and safe examination that should be used preferably in all clinical situations in which it will provide helpful information. This procedure seems to be reducing the frequency of cardiac catheterization, particularly for intracardiac masses and pediatric congenital heart disease.

POSSIBILITY OF FAILURE

Most clinicians recognize the primary use of echocardiography in the diagnosis of pericardial effusion, intracardiac masses, many stenotic valvular cardiac lesions, most forms of cardiomyopathy, some types of prosthetic valve dysfunction, and definition of the anatomy of complex congenital heart disease. Echocardiography is also recognized to be much more sensitive than ECG for the detection of left ventricular hypertrophy. The major limitation of this technique is the difficulty in obtaining a good study. Appropriate knowledge of the anatomy of the heart is needed by the technician or examiner in order to obtain a thorough examination, to analyze the dynamic pictures obtained during two dimensional echocardiography and to obtain the appropriate, representative still recordings. If there are questions as to whether echocardiography will answer a specific clinical question, the cardiologist who routinely does these examinations should be consulted. Imaging is poorer in older patients, especially those with chronic lung disease. Obesity, anatomic defects, chest trauma, and some prosthetic valves may cause inadequate images.

Radionuclide and contrast angiographic techniques currently seem to have the ability to define more fully global ventricular function, assess coronary artery disease, and identify regurgitant valvular cardiac lesions and intracardiac shunts in most patients.

The extent of left ventricular involvement in myocardial infarction as determined by regional wall motion seen on echocardiographic examination does correlate with infarct size as determined by enzymatic analysis, thallium scanning, technetium scanning, or pathologic examination. However, the echocardiogram tends to overestimate the infarction size, probably due to asynergy noted in nearby ischemic but viable myocardium. The more extensive the left ventricular involvement as judged by the wall motion index or the ejection fraction, the worse the prognosis. The predictive value of the echocardiogram in the post myocardial infarction patient appears similar to that of the ejection fraction determined by ventriculography.

The use of echocardiography to find a source of emboli in the heart has been popular in the past, but there is now ample evidence that the yield in this setting is low in the absence of clinical heart disease. Furthermore, incidental echocardiographic abnormalities found in the elderly may lead to the mistaken diagnosis of "embolic stroke" and inappropriate therapy may be used that could have substantial morbidity.

Measurements involving definitive quantitation of these conditions still require the more invasive procedure of cardiac catheterization. Contrast angiography or computerized tomography with contrast enhancement are still the best ways to define the location and extent of thoracic aortic dissection.

The procedure is sensitive for mitral valve prolapse, but specificity decreases when strict criteria are not employed in reading the images. Variants of normal that imitate mitral valve prolapse can cause false diagnoses.

CONTRAINDICATIONS

There are no contraindications to echocardiography although there are some conditions that limit the usefulness of this test. The examination is difficult or impossible to perform on patients with emphysema, chronic lung disease, or other pulmonary pathology. In the elderly, heart valves may be calcified, narrowing the intercostal spaces, and in thin patients, the bony anatomy may absorb the impulses; in obese patients, a decrease in reflected echoes is expected.

Heart failure may also make examination difficult because of the patient's inability to lie still for the required amount of time. Examination can be performed with the patient sitting up, but this is more difficult.

PATIENT EDUCATION

Patients should be told what the procedure is and what is hoped to be accomplished. A brief explanation of the transducer is helpful and patients should be informed that they will not feel, nor will they be harmed by, the electrical current emitted from the transducer.

The procedure is somewhat slow and can take 30 to 60 minutes. The patient will need to lie still during that time, although he may be asked to assume different positions during the examination. All clothing from the waist up will be removed and the transducer is held on the patient's chest while simultaneously observing the echoes displayed on the video monitor. The examiner must have both interpretive and technical competence if optimal results are to be obtained.

PREPROCEDURE PREPARATION

No specific preprocedure preparation is needed.

PROCEDURE

Electrocardiogram leads are usually attached to the skin before the procedure begins. A gel is used between the skin and the transducer (figure 7–1) to eliminate any air. The transducer is placed with care to avoid interference from the lung. Short bursts of high frequency sound waves are generated and sent through the chest tissue and the heart with a recording made of the echoes returning to the transducer. Care must be taken in the examination to obtain high quality recordings as the echoed sound waves are best received when the transducer is perpendicular to the structure being examined.

POSTPROCEDURE CARE

There is no specific postprocedure care needed.

COMPLICATIONS

Echocardiography has no risk or significant discomfort to the patient and can be repeated safely at intervals. Further discussion concerning the side effects of ultrasound are located in the appropriate section in chapter 58.

Echocardiographic results must be determined with the information obtained from the clinical examination of the patient. Since two-dimensional echocardiography often reveals minor morphologic and functional abnormalities that are not clinically apparent, there is great a likelihood of creating spurious disease. When this occurs in a patient with a typically innocent murmur, the patient is then labelled with a cardiac diagnosis and the morbidity of this "harmless" procedure becomes very great.

PATIENT QUESTIONS

Will this test hurt?

Echocardiography is a painless test in which sound waves are beamed through the chest to examine different parts of the heart. The only thing that the patient will feel is the slight pressure of the transducer that emits the sound waves. The procedure can be repeated many times without harmful effects.

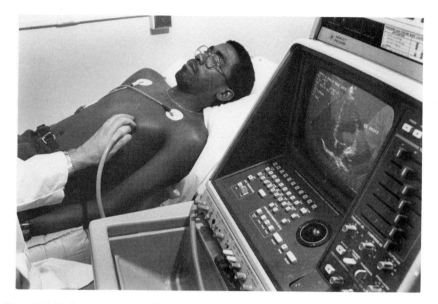

Figure 7–1. Performing an echocardiogram.

Will echocardiography tell me definitively whether I have mitral prolapse?

The M-mode and two-dimensional echocardiographic views can be very reveal-ing in the case of mitral prolapse. Classic late-systolic mitral valve prolapse as seen on the M-mode examination is sufficient to confirm the diagnosis. Only the coincident presence of a moderate-to-large pericardial effusion can produce a false-positive mitral valve prolapse pattern when later systolic prolapse is marked and classic. However, M-mode examination might fail to disclose a true, positive mitral prolapse echo if all three scallops of the posterior mitral leaflet are not carefully scanned. Specific criteria must be followed to evaluate the images obtained.

Two-dimensional echocardiography reveals unmistakable billowing in severe cases of mitral prolapse. Although this technique may more fully demonstrate valve thickening associated with myxomatous tissue, a well-done M-mode scan of the entire mitral valve is the most cost effective test in classic mitral valve prolapse.

If the patient is asymptomatic and an echocardiogram done for some other reason reveals classic marked prolapse, then the patient should be considered a prolapse patient. If the echo reveals a more subtle abnormality, such as bowing, the patient probably does not warrant the clinical classification of mitral valve prolapse.

In the patient with many symptoms (but few of the physical findings of mitral prolapse) and whose M-mode echo is equivocal for prolapse, the patient should have a careful two-dimensional study with thorough viewing of all three leaflets of the mitral valve. These may be equivocal in addition. At present, these situations are subjectively graded for mitral valve prolapse as not seen, possible, probable, and classic.

Will this test provide all the information needed about my heart so that I do not need any further examinations?

Echocardiography provides information about heart anatomy and function in several static and dynamic ways that are described above. Abnormalities must be correlated with clinical examination data. Although the echocardiographic evaluation is becoming more comprehensive with the addition of Doppler techniques, certain information about blood flow, coronary artery disease, and fine pressure measurements still require invasive radionuclide or catheterization studies. There is no guarantee that echocardiography will provide all the information needed to clarify a cardiac diagnosis.

CONSENT

Consent is not required for this noninvasive procedure.

SELECTED BIBLIOGRAPHY

Bansal RC, Tajik AJ, Seward JB, Offord KP: Feasibility of detailed two-dimensional echocardiographic examination in adults. *Mayo Clin Proc* 1980;55:291.

Bier AJ, Feigenbaum H, Kisslo J: Using echocardiography effectively. *Patient Care* 1988;Feb:22:18.

Nishimura RA, Miller FA, Callanan MJ et al: Doppler echocardiography: theory, instrumentation, technique and application. *Mayo Clin Proc* 1985;60:321.

Sahn DJ: Real-time, two-dimensional Doppler echocardiographic flow mapping. *Circulation* 1985;71:849.

8

Enzymatic Thrombolysis

RICHARD SADOVSKY AND DAVID H. GORDON

Pioneering clinical trials using mixtures of plasminogen and streptokinase for thrombolytic therapy have been in progress for 25 years. Streptokinase (SK) was recognized as the commercial mixture most superior to former preparations. Urokinase (UK), a substance of natural extraction prepared from urine and kidney cell, and lung adenocarcinoma cell lines in culture, was found later. Several therapeutic trials have shown that these agents are able to recanalize an obstructed artery or vein better than heparin by converting plasminogen to plasmin ("plasmin activation"). Plasmin possesses an affinity for fibrin and it lyses the fibrin mesh of the clot.

Acceptance of these agents has been slow. The fear of bleeding complications, high costs, and questions about efficacy as the main drawbacks. Dose-effect studies have been conducted poorly and little reliable pharmacologic data has been obtained.

In the 1980s, tissue plasminogen activator (t-PA) has become available. This is a new fibrin-specific thrombolytic agent. With the discovery of t-PA that interest in enzymatic thrombolysis has increased since it appears to have a higher affinity for fibrin and is able to more efficiently activate plasminogen on the fibrin surface. It is given by peripheral intravenous infusion. It is becoming clear that the fibrin selectivity of t-PA is influenced by the dose and duration of t-PA infusion. A recent competitor of t-PA is purokinase, or single-chain urokinase. The mechanism of this agent is unclear, but its efficacy appears to be high.

Enzymatic thrombolysis is a rapidly evolving therapeutic procedure and new agents are being developed and evaluated.

INDICATIONS

Both arterial and venous thrombi contain substantial amounts of fibrin, even though there is a great variety of structure in these fibrin networks. Recent research in the lysis of fibrin is helping to clarify the use of the enzymatic agents, with fibrinolysis requiring adequate levels of plasminogen and activator to be bound to the fibrin. A good thrombolytic agent should have high fibrin affinity, and should be stable in the systemic circulation allowing time for it to reach and penetrate through the thrombus.

The major applications of these thrombolytic agents include acute myocardial infarction seen within four hours of onset of persistent chest pain, electrocardiographic changes indicative of transmural ischemia, severe and acute pulmonary embolism, and proximal deep vein thrombosis (figure 8–1). These agents are also being used in graft thrombosis, and digital and pedal ischemia where Fogarty catheter procedures or bypass are not feasible.

Treatment in **acute myocardial infarction** must be urgent to prevent necrosis, whereas treatment of venous thromboembolism can be delayed for many hours while maintaining efficacy. Thrombosis does appear to be the major common pathologic event that creates the acute myocardial infarction in a majority of patients with the presence of chest pain and persistent ST segment elevation having a high predictive value for the developing stages of a transmural infarct. Reperfusion following occlusion must be done rapidly to salvage substantial portions of the damaged areas. The thrombolytic agent must be administered within 1 to 4 hours of the occlusive event. This is currently being done in many community hospital emergency rooms.

In addition, the size of the infarct remains proportional to the duration of arterial occlusion. Initial studies have demonstrated decreased mortality following thrombolysis up to 24 hours following an acute myocardial infarction, especially in patients having noncomplete occlusion as indicated by intermittent pain and mild ECG changes. Although it has been suggested that patients with inferior wall infarctions may not benefit from thrombolytic therapy, studies are showing increased life expectancy in second heart attacks in patients whose initial infarction was treated. SK has been the most frequently used agent in myocardial infarction because of cost factors. The use of UK appears to be

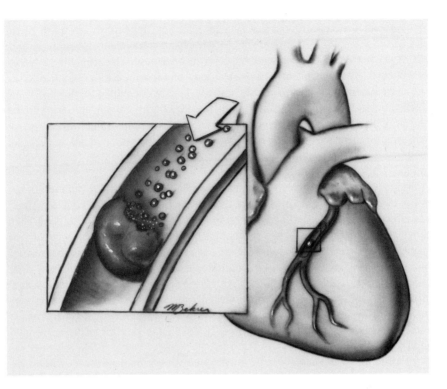

Figure 8–1. Coronary artery thrombus being lysed by enzyme therapy.

tolerated more easily by the body with fewer side effects, especially bleeding. Comparative reperfusion studies under way with t-PA show an efficacy equal, or slightly superior, to that of SK. Another cardiac use for thrombolytic agents is thrombosis on **prosthetic heart valves**.

With **acute pulmonary embolism,** heparin has been found to be effective in preventing thrombus growth, but it does not have direct thrombolytic action. Thrombolytic enzyme therapy for these patients remains in the exploratory stage because of bleeding complications, the lack of mortality differences, the higher costs, and the inertia of changing clinical practice.   There is also a lack of agreement between dosages, durations, and methods of administration. Accelerated recovery appears to occur with thrombolytic therapy, but evidence for long-term advantage over heparin therapy is less clear. Recommendations have been made about enzyme administration to resolve pulmonary emboli and studies in this area are currently under way. Urokinase, although more expensive, appears to be the better agent for this indication because of its natural origin and smaller unit dosage. The use of t-PA in pulmonary embolism is being explored since this "second generation" thrombolytic preparation appears to be more fibrin lysis specific and can be administered by peripheral intravenous infusion. Recent studies show t-PA to be somewhat superior to urokinase. Heparin should probably not be used concomitantly because it may increase bleeding complications.

The treatment of **deep venous thrombosis** has demonstrated the limited value of thrombolytic therapy with some accelerated recovery. Postphlebitic syndrome therapy with streptokinase has been shown to have some value. In any case, thrombolytic therapy should be restricted to relatively young patients with recent (less than 72 hours) proximal venous thrombosis. The use of t-PA for this condition has yet to be explored.

For the treatment of **acute limb ischemia,** local intraarterial instillation of SK or UK has been found more effective than intravenous treatment with decreased side effects. Intravenous administration of relatively high doses of SK have been shown to restore patency in two-thirds of recently (less than 72 hours) occluded arteries. This procedure is done only with extreme caution, however, because of the risks of bleeding or distal embolization with possibly fatal results. Low-dose (local) arterial infusions have been gaining greater acceptance with optimal thrombolysis and minimal complications. This procedure is currently being performed as a preliminary to vascular surgery. Recanalization of peripheral arteries has an advantage over that of coronary arteries in that it can be performed under less urgent conditions.

It should be noted, however, that the lesion causing the thrombosis will not be cured by thrombolytic therapy alone and may require concomitant angioplasty.

ALTERNATIVES

With the need for revascularization in cases of thrombus formation other procedures have been attempted. These procedures are generally aimed at achieving the same effect, which is dissolution of the clot and revascularization of the distal area when occlusion has occurred. This involves surgical intervention or the newer procedure, angioplasty. It should be noted that angioplasty is rarely, if ever, performed in the presence of fresh or subacute thrombus because of the danger of embolization. Emergency aortocoronary by-passes have been performed with acceptable levels of morbidity and mortality, but this technique has the logistical problems of requiring rapid access to the operating room and an appropriate team of surgeons.

Percutaneous transluminal coronary angioplasty (PTCA) has been used to revascularize the coronary arteries. This usually follows a prior thrombolysis, but it can be done without lytic therapy. The delay between the onset of symptoms and the procedure may be of some concern in the early minutes following occlusion. The success of PTCA relies on the clinician's experience but it has improved considerably with steerable catheter systems. It also appears to be more successful in cases in which there was a previously patent artery. Prospective randomized studies have demonstrated that PTCA alone or in association with thrombolysis is better than thrombolysis alone. Recent studies imply that the use of thrombolytic agents prior to angioplasty will permit more complete clot lysis, reducing the degree of residual stenosis and distal embolization. Immediate angioplasty does not appear to be superior to a delayed, elective procedure after successful thrombolytic reperfusion.

Embolectomy using a Fogarty catheter under local anesthesia has been used for acute arterial occlusions. This is preferable to thrombolytic therapy when it is clear that the hours or days required for thrombolytic therapy may jeopardize the limb. At the present time, thrombolytic therapy for arterial occlusion should probably be restricted to those situations in which arterial surgery has a low success rate or an unacceptable mortality and morbidity or in very peripheral vessels where surgery is not feasible, such as thrombosis in the femoropopliteal segment extending to the distal outflow tract and in patients in precarious conditions with high operative risks. Catheter embolectomy or percutaneous transluminal angioplasty is another option.

POSSIBILITY OF FAILURE

The stability of patients following enzymatic thrombolysis is an unresolved issue. Some investigators feel that with meticulous attention to anticoagulation following the procedure, patients will do well. Others emphasize the need for further procedures to remove the remaining obstruction.

In cases of poor reperfusion, or even in cases of successful reperfusion, a significant arterial lesion or clot may remain. This lesion may require subsequent percutaneous transluminal angioplasty, embolectomy, bypass surgery, or other procedure. Early reocclusion or recurrent ischemia after thrombolytic therapy of coronary arteries is encountered in 20% to 40% of patients who are successfully recanalized. Many patients are left with a high-grade stenotic lesion. The use of maintenance t-PA and the role of angioplasty following thrombolytic therapy is being studied.

CONTRAINDICATIONS

Patients who have undergone recent surgery or internal organ biopsy are ineligible to receive enzyme thrombolytic therapy because of the inability of the chemical to distinguish between "good" and "bad" clots. Other contraindications include active intracranial bleeding, trauma, pregnancy, or intracerebral processes that are likely to bleed. This latter category includes patients with prior history of cerebrovascular accident within the preceding three months. Some centers expand this contraindication to any history of cerebrovascular accident or transient ischemic attack.

Severe, uncontrolled arterial hypertension, diabetic hemorrhagic retinopathy, advanced age, endotracheal intubation, and any coagulopathy are also considered contraindications.

PREPROCEDURE PREPARATION

No single laboratory test predicts exactly the patient's propensity to bleed when treated with thrombolytic agents. Screening tests should be performed, if time permits, in order to eliminate patients with a predisposition to bleeding and with high levels of SK antibodies (if SK is going to be used). Prothrombin times (PT) and partial thromboplastin times (PTT) are generally measured, in addition to fibrinogen assays, blood cell counts, and determination of blood group.

Recently, t-PA inhibitor assays have been developed. Levels of this inhibitor appear to be elevated in patients with acute myocardial infarction. The importance of this finding has not yet been determined.

Premedication with steroids, antihistamines, and/or antipyretic medications have been used in various centers. Aspirin should be specifically avoided to prevent distortion of clotting factors.

PATIENT EDUCATION

The patient should understand the reason for using enzymatic thrombolysis and its possible complications. The patient can be told that if there is pain with the newly formed clot, it will be significantly diminished or may even disappear with the procedure. If a catheter is going to be used to instill the enzyme, the patient should be informed of the possibility of bleeding around the catheter and the formation of thrombus proximal to the catheter.

PROCEDURE

Intravenous administration of thrombolytic agents has been generally found to be unacceptable due to the complications caused by the systemic effects on fibrin clot formation and the resulting risks of hemorrhage. (However it has been used for patients with acute myocardial infarction based on the need for rapid administration immediately following diagnosis.) Initial studies of intravenous administration of SK in acute myocardial infarction demonstrate a 50% reperfusion rate compared to a 75% success rate when SK is infused into the coronary artery directly to the site of the clot. t-PA appears to be more fibrin lysis specific and is administered by intravenous peripheral infusion.

An easily compressible puncture site is chosen and a suitable catheter is introduced into the occluded vessel (as in percutaneous transluminal angioplasty) for delivery of the thrombolytic agent. Ideally, the catheter is inserted into the proximal part of the occluding thrombus. Repeated injections of the thrombolytic agent are delivered frequently while slowly advancing the catheter with or without a guide wire. Making holes in the thrombus with a wire will help the agent to permeate the clot. The procedure is continued until the thrombus is completely infiltrated and the distal lumen is reached.

The second, and more popular, scheme is a continuous infusion administered with the aid of an arterial infusion pump. The duration of treatment is determined by the individual's response. For a small thrombus, an infusion of limited duration (one to a few hours) may be sufficient to obtain lysis, but an extended clot may require several days to resolve. Progression of clot lysis can be followed by fluoroscopy or angiography via the catheter at regular intervals. The catheter is advanced when evidence for partial clot lysis is obtained. If no lysis occurs in 24 to 48 hours, the treatment is considered to have failed. The value of laboratory tests during thrombolysis is under investigation. Fibrinogen levels are generally measured during the procedure when long-term treatment is anticipated. Plasminogen activity and t-PA levels can be measured also. Ideally, this laboratory monitoring should be able to scrutinize the thrombolytic effectiveness of the drug and to predict bleeding or rethrombosis. For example, low fibrinogen levels have been associated with better clot dissolution during SK therapy. The predictive value of platelet studies is presently unclear. Prolongation of the thrombin time to greater than 5 times control means that the patient is probably predisposed to bleeding. Blood counts are also taken. If the fibrinogen level drops below a critical point, the treatment procedure must be discontinued.

There is disagreement as to whether to stop or continue the concomitant use of anticoagulants during thrombolytic therapy. Some cardiologists feel that the heparin infusion must be continued throughout enzymatic thrombolysis of coronary vessels in order to decrease the potential of reocclusion and thrombus formations proximal to the catheter tip.

POSTPROCEDURE INFORMATION

After treatment with thrombolytic enzyme preparations, patients are maintained on anticoagulant therapy for varying amounts of time using coumarin or combinations of aspirin and dipyridamole.

Patients who have been treated for recent coronary artery occlusion should be kept on anticoagulants for approximately 2 months, since this is the period needed for a damaged endothelium to regenerate.

COMPLICATIONS

The use of streptokinase, a bacterial protein that is recognized as foreign to the body, can result in allergic reactions in approximately 5% of the cases. The most common are fever and drug rash; anaphylactoid shock occurs rarely. Hypotension has been reported in up to 15% of the patients, some of whom require vasopressor support.

The ability of thrombolytic enzymes to differentiate between "good" and "bad" clots is not dependable. Most complications occur because of the inability to maintain general hemostasis with ultimate hemorrhagic side effects. Local bleeding from the arterial puncture site occurs in 10% to 30% of the patients, but it is usually minor and can be controlled by prolonged compression. Major hematomas or retroperitoneal hemorrhage occasionally requires blood transfusion. Remote bleeding has been reported to occur in 3% to 5% of the treated patients and can be life threatening if intracranial bleeding or severe gastrointestinal or hemorrhage occurs. Catheter manipulation itself has the complications of thrombosis, wall dissection, or vessel spasm.

The use of thrombolytic agents in patients with acute pulmonary embolism has the major complication of bleeding with the rate being around 5% in t-PA-treated patients and around 27% in those treated with UK. It is unclear as to whether this difference is due to intrinsic chemical properties of the enzyme being used or the different skill in managing patients receiving lytic therapy. In neither case does the degree of fibrinogen depression (which indicates a systemic lytic state) correlate with the severity of bleeding.

When used in patients with acute myocardial infarction, the risk of life-threatening bleeding (including intracranial bleeding) has been found to be as low as 0.5% when limited doses of t-PA are used. When concomitant heparin therapy is given, the intracranial bleed rate increases to above 1.0%. Bleeding complications from tPA appear to be dose related and exacerbated by concomitant heparin therapy. Low-dose (minidose) heparin may be used, but this is controversial. Additional complications include reperfusion arrhythmias such as ventricular premature beats, accelerated idioventricular rhythms, ventricular fibrillation, hemorrhage and/or cardiac rupture at the infarct site, and intracranial bleeds. "Reperfusion" arrhythmias can be decreased by preventive administration of intravenous lidocaine.

When SK has been used for treatment of venous thrombosis, hemorrhagic complications were found to occur about 3 times as often as with heparin. The frequency of recurrent hemorrhagic accidents with SK requiring blood transfusions is around 3% to 4% with some studies reporting a death rate as high as 1%. The use of UK seems to be as successful as SK, and with a lower hemorrhagic risk, but the duration of treatment has to be longer, which markedly increases the cost.

The use of thrombolytic agents for resolution of clots on prosthetic heart valves carries the major risk of embolism. Small emboli can result in permanent brain damage with hemiplegia. For this reason, treatment of prosthetic valve clots with thrombolytic agents should be restricted to critically ill patients who are too sick to undergo emergency surgery.

The use of thrombolytic agents for treatment of acute arterial occlusion has been shown to result occasionally in showers of small emboli that may cause transient pain or areas of localized ischemia.

PATIENT QUESTIONS

Should I have thrombolytic enzyme therapy following my heart attack?

The value of enzymatic clot dissolution following acute myocardial infarction is limited to a narrow spectrum of patients because the time interval between thrombosis and infarction is relatively narrow. These are patients whose heart attacks have occurred within a few hours as evidenced by both chest pain and ECG changes demonstrating persistent ST segment elevation; they have developed complications of myocardial dysfunction, and have no contraindications. Most clinical studies have confirmed that the earlier the reperfusion is achieved, the less myocardium is lost. At present, a precise cut-off point, after which reperfusion is of little or no value, cannot be given. Reperfusion within 4 to 6 hours appears to be optimal. Whether this procedure should be urged for all patients with acute myocardial infarctions is unclear because the effect of intracoronary thrombolytic therapy on mortality is not yet conclusive.

Will the use of enzyme therapy prevent this blockage from occurring again?

It should be stressed that resolution of occlusion by thrombolytic enzyme therapy does not eliminate the underlying cause of clot formation. If the cause was a prosthetic valve, infection, vascular spasm, atherosclerotic plaque, or injury, lysis of the clot alone will not prevent a recurrence of the clot. Approximately 10% to 20% of reperfused arteries undergo rethrombosis despite anticoagulant therapy. The underlying pathology needs to be corrected with either medication or additional interventional procedures such as angioplasty.

Does it make a difference which enzyme is used?

T-PA appears to be somewhat more effective, usable in lower doses, and causing fewer side effects such as hypotension, than do the other enzymes that are more readily available. In addition, the half-life of t-PA is several minutes while that of streptokinase is several hours. This would mean that if surgery is required following enzymatic thrombolysis, the patient would have a significantly shortened impairment of coagulation if t-PA is used. The cost of t-PA, however, has limited its use and less expensive thrombolytic agents are being utilized. Recently, severe bleeding episodes, in particular intracranial hemorrhage, have been reported in the t-PA.

CONSENT

Informed consent should be obtained when practical from the patient or the family. In the situation of acute myocardial infarction, time may be critical. In these cases, attempts should be made to obtain consent by phone and document that clearly in the patient's chart.

SELECTED BIBLIOGRAPHY

Cella G, Palla A, Sasahara AA: Controversies of different regimens of thrombolytic therapy in acute pulmonary embolism. *Sem Throm Hemostasis* 1987;13:2:163.

Connors ML: Thrombolytic therapy. *J Cardiovasc Nurs* 1987;Feb 1:2:59.

Crabbe SJ, Cloninger CC: Tissue plasminogen activator: a new thrombolytic agent. *Clin Pharm* 1987;May 6:5:373.

Kennedy JW: Thrombolytic therapy for acute myocardial infarction. *Heart Lung* 1987;Nov 16:6:2:740.

Marder VJ, Sherry S: Thrombolytic therapy: current status. *N Engl J Med* 1988;June 318:23 and 24:1512 and 1585.

Topol EJ: Thrombolytic therapy for myocardial infarction. *Pract Cardiol* 1988;Mar 14:3:53.

9

Percutaneous Transluminal Angioplasty

DAVID H. GORDON

Percutaneous transluminal angioplasty (PTA) is a nonsurgical method for opening narrowed or occluded vessels using a catheter introduced through a major peripheral vessel as a dilating tool. A balloon inflated within the lesion enlarges the intravascular diameter and increases the blood flow. Percutaneous transluminal coronary angioplasty (PTCA) entails introduction of the catheter to the area of stenosis within a coronary artery. Both procedures are invasive and have a risk of morbidity and mortality.

New devices under development for PTA include atherectomy catheters, laser balloon systems, "hot-tip" lasers, vascular stents and atherolytic wires.

INDICATIONS

Indications for PTA in the extremities involve a combination of clinical and angiographic findings. Percutaneous transluminal angioplasty is indicated only in patients who are symptomatic. The demonstration of a stenosis on arteriography is rarely considered an indication for the procedure. The use of prophylactic procedures in the extremities is discouraged because of the risk of injury to the vessel wall, embolization, or occlusion. Specific indications include (1) the presence of intermittent claudication adversely affecting the patient's life style, (2) the presence of rest pain, (3) the presence of ulceration or poor wound healing following a surgical procedure, and (4) the presence of impending or overt gangrene.

Additional use of PTA as a complement to surgery include (1) correction of an iliac lesion to assure flow to a femoropopliteal bypass, (2) attempt to salvage a limb prior to amputation by increasing the inflow, and (3) correction of postoperative strictures in patients with anastomotic stenosis in bypass grafts.

PTA is ideally performed as an alternative to surgery in symptomatic patients with short, isolated stenoses. It is also indicated in symptomatic patients who have short life expectancies, those who are morbidly obese, and those who are otherwise poor operative risks. Major vessels for which PTA is indicated include the aorta and its bifurcation, the iliac arteries, the common femorals, the superficial femorals, the popliteals and distal runoff vessels, and visceral vessels such as the renal and superior mesenteric arteries (figures 9–1, 9–2, and 9–3.).

Indications for PTA of the renal artery include the correction of proved renovascular hypertension in patients who have underlying renal artery stenosis and for preservation of renal function associated with renal artery disease.

PTCA has been used in both symptomatic and asymptomatic lesions that may be proximal or distal, single or multivessel, calcified or noncalcified, concentric or eccentric, partially or totally occluded.

PTCA has recently been used in conjunction with intracoronary thrombolysis in acute unstable patients with coronary artery disease. Criteria include chest pain that is not easily controlled with medication or electrocardiographic changes consistent with coronary insufficiency. Patients selected for PTCA should be suitable candidates for surgical revascularization in the event that the dilatation results in a major complication that requires surgical intervention.

With the decreasing rate of complications and the increasing success rate of PTCA, the procedure is now often recommended for patients with minimal symptoms who have high-grade proximal stenosis, if results of functional tests are abnormal, or if the patient is young and active. Some patients with coronary occlusions (previously considered a contraindication to PTCA) can now be successfully treated. Some coronary artery bypass graft patients whose symptoms recur after surgery are being considered for PTCA instead of a second bypass. The indications are the same as those already described for initial angioplasty. Good candidates are those with small focal lesions in no more than two or three vessels. If grafts are involved, it is desirable that they be less than five years old and only partially blocked. Angioplasty becomes less of an option as the disease becomes more diffuse.

PTCA may be used during acute infarction because of (1) more rapid reperfusion time when compared to intracoronary thrombolytic therapy, (2) relief of the

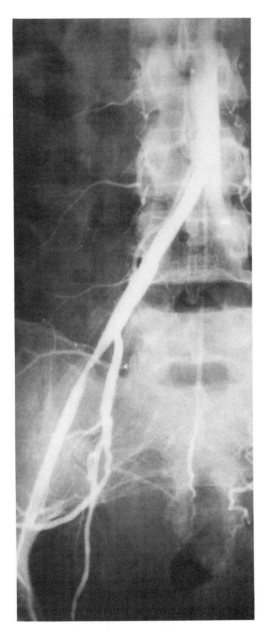

Figure 9–1. Narrowing of the right external iliac artery.

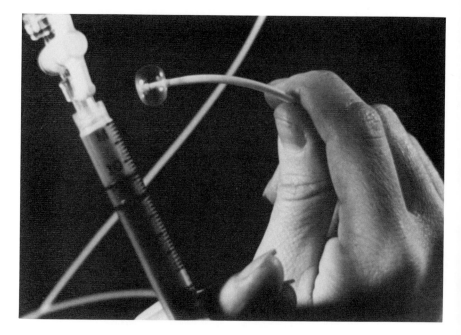

Figure 9–2. Testing the balloon catheter.

underlying atherosclerotic stenosis, and (3) a fairly high success rate for patients for whom thrombolytic therapy has failed. PTCA may be used as sole treatment for acute myocardial infarction, but is usually used in combination with thrombolytic therapy. At present, a large percentage of patients with acute myocardial infarctions may not be candidates for PTCA as a definitive therapy because of complex and extensive multivessel coronary disease. For these patients, thrombolytic therapy is the most appropriate initial intervention. Certain subgroups may benefit from early PTCA such as those for whom thrombolytic therapy fails, in patients for whom systemic lytic therapy might be contraindicated, and patients with severe, uncontrolled hypertension. PTCA should be used for revascularization rather than reperfusion, and scheduled generally 72 hours or more after thrombolytic therapy.

ALTERNATIVES

Peripheral arterial lesions can be treated by surgical endarterectomy, sympathectomy, or medical regimens. Endarterectomy has the complications of any surgical procedure and requires general anesthesia. Sympathectomy also has undesirable side effects and has been recently discredited as treatment for arterial disease. Medical regimens have been found to be of questionable value in arte-

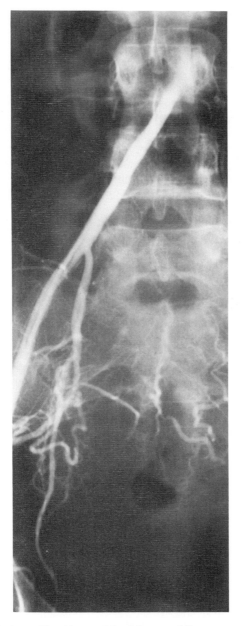

Figure 9–3. Post-angioplasty widened lumen of the right external iliac artery.

rial disease with distinct lesions. The therapeutic plan for each patient and each lesion requires individualized consideration.

PTCA is rapidly becoming the treatment of choice for patients with single-vessel disease and severe angina. For patients with multivessel disease, PTCA should be compared with bypass surgery. These trials are in progress and may determine the relative efficacy of PTCA versus coronary bypass graft surgery. Because PTCA is inherently less invasive than bypass surgery, it is being done in elderly patients and in persons with poor left ventricular function, renal failure, or severe pulmonary disease, which renders them unsuitable or at high risk for a surgical procedure. Some centers are using PTCA to treat patients with as many as 10 coronary lesions in one sitting. It must be kept in mind, however, that the potential for complete revascularization is less with PTCA than with bypass grafting.

The role of PTCA in the patient with acute myocardial infarction is being evaluated in comparison to thrombolytic therapy. PTCA may be used if thrombolytic therapy fails or is contraindicated, or if residual stenotic lesions are present.

Newer techniques that may replace or complement percutaneous transluminal angioplasty include laser angioplasty (hot and cold tip), which is useful to establish a lumen in a thrombosed vessel prior to PTA and to "glaze over" the roughened intimal surface post-PTA.

An atherectomy catheter is now being investigated that physically removes small chunks of atheroma from the superficial femoral artery and the iliac vessels. Rotating atherolytic wires may have promise in literally "roto-rootering" arterial stenosis. Endovascular stents delivered percutaneously show promise in maintaining patency of vessels post-PTA or postatherectomy.

Angioscopy, which is direct visualization of the vessel lumen, shows potential for both the diagnosis and treatment of endovascular problems. It is performed currently by surgical cutdown and requires a dry field, mandating interruption of blood flow to the area being investigated.

CONTRAINDICATIONS

PTA of the extremities is contraindicated in certain specific situations. These include (1) patients with ulcerated plaques and the clinical manifestations of blue-toe syndrome in whom PTA is likely to precipitate embolism and in whom the problem of recurrent emboli will not be resolved, (2) patients with aneurysms coexistent with stenoses of the vessel, (3) patients with embolic occlusion, (4) patients with long complete blocks of the iliacs, (5) patients with recent, complete occlusion of the vessel, in whom PTA may cause distal embolization and poor resolution of the recent thrombus, and (6) patients who have a major branch that originates at the level of the proposed dilation.

Contraindication for PTCA include (1) diffuse atherosclerosis, (2) lesions in severely tortuous vessels, (3) total occlusion for more than 3 months, and (4) left main artery stenosis. The degree to which these latter contraindications should be considered depends largely on the skill and experience of the cardiologist performing the procedure.

PREPROCEDURE PREPARATION

The proper selection of patients requires a team approach.   Generally, prior measurements are made of the extent of the lesion using angiography, plethysmography, or Doppler scan techniques.

PATIENT EDUCATION

Some studies have shown that patients who receive information about visual, auditory, and tactile sensations in addition to information about procedural activities had lower distress ratings and less anxiety. The sympathetic response demonstrated by frightened patients can have a significant effect on cardiac function. Brief explanations about the possible need for surgery if the procedure is unsuccessful is important, as is discussion of the postprocedure course.

The patient should be assessed to determine what effect the abrupt change in lifestyle will have on those who have been restricted because of angina, claudication, or other symptoms. Patients should be given a realistic understanding of the benefit of the procedure and the need to continue to modify risk-causing behavior such as smoking and obesity.

PROCEDURE

Early (PTA) catheters were of a single diameter, causing forward, shearing forces that had the potential to cause distal embolization. Later catheters were used coaxially with graduated, gradually tapered tips. These produced more laterally directed force and decreased the risk of embolization. These catheters are used today only when firm lesions are encountered through which the balloon catheter cannot be advanced.

Newer balloon catheters allow dilation up to 2 cm on an 8F double-lumen catheter, which renders obsolete the catheters being used previously. Teflon-coated guide wires, with or without platinum tips, were developed for initial introduction through the lesion with minimal damage to the artery and lower thrombogenic potential.

The procedure requires about 1 to 2 hours, depending on its complexity and is done under local anesthesia. Drugs are used during PTA primarily to prevent thrombosis and spasm. The catheter is flushed with a small amount of heparin, which provides anticoagulation. The amount of heparin used, however, must be carefully controlled to prevent severe hematomas at the site of catheter insertion.

Spasm is a frequent occurrence during PTA of the renal, popliteal, and runoff vessels. This is caused by mechanical stimulation of the vessel walls. Calcium channel blockers are effective in preventing and reversing spasms and may be administered intraarterially. An alternative approach is to administer sublingual calcium channel blockers 15 to 30 minutes prior to the procedure. Intraarterial nitroglycerin has an additive effect with the calcium channel blockers and can effectively prevent and control spasm.

In the extremities, for iliac lesions the diagnostic retrograde puncture is utilized for PTA following angiography. For superficial femoral artery lesions, the femoral artery is punctured downhill, and the guide wire is inserted into the superficial femoral artery. Once the stenosis has been crossed by the guide wire, the balloon catheter usually passes easily over the guide wire. Alternatively an axillary approach can be used to dilate lesions in the mesenteric, renal, iliac, common femoral, and the superficial femoral arteries.

PTCA involves percutaneous puncture and passage of a catheter along a guide wire into the narrowed section of the artery, where the catheter's balloon is inflated. A pacemaker catheter is usually placed in the right ventricle and can be used at any time that bradyarrhythmias require pacing. Under fluoroscopy, the physician continuously observes the effect of the balloon dilation on the atherosclerotic narrowing. Repeat angiographic films are made of the artery to confirm dilation. The lumen at the distal end of the catheter measures intraluminal pressure, allowing a recording of the change in flow following the procedure.

POSTPROCEDURE INFORMATION

Careful postangioplasty management is very important to the long-term success of the procedure. Following PTA of the extremity, the patient should be on strict bed rest for 6 hours and should be cautioned not to bend the limb at the puncture site. The condition of the peripheral pulses is monitored regularly for 24 hours, and the puncture site is checked for hematoma. At most centers, patients receive either 48 hours of subcutaneous heparin or are started on aspirin or dipyrimadole. These drugs are frequently continued for 3 months to a lifetime. Long-term coumadin is reserved for patients who have extensive distal disease and poor runoff.

In addition, patients are encouraged to stop smoking and to become involved in a graduated exercise program tailored to their condition. Noninvasive plethysmography and/or Doppler scan studies can be used to follow alterations in hemodynamics following the procedure.

Patients should be reminded that PTA is a palliative treatment. Atherosclerosis remains a total body disease that is currently treated but not cured.

Following PTA of the renal artery, the blood pressure must be closely monitored for 24 hours. Anticoagulation is handled as described for procedures involving vessels of the extremities.

COMPLICATIONS

PTA is an invasive procedure. Complications can be expected in 5% to 15% of the patients. Most of the complications are minor and can be managed with conservative therapy. However, surgical management will be required in 1% to 3% of cases. Complications can occur at the puncture site, angioplasty site, distal to the procedure, or can be systemic in nature.

Puncture site complications are the most common—most frequently, hematoma related to multiple attempts, the size of the balloon, or hypertension. The use of anticoagulants further complicates this problem. Other complications can include bleeding into an undetected location such as the retroperitoneal space, the development of a large hematoma or false aneurysm, and nerve injury secondary to compression by a hematoma.

Angioplasty site complications include occlusion of the vessel due to subintimal dilatation, intimal flaps, spasm, or thrombosis. These problems can usually be resolved although they may require a delay in the performance of the angioplasty. Care should be taken to protect major vessels and collaterals near the angioplasty site.

Distal embolization occurs in up to 5% of cases. In most patients it will be of no clinical significance. A few cases will require surgical embolectomy. Care needs to be taken to avoid dilating fresh thrombi. Spasm in a distal vessel may result from mechanical stimulation or from the pain caused by the injection of contrast material.

Other complications include transient renal insufficiency caused by the contrast material. This can be minimized by keeping the patient well hydrated. Death is a rare complication, but systemic complications in patients with severe diffuse vascular disease can occur.

Complications of PTCA occur in approximately 10% of patients and consist of coronary dissection, occlusion, arrhythmia, infarct, and death. A surgical bypass team should be available during angioplasty because of the possibility of sudden occlusion of the vessel secondary to a spiral dissection or vascular occlusion due to plaque embolization.

Other serious complications include coronary spasm and thrombus formation. Spasm responds to nitroglycerin or calcium channel blockers. Thrombus responds to recrossing and redilation of the lesion or thrombolysis. Myocardial infarction has been found to occur in 2% to 5% of cases. Acute coronary events are more common in women and in patients with unstable angina.

PATIENT QUESTIONS

Will this procedure help me and be safe for me?

Patient selection for percutaneous transluminal angioplasty requires close scrutiny of the anatomic lesions. The "ideal anatomy" for a successful and safe procedure includes single, proximal, discrete, or subtotal lesions. During the early experience at any medical center, procedures should be restricted to patients with ideal anatomy. In patients with diffuse or multivessel disease, the likelihood of success will decrease. Today's success rate for single vessel and multivessel coronary disease is greater than 90% at centers that perform adequate numbers of the procedure to gain the necessary expertise. Iliac PTA produces successful results (5 year patency) ranging around 80%. Superficial femoral procedures yield 60% to 70% 5-year survival rates. The objective should be optimal medical care, not optimal dilation statistics.

What happens to me over the long term following coronary artery angioplasty?

Long-term prognosis following PTCA is difficult because the procedure was developed quite recently. In most patients with unsuccessful dilation, the procedure is commonly followed by cardiac bypass surgery. The long-term outcome is probably related to the completeness of revascularization. Initial statistics show clear relief of symptoms in patients who had complete revascularization and a lower incidence of the need for coronary bypass surgery.

Return-to-work statistics for patients with coronary artery disease have been disappointing following coronary bypass surgery. However, patients with successful transluminal dilation have been shown to return to work sooner than those having coronary bypass grafting. The absence of chest pain after the procedure is a good indicator of the ability to return to work.

The major problem associated with PTCA is restenosis. This occurs in about 25% to 35% of cases and usually becomes evident 6 to 8 months following the initial procedure. Recurrence of symptoms after 6 to 12 months following the procedure is usually due to progression of disease elsewhere.

What is the possibility that I will restenose following PTCA and that an additional procedure will be needed?

The risk factors for restenosis in PTCA include male gender, diabetes, cigarette smoking, hyperlipidemia, long eccentric lesion, inadequate dilatation in which a hemodynamically important lesion is left behind, dilation of bypass graft stenoses, left anterior descending arterial lesions, and absence of prior myocardial infarction. Much of the variability remains unexplained. The role of platelet aggregation and the concomitant proliferation of intimal smooth muscle cells may be involved. Medication regimens including warfarin sodium and nifedipine aimed at decreasing the rate of restenosis have been ineffective. Trials of other antiplatelet medications are currently in progress. Restenosis is usually amenable to a second PTCA, which is recommended as soon as the restenosis is identified because the less the stenosis, the easier it is to redilate. Second-time PTCA is highly successful and the chance of restenosis is no higher than it is with first-time angioplasty.

Should I have PTCA simply to decrease the dosage of my medications and to avoid their side effects?

In patients whose symptoms are reasonably well controlled with medication but who may have undesirable medication side effects that interfere with an active lifestyle, PTCA can be considered. The procedure will not increase their life expectancy, but it can eliminate the need for medication and allow them to be fully active. The use of PTCA for this indication is controversial, but is becoming more widely accepted, especially among men in their thirties.

Will I be awake during the procedure, and if so, what will I feel?

Yes, the patient will be awake to assist the physician by turning taking deep breaths, coughing or making any other required movements. The patient may have some pain when the balloon is inflated at the site of the lesion or in the muscle being perfused by the involved artery. Any pain should be reported to the physician during the procedure.

CONSENT

Informed consent is ethically and legally prudent and should include (1) reasons for recommending the treatment; (2) potential risks or hazards specifically listed; (3) details of the procedure to be done; and (4) available alternatives and their risks.

SELECTED BIBLIOGRAPHY

Detre K: Percutaneous transluminal angioplasty in 1985–1986 and 1977–1981 *N Engl J Med* 1988;Feb 4:318:5:265.

Gardiner GA: Complications of transluminal angioplasty. *Radiology* 1986;April:159:1:201.

Holmes DR, Vliestra RE: Percutaneous transluminal coronary angioplasty: current status and future trends. *Mayo Clin Proc* 1986;Nov:61:11:865.

Lemarbre L, Hudon G, Coche G, Bourassa MG: Outpatient peripheral angioplasty: survey of complications and patient perceptions. *AJR* 1987;June:148:6:1239.

Scobie TK: Current status of transluminal angiography. *Can J Surg* 1987;May:30:3:175.

10

Stress (Exercise) Testing

RICHARD SADOVSKY

Stress testing (exercise testing) offers data about cardiovascular function during activity. Exercise increases the myocardial demand for oxygen, and the cardiovascular response is measured while the patient performs a measurable and reproducible amount of exercise. A disparity between the oxygen demand and supply of the heart results in electrocardiographic changes, the most common being ST segment depressions. Other changes can be rhythm abnormalities, conduction defects, and voltage variations.

Two protocols for stress tests are used: one is the submaximal or limited-goal examination that terminates automatically when the patient reaches a specific physiologic goal; the other is a maximal or symptom-limited test in which the patient continues to exercise and be monitored until moderate symptoms develop. The latter type of evaluation involves fewer false negatives and gives more information about cardiac function and ischemia.

Routine graded exercise testing can be augmented by thallium imaging, radionuclide ventriculography, Doppler ultrasound measurements of the peripheral circulation, two-dimensional echocardiography, and Doppler ultrasound estimations of changes in the ejection fraction. Thallium imaging has been well standardized and provides indirect information about coronary circulation.

INDICATIONS

Stress testing is helpful in diagnosing ischemic heart disease. This is true in both symptomatic and asymptomatic patients and is valuable in determining the cause of chest pain not clearly identifiable as cardiac.

The assessment of the effect of surgical and medical intervention in patients with coronary artery disease is possible with stress testing. The procedure permits evaluation of antiarrhythmic or antianginal therapy.

Exercise tolerance can be evaluated and is useful prior to starting a cardiac rehabilitation program in the patient with known cardiac disease, the patient with chronic pulmonary disease, and even the asymptomatic patient who is planning to initiate an exercise program.

This type of functional cardiovascular evaluation helps to determine if the cardiovascular system's ability to transport oxygen is a factor in limiting the patient's performance. For this evaluation, it is valuable to continue to maximal effort (not just 85% to 90% of maximum) unless abnormalities are demonstrated. If the tests do not proceed to maximum, a significant number of abnormalities may be missed. In addition, functional tests are generally done with the patient on all their medications since exertional activities in the future will take place with the patient on the medications. Of course, if the patient develops moderately severe symptoms during the test, the procedure is terminated.

Submaximal stress testing in the early weeks following myocardial infarction (MI) may be helpful in determining the patient's prognosis and providing the patient with a posthospital exercise prescription. The use of stress testing for functional and long-term management purposes is clearly established. Recent data also show that stress testing in the post-MI patient can greatly assist in the noninvasive determination of the anatomic extent of coronary artery disease and in preparation of the post-MI exercise prescription and determination of prognosis.

In asymptomatic patients, the absence of clinical trials of available therapy in the "high-risk" patients defined by exercise testing leaves some uncertainty between the information resulting from stress testing and the results of management decisions based on this information.

The diagnosis of a positive stress test is ST segment depression of 1 mm or more persisting for at least 80 msec. A greater than 2 mm upsloping ST segment is also considered abnormal if it lasts for greater than 80 msec from the J point (the junction of the QRS and the ST segments). Chest pain in association with ST segment depression is strongly suggestive of coronary artery disease. Other criteria used to determine abnormality in the stress test include a fall in blood pressure and the R wave amplitude, which should decrease in the normal response to exercise. ST segment elevation may indicate dyskinetic left ventricular wall motion or severe transmural ischemia. Since ST segment depression may be seen only during recovery, continued recording of the ECG even after the stress test has ended is an essential part of the examination.

Graded exercise testing may be used also to uncover arrhythmias. An ambulatory ECG is probably more sensitive in arrhythmia detection, but standard exercise testing may provide the answer more quickly.

ALTERNATIVES

Despite the advent of radionuclide exercise tests, which are more sensitive and specific for diagnoses than is the stress test, many physicians still use stress testing for functional testing. The stress test serves as a useful, noninvasive supplement to assess performance. It can be frequently repeated, it is one-third the cost of the radionuclide tests in most institutions, can be modified to suit the circumstances, and will provide valuable information concerning work evaluation and exercise prescription.

Further description of cardiac imaging using radionuclide techniques is in the chapter on radionuclide techniques.

POSSIBILITY OF FAILURE

The predictive value of this test for coronary insufficiency varies in different situations. False negatives and false positives can occur and further testing such as thallium imaging and stress testing, exercise with multiple-gated acquisition scanning, or coronary angiography may be necessary.

False-positive tests can be caused by digitalis or hypokalemia inducing ST segment depression, aortic stenosis, left ventricular hypertrophy, mitral valve prolapse, and occasionally heavy glucose ingestion just prior to the stress test, which may cause potassium fluxes in the cells resulting in transient hypokalemia and ST segment depressions.

False negatives occur most commonly in a submaximal stress test in which the maximal heart rate obtained is less than 85% of the predicted rate. A false negative can also occur if too few leads are recorded, in patients with previous myocardial infarctions, and in patients taking nitrates or propranolol.

The use of stress testing to identify potentially important arrhythmias is probably less valuable than 24 hour ambulatory electrocardiography.

CONTRAINDICATIONS

A stress test is contraindicated in patients with untreated hypertension, rapid atrial arrhythmias, second or third degree heart block, unstable angina or angina

at rest, acute cardiac conditions such as myocarditis or uncompensated congestive heart failure, severe valvular disease, an abnormal resting ECG, hypokalemia, severe lung disease, and congestive heart failure. Certainly, stress testing
should not be done in patients with any acute noncardiac illness, including
infection, pulmonary embolism, and myxedema.

PREPROCEDURE PREPARATION

A complete history and physical examination should precede stress testing. A
resting cardiogram should be performed to look for ECG abnormalities at rest.
A review of the patient's medications should be done to determine if any of them
will affect the cardiac response during the stress test and decrease the ability of
the procedure to identify myocardial dysfunction. If the purpose of the test is to
determine myocardial ischemia, medications that blunt the myocardial rate response to exercise should be halted. These might include digitalis, which would
need to be terminated at least 7 days prior to the test, beta-blockers, at least 48
hours before the test, and nitrates, at least 24 hours before.

PATIENT EDUCATION

Patients are often fearful of undergoing stress tests either because of the fear of
chest pain and other alarming symptoms or fear of concern over possible heart
disease or even having a heart attack. Telling the patient what to expect before
the test helps to relieve much of the anxiety. The treadmill should be described
as a belt that moves at varying speeds and can be tilted to increase the exertion
needed to walk. The patient should be informed that a physician will be present,
the blood pressure and pulse rate will be monitored closely, and the patient will
be able to terminate the procedure at any time that discomfort is experienced.
Fatigue, slight breathlessness, and sweatiness may occur, but these symptoms
are rarely evidence of impending cardiac events.

The patient should be told to avoid strenuous activity for at least 12 hours
before the procedure and to get a full night's sleep before the test. Either a light
breakfast or lunch or nothing at all should be eaten for at least 3 hours prior to
the test and coffee, tea, cola drinks, alcohol, and any other caffeine-containing
beverages should be avoided. The patient should be told to dress comfortably
with light weight, loose clothing and rubber soled shoes. Men generally do not
wear shirts during the test and women generally wear a light patient gown with a
front closure. All medications should be taken if not specifically proscribed by
the physician.

PROCEDURE

Stress testing is performed in a well-equipped exercise laboratory supervised by a trained professional. The ECG is monitored throughout the test and during the recovery period. The laboratory should be equipped to handle any emergencies that may arise. A baseline ECG is always done to check for abnormalities. In addition, the resting blood pressure is recorded and the heart is examined for auscultory evidence of disease.

A number of different procedures are available for stress testing. The common procedures utilize either steps, bicycle ergometer, or a treadmill with the latter being the most commonly used parameter in the United States (figure 10–1). The principles and the interpretation of the results are the same regardless of the method used.

There are a variety of protocols for using the treadmill. Most of these use continuous activity in progressive stages of three minutes' duration. Each stage provides greater exertion in terms of speed of the treadmill and the grade of the incline. The most commonly used protocol is the Bruce protocol, which is a maximum, symptom-limited protocol in which the patient exercises until chest pain, fatigue, or other symptom requires the test to be terminated. The other type of protocol, used less commonly, is a maximum heart rate limited protocol, in which the test is terminated at a certain percentage of predicted heart rate or when a predetermined work load is achieved. Treadmill and arm exercises are the most widely used modes of exertion. However, treadmill exercise is clearly preferable because it results in a significantly higher mean systolic oxygen consumption and systolic blood pressure.

The blood pressure is monitored throughout the test and an ECG is continuously recorded. The target heart rate is 90% of the maximal heart rate predicted by age. This targeted rate may vary depending on the patient's age and other related medical conditions. As the test proceeds, the patient is gradually stressed at higher levels by increasing the speed and angle of the treadmill every three minutes. Common responses to maximal exercise are dizziness, light headedness, leg fatigue, dyspnea, diaphoresis, and a slightly ataxic gait. In a submaximal examination, the test is terminated when the target heart rate is achieved when the patient complains of pain or shortness of breath, when the exercises can no longer be tolerated, or when ECG changes occur. The indications for termination of stress testing are well established to prevent danger to the patient.

Other modes of exercise stress testing are available for use in obese patients, those who have peripheral vascular disease or orthopedic problems, and patients who cannot walk on the treadmill for any other reason.

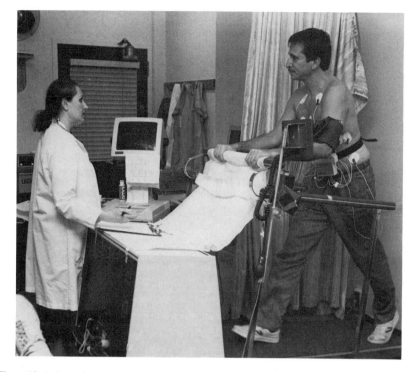

Figure 10–1. Stress (exercise) test in progress.

POSTPROCEDURE INFORMATION

It is appropriate that a member of the family accompany the patient to the test and be prepared to assist the patient home. If no one is available, the patient should remain in the doctor's office for an hour after the procedure then resuming normal diet habits at that time.

The patient should avoid taking a hot or very warm shower within two hours of the test in order to avoid dizziness and possible fainting.

Generally, there are no after effects of this procedure.

COMPLICATIONS

Possible complications include arrhythmias, myocardial infarction, and hypertension. The risk of myocardial infarction during stress testing is less than 1 in 500; the risk of death is less than 1 in 10,000. Ventricular fibrillation, if it does occur, is more likely to occur in patients with exertional hypotension. Noncardiovascular complications include musculoskeletal trauma and retinal detachment.

PATIENT QUESTIONS

Will this stress test cause me any harm?

Stress tests are performed under the supervision of a physician. The heart is exerted in a slowly increasing manner with constant monitoring of the pulse, blood pressure, and the electrocardiogram. The examination will be terminated immediately if the patient has moderately severe symptoms or if any myocardial changes are noted on the electrocardiogram. The precautions taken make the risks of stress testing acceptable.

Will the test provide definite information about poor blood supply to the heart muscle?

One must ask whether stress testing will provide the information necessary to guide clinical decision making. The combination of chest pain and ST segment depression during the electrocardiogram taken with stress testing has a higher predictive value for ischemia than either chest pain or ST segment depression alone. ST segment changes can be accurately measured and evaluated by skilled physicians. These results have good predictive value. There is, however, a possibility of false-positive and false-negative tests. A stress test with radionuclide scanning is somewhat more sensitive (lower false-negative rate). Further testing may be needed to clarify myocardial blood supply after stress testing is performed. The role of the stress test in clinical decision making is currently under study.

Should a stress test be done prior to beginning an exercise regimen?

Stress testing is well able to evaluate functional cardiac capacity. The screening of asymptomatic patients for latent coronary atherosclerotic disease is controversial. Determining whether a specific patient requires stress testing prior to an exercise regimen is a highly individualized decision. Patients over age 35 who have several risk factors for cardiac ischemic disease such as hypertension, smoking, hypercholesterolemia, and family history of coronary artery disease, or who have moderate to severe pulmonary disease may be candidates for stress testing to determine functional limits. This information can be used to construct optimal aerobic exercise programs. Stress tests can be used to determine changes in functional limits following exercise programs or periods of illness.

Should a stress test be done following a myocardial infarction?

Submaximal stress tests in early weeks following myocardial infarction appear to be safe in selected groups who have not suffered any major complications such as congestive heart failure, hypertension, left ventricular dysfunction, or other significant electrocardiographic abnormalities, or those who have suffered an unstable form of non-Q wave infarction. These tests have been done as early as 3 weeks post-infarction. Potential benefits could include (1) promotion of patient self-confidence; (2) determination of posthospital exercise prescription; (3) detection of arrhythmias; and (4) determination of posthospital prognosis. However, the practical value of the apparent psychological benefits and of the exercise prescription information in a patient not participating in a formal exercise rehabilitation program is unclear. More study needs to be done in this area.

Am I too old to have a stress test?

As in all medical testing, patients must be evaluated as individuals, not as members of an arbitrary age group. There is no evidence that age alone increases the risk of stress testing. However, reduced functional capacity in the aged do frequently limit stress test performance. Special protocols have been developed that allow for the testing of the elderly patient with limited functional capacity giving information that can be used in medical, surgical, and exercise therapeutic interventions.

CONSENT

Informed consent statement is needed.

SELECTED BIBLIOGRAPHY

American College of Cardiology/American Heart Association Task Force on Assessment of Cardiovascular Procedures. Guidelines for exercise testing. *J Am Coll Cardiol* 1986;8:725.

Beller GA; Radionuclide exercise testing for coronary artery disease. *Cardiol Clin* 1984;2:367.

Cintron G: Modifiers of exercise-induced S-T segment changes. *Cardiol Clin* 1984;2:349.

Gubin SS, Judge RD: Graded exercise testing. *AFP* 1987;Apr:35:4:123.

McHenry PL: Role of exercise testing in predicting sudden death. *J Am Coll Cardiol* 1985;5(6 suppl):9B–12B.

11

Vein Stripping and Ligation

RICHARD M. STILLMAN

Varicose veins are tortuous, dilated, elongated superficial veins of the lower extremities. They occur in about 15% of the world's population. Aggravating factors associated with increased incidence of varicose veins include female sex, multiparity, a lifestyle or job requiring prolonged standing or sitting, obesity, chronic low-fiber diet, and chronic use of constrictive garments.

Varicose veins may be primary or secondary. Primary varicose veins result from valvular incompetence in the superficial venous system or in the communicating veins. This produces a cascade effect by allowing pooling of blood distal to the incompetent valve, causing dilatation at the next valve, resulting in sequential valvular incompetence. Secondary varicose veins are those resulting from problems with the deep venous system. Of these, the majority are due to recanalization of a thrombosed deep venous system with resultant valvular incompetence. In rare cases, the superficial varicosities are actually the collateral pathways around an occluded deep venous system. In this latter case, removal of the varicose veins is, of course, contraindicated. Most patients with varicose veins require no specific treatment. When intractable symptoms occur, varicose vein stripping should be considered.

INDICATIONS

The mere presence of varicose veins is not an indication for varicose vein removal. About 15% of the world's population has some varicose veins, and in the vast majority of cases these are harmless and require no treatment. However, there are several indications for removal of varicose veins. Most varicose vein operations are performed for cosmetic reasons. Other operative indications are bleeding or hemorrhage from a varicose vein, ankle or leg ulceration due to the varicose veins, severe skin changes, burning, itching due to the varicose veins, attacks of inflammation or clotting (thrombophlebitis) of the varicose veins, or very large varicose veins (which are at risk for developing any of these complications).

In the procedure of vein stripping, some or all of the varicose veins will be surgically removed. This will help alleviate symptoms such as heaviness of the legs occurring at the end of the day, darkening of the skin of the leg and ankle, ankle ulceration, bleeding from the veins, dermatitis and skin irritation, and cosmetic deformity.

ALTERNATIVES

An alternative to surgical removal of varicose veins is injection sclerotherapy. This involves repeated injections of a sclerosing agent (usually 3% sodium tetradecyl sulfate) directly into the varicose veins. This agent will cause the walls of the vein to seal together by fibrosis, obliterating the vein's lumen. Although this method can effectively eradicate small leg varicosities, it is ineffective with large varicose veins or those located in the thigh. Also, both systemic and local allergic reactions can occur. Furthermore, sclerosed veins often recanalize and recur within several months. For these reasons, injection sclerotherapy is best reserved for minor leg varicosities or varicosities that persist or recur after surgical vein stripping.

CONTRAINDICATIONS

Surgical stripping of major varicose veins requires general or regional anesthesia, and is therefore contraindicated if the patient cannot tolerate anesthesia. Removal of minor varicose veins may be performed under local anesthesia. Removal of varicose veins is also contraindicated in the presence of deep venous thrombosis. In this case, the varicose veins are collaterals to the occluded deep system, and removal of the varicosities would result in severe leg edema. If deep vein thrombosis is suspected by history (leg edema, calf pain, prior venous thromboembolism), physical examination (calf tenderness, edema, positive Homans' sign) or by the results of noninvasive venous flow testing, venography is performed prior to vein stripping. Varicose vein stripping is not performed while there is an infected ankle ulcer. In this case, topical treatment of the ulcer is instituted and continued until the ulcer is clean and granulating, at which time vein removal and skin grafting of the ulcer may be considered. Removal of varicose veins is rarely, if ever, indicated during pregnancy. This is because varicose veins that occur or become exacerbated during pregnancy usually return to normal or their prepregnancy condition after delivery.

PREPROCEDURE PREPARATION

History and physical examination should rule out deep vein thrombosis. Preferably, noninvasive vascular testing with Doppler flow and plethysmography should be performed to evaluate the possibility that the varicose veins are secondary to deep vein thrombosis. If there is any doubt, venography should be performed if it is not contraindicated.

The nature of the proposed procedure should be discussed with the patient. In order to minimize the chance of postoperative infection, the patient should be advised to shower twice on the day prior to surgery and once the morning of surgery. The surgeon may suggest use of an antibacterial skin cleanser (e.g., Hibiclens®, or Betadine®). The surgeon may decide to have the patient's legs and, possibly, groin areas shaved before surgery. The surgeon or an assistant will use an indelible marker to trace on the skin the distribution of the veins the surgeon intends to remove. The patient should take an active role during this mapping, especially if the vein stripping is being performed for cosmetic reasons. For each vein to be removed, there will be at least one surgical scar. The patient must weigh the cosmetic deformity of persistent varicose veins against the cosmetic deformity of the surgical scar. The night before to surgery, the patient will meet with the anesthesiologist, to determine the type of anesthesia. Unless local anesthesia, only, is to be used, the patient must take nothing by mouth for at least 8 hours prior to surgery (usually, nothing after midnight). Preanesthetic medications may be ordered to sedate the patient or to minimize upper aerodigestive tract secretions. These may cause the patient to be sleepy and the mouth to feel dry just prior to the operation.

PATIENT EDUCATION

The patient should be informed of the risks, benefits, and alternatives of varicose vein stripping. The patient should be told why varicose vein surgery is indicated. If there is no definite medical indication, the patient should be advised that varicose veins are common, and that surgical removal is not medically necessary.

PROCEDURE

The operation is usually performed under general or spinal anesthesia, although local anesthesia may be used for limited stripping of small areas of varicose veins. The patient will be supine for removal of the greater saphenous system and tributaries, prone for removal of an isolated varicose lesser saphenous system. Using multiple surgical incisions (usually transverse), the surgeon will isolate each vein, introduce an intraluminal stripper into the distal end of the vein, retrieve it from the proximal end of the vein, and then avulse the entire vein. In order to minimize the number of incisions required and, therefore, the postoperative scars, most vein branches are not ligated, and hemostasis relies upon surrounding tissues, application of a compression dressing (elastic bandage), and leg elevation. Large tributaries, isolated superficial varicosities that do not attach directly to the greater or lesser saphenous vein, and major perforating veins will be approached through separate incisions, surgically dissected free, ligated, and removed (figure 11–1).

The incisions are closed with sutures or with skin tapes, and a sterile dressing is applied. Elastic bandages are wrapped over the dressings. The legs are maintained in an elevated position in the recovery room to diminish subcutaneous bleeding from unligated vein branches.

POSTPROCEDURE INFORMATION

The patient may have some postoperative incisional pain and may therefore require some assistance for several days or even weeks. Most patients, however, are able to resume normal activities the day following surgery.

COMPLICATIONS

The patient and the surgeon should be aware of the risks of bleeding, infection, recurrence or persistence of varicose veins, poor wound healing, scar formation, pain or numbness around the surgical incisions, bruising around and between the incisions, and ankle ulceration. The patient should understand that there will be some postoperative incisional pain that may require treatment with analgesics. Depending on the patient's employment and tolerance to pain, postoperative pain may delay return to work for several days or weeks postoperatively.

Mortality is very low. Morbidity includes approximately 10% recurrence rate, and 1% rate of wound infection. Many patients will note numbness or pain near the incisions. There will be ecchymosis of variable magnitude depending on the number and size of veins removed. Postoperative deep vein thrombosis occurs in less than 1% of cases.

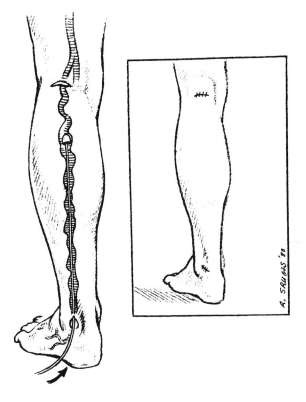

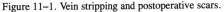

Figure 11–1. Vein stripping and postoperative scars.

PATIENT QUESTIONS

What causes varicose veins?

Varicose veins result from increased pressure in the veins of the legs. This may be due to absent or malfunctioning valves, a condition that may be hereditary. The problem may be exacerbated by chronically increased intraabdominal pressure (for example, pregnancy, or chronic constipation). Varicose veins may be a long-term result of clots in the deep veins, but varicose veins themselves do not imply that clots are present at this time.

What symptoms result from varicose veins?

Varicose veins may result in a sensation of heaviness of the legs, darkening or thickening of the skin around the inner ankle, breakdown of skin and soft tissues around the inner ankle (ulceration) or just cosmetic unsightliness. Not every small spidery vein is a varicose vein.

What does the doctor look for on examination?

Physical examination will determine the particular system of veins involved, whether your symptoms are actually a result of the varicose veins, and whether further studies are indicated.

What further studies may be indicated?

Further studies may involve listening to blood flow with an ultrasound stethoscope (Doppler) or measuring blood flow with two blood pressure cuffs attached to a special machine (Plethysmography).

How are varicose veins nonsurgically treated?

Many need no treatment. If treatment is indicated, it is directed toward lowering the high pressure at the ankle as follows:

1. Sleep with the foot of the bed elevated above heart level. Six-inch blocks or old telephone books placed under the foot of the bed work nicely.
2. Exercise with a program of walking (1 to 2 miles daily), jogging, bicycle riding, swimming. Exercise increases flow in the deep veins. If you have a heart or lung problem, check with your doctor before starting any exercise program.
3. Avoid prolonged sitting or standing. If you must stand for a prolonged period of time, periodically exercise by extending your feet and standing on your toes. This contracts the muscles of the calf and increases flow in the deep veins.
4. Use elastic stockings, either ready made, or specially prescribed by the doctor and obtained from a surgical supply store.
5. To lessen the chances of skin breakdown (ulceration), avoid dry skin. A warm bath daily followed by the application of moisturizers is a good idea.

Do I need an operation?

Unless you have a nonhealing ulcer, severe cosmetic problems, or have had infection, bleeding, or clotting of varicose veins, an operation is usually not mandatory. It is purely elective, and whether to operate is a matter that you should feel free to discuss. It is your decision.

CONSENT

Varicose vein stripping and ligation is a surgical procedure, and as such it requires signed, witnessed, informed consent. Risk, benefits, and alternatives should be discussed.

SELECTED BIBLIOGRAPHY

Keith LM Jr, Smead WL: Saphenous vein stripping and its complications. *Surg Clin North American* 1983;63:1303.

Sladen JG: Compression sclerotherapy: preparation, technique, complications, and results. *Am J Surg* 1983;146:228.

Tolins SH: Treatment of varicose veins: an update. *Am J Surg* 1983;145:248.

12

Venography

DAVID H. GORDON

Venography is the study of the venous structures of the body. This procedure is used to evaluate peripheral venous disease as well as pelvic and abdominal pathology. Venography is considered contrast radiography because of the use of injected contrast material to visualize the lumen of the veins and the course of the vessel. Both intraluminal and compressing extraluminal problems can be detected. This examination is clearly the most effective way to evaluate venous disease.

INDICATIONS

The basic type of **venogram** is the peripheral or lower leg-venogram, although venography is also done in the upper extremities. The most common indication for peripheral venography of the lower extremity is for the evaluation of deep venous thrombosis (DVT). The second indication is in the evaluation of varicose veins to establish patency of the deep venous system (figure 12–1). The third is for the evaluation of uncommon anomalies such as Klippel-Trenaunay syndrome and also to evaluate patency of veins in relation to nearby masses or tumors.

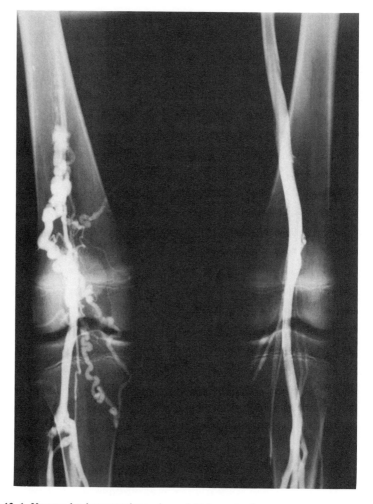

Figure 12–1. Venography demonstrating varicose right femoral vein.

When performing venography of the lower extremities, anatomy of both the deep and superficial venous systems will be defined and delineated. In addition, intraluminal filling defects or thrombosis of the deep venous system will be demonstrated. In place of thrombosed vessels, collateral vasculature will be opacified.

Indications for upper extremity venography include determining patency of the veins prior to insertion of access grafts or fistulas, or the evaluation of a swollen arm. Entities such as stress axillary vein thrombosis, or metastatic disease may be responsible for upper extremity venous occlusion. It is necessary to document whether the vein is actually thrombosed or merely extrinsically compressed.

Indications for visceral venography include pelvic vein thrombosis and a search for sources of pulmonary emboli. Lower extremity venography may reveal the external ileo-femoral veins in a careful study, but if involvement of the internal iliac veins are suspected, they must be opacified by catheter contrast insertion. Renal venography is performed to determine the presence of renal vein thrombosis although ultrasound and computerized tomography (CT) scanning should be done initially since they are less invasive examinations. Hepatic vein studies are done to evaluate for Budd-Chiari syndrome and for the assessment of portal hypertension and to obtain hepatic vein pressures. CT scanning and magnetic resonance imaging (MRI) should be considered preliminary tests in the evaluation of hepatic vein congestion.

ALTERNATIVES

Multiple noninvasive tests for the delineation of the lower extremity veins have been described in the literature and are currently employed. These include impedance plethysmography, nuclear scanning, ultrasound, and radionuclide venography. Considering whether these less invasive procedures should be performed involves careful evaluation of several factors. Among the most important factors is whether a capable laboratory for the performance of these procedures exists. In general, although they are less invasive than venography, they are also less specific and less accurate. In the case of deep venous thrombosis, which is a potentially life-threatening situation, venography is by far the most appropriate examination to obtain maximum information that will permit optimal therapeutic decisions. It is well known that clinically assessing deep vein thrombosis and differentiating it from other clinical problems such as cellulitis is very difficult.

Radionuclide venography is of some value in defining gross patency of the deep venous system, but it will not reveal nonobstructing lesions. A variant of nuclear studies that utilizes labelled fibrinogen for clot may be useful to define the presence of a thrombus but requires a minimum of 24 hours to perform.

Plethysmography is of some value in the calf veins but it is of less value in the thigh veins and valueless in the pelvis. Doppler ultrasound with compression is of value in the thigh but is a very new modality in terms of defining deep venous thrombosis and it will require further experience and followup. This technique may replace venography in the future as the delineation of thrombus in thigh veins is the vital information needed when combined with followup studies to rule out propagation from calf veins.

POSSIBILITY OF FAILURE

As stated above, the contrast venogram is the "gold standard" and, if the examination is properly performed, further studies should not be needed. Utilization of tourniquets to force circulation into the deep venous system and tilting the patient into the semierect position will markedly aid in producing complete diagnostic studies of the lower extremity veins.

CONTRAINDICATIONS

The major contraindications to the performance of venography are the presence of compromised renal function, the history of previous reaction to intravenous contrast administration, and congestive heart failure.

The risk of venography in the patient with compromised renal function can be handled by first using the less-invasive screening examinations. Depending on the information obtained, contrast venography may not be necessary. If venography is clearly needed, then the patient should be well hydrated to maximize renal function.

Allergic reactions can be handled by careful monitoring of patients with an ECG, prior administration of prophylactic steroids, and having anesthesia support on stand-by to deal with any serious allergic reactions. In addition, pretreatment with antihistamines may be of value in reducing reactions.

Fluid overload and congestive heart failure can be handled by treating the cause of heart failure and by dialyzing excess fluid if the patient is in chronic renal failure.

Contraindications to catheter venography are the same as those of peripheral venography.

PREPROCEDURE PREPARATION

Preparation involves physiologically preparing the patient to handle the contrast load and managing any of the contraindications noted above. Elevation of a swollen leg will be valuable for reducing edema permitting easier access to the vein. Tissue edema can also be reduced by wrapping the leg in elastic bandages.

PATIENT EDUCATION

It is important to inform the patient that the procedure will be uncomfortable and even painful, especially if the ionic contrast agents are used. Because of the much greater expense involved in the use of nonionic contrast agents, it is not currently feasible to use this clearly superior contrast material for all patients.

Nausea and vomiting may occur with injection of contrast and occurs in up to 25% of all patients who have venography.

Procedure

Venography is generally performed as an outpatient procedure and consists of placing a small needle into a superficial dorsal foot vein (or the hand) and being certain that it is within the lumen of the vessel. The needle is anchored with tape with the point of the needle visible so that contrast material extravasation will be immediately recognized. The patient is asked to tell the radiologist about the onset of any pain so that the procedure can be terminated if necessary.

Once the needle has been well seated in a vein, the patient is turned to a semi-erect, nonweight-bearing position with the leg to be studied dangling dependently while the other leg is supported on a box that elevates the patient from the base of the table. A tourniquet may be applied tightly around the ankle to force contrast into the deep venous system. This procedure can be generalized to venography of the upper extremity with the upper extremity being suspended above the heart allowing the gravitational flow of the contrast material into the heart. The use of a catheter allows more proximal dye insertion allowing visualization of the brachiocephalic vein.

Contrast is injected, either by hand or by a drip infusion, while carefully monitoring the tip of the needle and frequently aspirating back to be certain that the contrast is going into the vein. Approximately 60 to 80 cc of contrast material is injected and then lower leg is filmed in at least two projections. Further aliquots of 20 cc of contrast material are injected with further filming over the thigh and the pelvis.

After approximately 100 cc of contrast is administered, the patient is returned to the supine position and an additional film of the pelvis is taken. Finally, the head is tilted into a dependent (Trendelenburg) position and heparin is injected into the vein to decrease the incidence of postvenography phlebitis.

Catheter venography is used to evaluate the pelvic and abdominal veins. This requires insertion of a catheter in order to deliver the contrast material in more concentrated amounts to the vein being studied.

POSTPROCEDURE INFORMATION

Patients do not need to be accompanied by another person to the examination and will be able to leave the testing site on their own. It is advisable, however, that patients who require more than the usual amount of support should be accompanied to the examination.

Following the examination, patients may urinate frequently for several hours while the contrast is excreted into the urine. There may be some pain at the puncture site. Signs of postvenography phlebitis include erythema, swelling, and severe pain and these should be watched for. The patient should contact the physician if any of these symptoms occur. Any expanding hematoma should be compressed by direct pressure.

COMPLICATIONS

Risk factors for complications include advanced age, acute systemic illness, ischemic cardiovascular or cerebral disease, asthma, diabetes, multiple myeloma, preexisting renal disease, dehydration, coagulopathy, hypertension, and valvular heart disease.

Complications of angiography occur in just over 1.5% of the cases and mortality is reported to be between 0.03% and 0.05%. Good communication between the referring physician and the angiographer is essential to avoid complications.

Many of the risks of angiography are related to the risks of iodinated contrast material. This risk increases in proportion to the quantity of dye used, the duration of exposure, and the concentration of the contrast material. Hematologic effects can include red blood cell hemolysis and increased thromboembolic phenomena. Cardiopulmonary effects can include a greater susceptibility to arrhythmias and to vasovagal bradycardia with hypotension. Potential neurotoxic effects of the dye include seizures, paresis, and cortical blindness. Renal toxicity, directly related to the total dose, includes dehydration and hypotension.

Hypersensitivity reactions may be minor: self-limiting problems such as itching, urticaria, nausea, or vomiting. More significant responses include vasovagal reaction with hypotension, and mild bronchospasm. Severe contrast reactions are generally idiosyncratic and are not dose related. Patients are often premedicated with steroids or antihistamines if there is a history of prior contrast reactions.

Angiographic complications from catheterization include hemorrhage, thrombosis, thromboembolism, and vascular wall damage. Puncture-site bleeding is the most common complication and occurs more often in the patient with a coagulopathy.

Other consequences of venography include transient or occasionally prolonged renal failure caused by the nephrotoxicity of the contrast material. Hydration will reduce the incidence of this complication. Post-venography phlebitis occurs in 5% to 50% of the patients with the lower number being more accurately reflective of centers doing large numbers of procedures. Phlebitis is a much less common complication following studies of the upper extremity. It can be treated with elevation and soaks, rarely progressing on to an iatrogenically induced deep venous thrombosis.

Extravasation of contrast into the tissue is a feared complication that should not occur. If extravasation occurs in the presence of peripheral arterial disease a slough may occur and skin grafting may be required.

Catheter venography may result in the problems related to the puncture of a femoral vein such as hematoma formation, major vein thrombosis, and even pulmonary embolism. This, however, is quite rare. Intimal dissections have occurred during venous catheterization, which is less likely if an atraumatic guide is used to lead the catheter.

PATIENT QUESTIONS

Will venography hurt?

The test will be uncomfortable at best, if not painful. The pain will be crampy in nature for about two minutes and the patient will not be able to move the leg during the procedure. The radiologist performing the procedure should be informed if the pain becomes significant. For patients sensitive to discomfort, the nonionic contrast can be used. If an iodinated contrast material is used, the patient should be alerted to the possibility of an unpleasant taste in the mouth as the contrast material circulates through the body.

Will I be able to walk after the test?

The patient is permitted to ambulate after venous stasis has been obtained. This procedure can be done safely as an outpatient. Although it is often helpful to have someone accompany the patient home after the venogram, this precaution is not necessary.

Where does the dye go after the injection?

The contrast material is excreted in the urine and is both colorless and odorless. Increased frequency and quantity of urine is to be expected for several hours following the examination. Self-limited pyrogen reactions consisting of fever and chills have been reported, but if a reaction to the contrast material does not occur in the first hour, it is unlikely that any delayed allergic reactions will occur.

Will this test affect my varicose veins or make them worse?

There is no evidence that venography can cause either superficial or deep varicose veins to get worse. In addition, there is no evidence that venography will cause varicose veins. The patient should be reassured that venography has no cosmetic side effects.

CONSENT

Informed consent must be obtained for all contrast vascular studies. The patient must be informed of all the potential complications.

SELECTED BIBLIOGRAPHY

Bettman CF: Noninvasive and venographic diagnosis of deep vein thrombosis. *Cardiovasc Intervent Radiol* 1988;11Suppl:S15.

Cardella JF, Young AT, Smith TP, Darcy MD, Huinter DW, Casteneda-Zuniga WR, Knighton D, Nelson D, Amplatz K: Lower extremity venous thrombosis: comparison of venography, impedance plethysmography, and intravenous manometry. *Radiol* 1988;Jul 168:1:109.

Gomes AS, Webber MM, Buffkin D: Contrast venography vs. radionuclide venography: a study of discrepancies and their possible significance. *Radiol* 1982;Mar 142:3:719.

Naidich JB, Feinberg AW, Karp-Harpman H, Karmel MI, Tyma CG, Stein HL: Contrast venography: reassessment of its role. *Radiol* 1988;Jul:168:1:97.

II
Hematopoietic System Procedures

13

Bone Marrow Aspiration, Biopsy, and Transplant

RICHARD SADOVSKY

Bone marrow can be removed by aspiration or by needle biopsy. Aspiration involves extracting a liquid solution in which marrow segments are suspended, while needle biopsy removes a core of marrow tissue in a block. These two techniques can be used simultaneously or alone.

Bone marrow transplants have become more common. Marrow transplantation is a lengthy procedure requiring identification of an appropriate donor, obtaining of marrow from the donor, intravenous administration of the marrow into the recipient, and monitoring of the recipient during the period needed for the marrow to begin to regenerate. This procedure is readily available and ongoing investigation into improved techniques is improving survival rates.

INDICATIONS

Bone marrow is the major site of blood cell production. By examination of this tissue, reliable diagnostic information can be obtained about blood conditions. Primary bone disorders that can be revealed include diseases of all the blood cell lines such as leukemias, thrombocytopenias, and aplastic, hypoplastic, and pernicious anemias. Secondary disorders such as granulomatous disease, metastatic tumors, and myelosuppression secondary to chemotherapy can be evaluated by this technique. Aspiration is helpful primarily for cytologic diagnoses.

Most operators advocate performance of a biopsy along with aspiration. The biopsy allows a better assessment of cellularity and is essential when the aspiration has failed or in cases where marrow infiltration has occurred. Specific indications for biopsy include (1) failure to aspirate marrow, (2) myeloproliferative syndrome, (3) metastatic neoplasia, (4) acute leukemia leading to a dry tap, (5) staging and followup of patients with lymphoma, (6) granulomatous disorders, and (7) lead poisoning.

Bone marrow transplants are becoming more common and are being used for patients with hematologic cancers, aplastic anemia, immunologic deficiency diseases, and diseases of inborn errors of metabolism. Primary-care physicians must be prepared to discuss bone marrow transplants with patients because the decision as to whether to undergo marrow transplant is often made before the patient goes to a transplant center. The patient expects the primary-care physician to participate in the process. With information changing rapidly, consultation with an oncologist or hematologist might be helpful. If transplant is being considered, families should be urged to visit transplant centers before making the decision.

Patients with aplastic anemia should be considered for transplant early in the course of disease before multiple transfusions sensitize the patient to relatively minor transplant antigens.

ALTERNATIVES

Radioisotope scanning can be used to locate areas of abnormal marrow. A diagnosis cannot be made because of the lack of tissue, but scanning can help the physician determine an appropriate site for marrow aspiration and biopsy.

Chemotherapy is the alternative to marrow transplant for the control of certain blood disorders. The choice between marrow transplantation and chemotherapy is a difficult one. New data are available continuously and need to be considered. For example, in patients under 30 years of age with acute nonlymphoblastic leukemia in first remission, marrow grafting is the therapy most likely to result in a cure. For patients over 30 years, the treatment of choice is more debatable. The risk of early death from marrow transplant must be weighed against the long-term survival and cure rates.

POSSIBILITY OF FAILURE

Aspiration and/or biopsy of the marrow is the definitive way to learn about the morphology of the blood system and its forming elements. Aspiration alone is limited in its inability to provide positive diagnostic information in patients with granulomatous disease, myelofibrosis, and infiltrative diseases of the marrow.

Bone marrow transplantation may be rejected by the recipient resulting in nonresolution of the initial disorder and perhaps the addition of new problems such as sepsis or increased autoimmune difficulties.

CONTRAINDICATIONS

There are no absolute contraindications to aspiration and biopsy, although the procedures should be performed carefully in patients with severe bleeding disorders. The procedure is best performed on patients with prolonged bleeding time as inpatients so that appropriate observation can be made for 24 hours. Thrombocytopenia is generally not associated with significant bleeding. The presence of disseminated intravascular coagulation makes bone marrow biopsy a risky procedure. Patients with hereditary coagulation factor deficiencies can have bone marrow procedures after being covered by the appropriate component. Anticoagulation therapy should be stopped and adequate hemostatic status regained before the procedure is performed.

There are no known contraindications to marrow transplant assuming an appropriate donor can be found.

PREPROCEDURE PREPARATION

The patient should be evaluated for prior history of hypersensitivity to local anesthesia. Blood testing for a bleeding disorder should be performed. Anxious patients can be given a mild sedative and an analgesic prior to the procedure.

Marrow transplantation requires scrupulous tissue antigen typing and leukocyte culturing through blood testing. Once a donor has been found, the recipient is prepared with appropriate immunosuppressive medications including agents such as cyclophosphamide, cytosine arabinoside, busulfan, and/or methotrexate. Total body irradiation may be used in addition to enhance the immunosuppressive effects of the chemotherapy. Newer techniques of total lymphoid irradiation are in the experimental stage. When marrow transplant is performed to reconstitute lymphopoiesis in patients with severe immunodeficiency, or when a patient is receiving a syngeneic transplant, an immunosuppressive regimen may not be required prior to the procedure.

Baseline studies of the marrow recipient include a large number of chemical and bacteriological tests that are done on admission to the hospital.

PATIENT EDUCATION

The patient should understand the procedure of aspiration and/or biopsy and its appropriate indications. There is no need to restrict food or fluids before the test and often the procedure is performed as an outpatient. The procedure takes 5 to 10 minutes and the test results are usually available within 1 day. The site to be used for the procedure should be discussed.

Prior to bone marrow transplantation, the risks and benefits of the procedure should be discussed. The patient should understand that compatible tissue types are found for only half of the potential recipient candidates.

PROCEDURE

The patient is positioned in such a way as to make the aspiration or biopsy site easily accessible. The skin is cleansed with an appropriate antiseptic solution and a local anesthetic is injected. The aspiration is done inserting the needle through the skin and, with a twisting motion, the needle is advanced through the subcutaneous tissue and into the bone cortex (figure 13–1). The stylet is removed from the needle, a syringe is used to aspirate a small quantity of the marrow, and the needle is withdrawn. Pressure is then applied to the site for several minutes, the site is cleaned and covered with a sterile bandage. Slides of the marrow aspirate must be prepared immediately to allow clear examination of the cells.

Needle biopsy involves a similar twisting motion to insert the needle into the bone cortex. The trephine tip of the biopsy needle allows removal of a plug of marrow tissue. The needle is then withdrawn and the plug is expelled into an appropriate fixative solution. The biopsy site is cleaned and covered. In rare instances, the biopsy must be performed under general anesthesia when a larger amount of tissue is needed.

Bone marrow transplants are either autologous (the patient receives his or her own stored marrow), syngeneic (between identical twins), or allogeneic (between two persons of different genetic origin but within the same species). Marrow is obtained from the appropriate donor under general or spinal anesthesia by multiple aspirations performed at the anterior and posterior iliac crest. The marrow is intravenously infused into the recipient at the same rate as red blood cells would be given. These patients remain in the hospital for at least 2 to 4 weeks because of the complete lack of marrow function during this period.

POSTPROCEDURE INFORMATION

The biopsy site should be observed for bleeding, inflammation, and infection. Signs of hemorrhage and infection, such as rapid heart rate, fever, severe pain, loss of mobility, or general malaise should be reported to the physician. The patient may return to normal activities and shower 24 hours after the procedure. The puncture site can be uncovered after the same period. Slight soreness in the area of the biopsy may be present for several days.

The patient who has received a bone marrow transplantation is observed in the hospital until clear signs of marrow regeneration are present. On discharge,

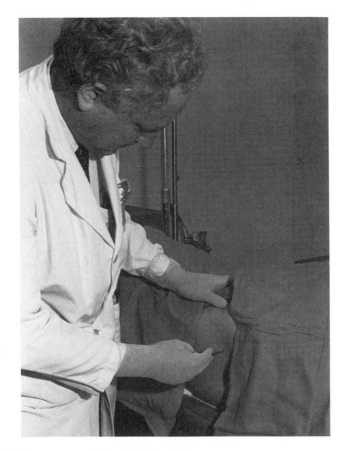

Figure 13–1. Bone marrow aspiration at the iliac cerst.

the patient must be observed for signs of infection and must be encouraged to eat properly. Parenteral nutrition should be provided if needed. Multivitamin therapy is often recommended. Visitors can be permitted after the first few weeks, but sick people and children should be avoided initially. Exercise, good pulmonary toilet using breathing exercises, appropriate antibiotic therapy, and emotional support are important factors in the health of the marrow recipient. Medications containing aspirin should be avoided.

COMPLICATIONS

Complications following marrow aspiration or biopsy are rare. Bleeding or infection has occurred, but in only very rare cases. The latter occurs more frequently in patients who are receiving immunosuppressive medications. The puncture of nearby structures is exceedingly rare.

The major dangers of marrow transplantation include infusion problems such as fluid overload, emboli, reactions to the white cells in the marrow, and bacterial contamination of the marrow. The patient prepared with cyclophosphamide may experience nausea and vomiting. Total body irradiation may cause nausea, vomiting, diarrhea, fever, parotitis, stomatitis, alopecia, and sterility. The frequency of side effects can be diminished by fractionating the doses of radiation. Fevers may also occur, but generally subside within 4 to 6 hours.

Graft-versus-host reactions can occur causing damage to the skin, liver, and gastrointestinal tract. These can range in severity from a mild rash to severe liver involvement with high mortality. The occurrence and course of graft-versus-host disease (GVHD) is difficult to predict, although recent studies imply higher risk with advancing age. Patient sex, marrow cell dose, and use of laminar flow rooms do not seem to correlate with GVHD. The symptoms of GVHD may begin as early as 10 days following the transplantation or as late as 18 months after the procedure. Graft rejection is slightly more common in patients who have received multiple transfusions prior to the transplant. Prophylactic use of cyclosporine A appears to decrease the frequency of both graft rejection and graft-versus-host reactions when adequate cyclosporine concentrations are achieved. The combined use of cyclosporine and methotrexate in patients with severe aplastic anemia seems to lower the incidence of GVHD even further.

PATIENT QUESTIONS

In what location will the aspiration and biopsy be performed?

Common sites for aspiration and biopsy include the posterior superior iliac spine, the sternum, the spinous processes, and the tibia. The posterior superior iliac spine is the most commonly used site in adults since no vital organs are located nearby. The sternum site involves the greatest risk, but is often used because it is near the surface, the bone is thin, and the marrow cavity contains numerous cells. The spinous process is preferred if the other sites do not contain marrow, and generally the third or fourth lumbar vertebra is the chosen site. The tibia is the site of choice for children under 1 year of age and the procedure is done just below the tibial tuberosity.

Will I feel pain during the aspiration and biopsy?

Aspiration of bone marrow can cause sharp pain although careful technique makes this rare and most patients report only slight discomfort. Biopsy of the marrow appears to cause less discomfort: The physician should try to allay anxieties before the test, administer adequate local anesthesia, and use careful technique.

How long does it take to determine whether a marrow transplantation has been successful?

After a period of 2 to 4 weeks, the granulocyte count begins to rise in the peripheral blood. This is usually followed by a rise in the platelet and red cell count. A marrow aspiration can be done to confirm the regeneration of the bone marrow. The patient can go home when the granulocyte count reaches 500 to 1,000 per mm^3 and no sign of infection is present.

What are the risks to marrow donors?

The potential risks to the donors include the problems associated with anesthesia, as well as bleeding, rare instances of infection, and slight postoperative discomfort. Donor marrow is readily regenerated, and the incidence of life-threatening complications in donors is extremely low. Hospitalization time for the donor is generally less than three days and is proportional to the degree of discomfort at the donation site. Ferrous sulfate may be ordered for a few months after donation to prevent anemia.

CONSENT

Informed consent is required for bone marrow aspiration and/or biopsy. Multiple informed consents may be necessary for bone marrow transplants depending on how the procedure is managed at the institution where the procedure is performed. Consents may be necessary for the radiation, the chemotherapy, and for the marrow transplantation.

SELECTED BIBLIOGRAPHY

Barrett AJ: Bone marrow transplantation. *Cancer Treat Rev* 1987;Dec 14:3–4:203.

Burkhardt R, Frisch B, Bartl R: Bone biopsy in haemotological disorders. *J Clin Pathol* 1982;Mar:35:3:257.

Datz FL, Taylor A, Jr: The clinical use of radionuclide bone marrow imaging. *Semin Nucl Med* 1985;Jul 15:3:239.

Knowles S, Hoffbrand AV: Bone marrow aspiration and trephine biopsy. *Br Med J* 1980;July 26:281:6235:280.

Westerman MP: Bone marrow needle biopsy: and evaluation and critique. *Semin Hematol* 1981;Oct 18:4:293.

Wiley FM, House KU: Bone marrow transplant in children. *Semin Oncol Nurs* 1988; Feb 4:1:3140.

14

Transfusion

RICHARD SADOVSKY

Blood is a complex fluid containing cellular components and plasma. Advanced technology has made it possible to separate these elements, permitting the physician to choose the appropriate component for his patient while leaving the other portions of the collected blood unit to be used by other patients for their specific clinical needs.

INDICATIONS

Transfusions of blood or blood products are done for patients with evidence of sudden or chronic blood loss, for preoperative patients, and for patients with abnormally low levels of coagulation factor. Transfusion involves the intravenous administration of blood or blood products with the aim of having the recipient be able to utilize the exogenous material as their own. Transfusion of various blood components are administered as needed.

ALTERNATIVES

In most situations, there is no substitute for blood or blood products. Saline or albumin infusions can be used for volume expansion in certain circumstances of minimal intravascular volume depletion with adequate red blood cell (RBC) mass.

CONTRAINDICATIONS

There are no absolute contraindications to transfusion of blood or blood products. In patients with a history of transfusion reaction, appropriate precautions should be taken to prevent a similar reaction if transfusion is again indicated.

PREOPERATIVE PREPARATION

There is no preprocedure preparation with the exception of the typing and cross-matching of the patient's blood with the blood to be transfused.

PATIENT EDUCATION

The patient should be informed of the reason for the transfusion, that the transfusion will be given intravenously, and that any feeling of malaise, fever, or pain at the site of the intravenous catheter or needle should be reported. The patient should be told what products are being transfused, how many "bags" are involved, and how long the transfusion will take.

PROCEDURE

Fresh serum obtained within 48 hours is needed for the crossmatch. The laboratory determines ABO and Rh typing and screening for irregular antibodies. A donor of the same ABO and Rh type is chosen and a crossmatch is performed. If there is a compatible crossmatch and no unexpected antibodies, the blood should be available for transfusion within 1 hour. The detection of irregular antibodies can delay the availability of compatible blood.

The crossmatch is like a minitransfusion in the test tube. The donor and recipient blood are mixed together exposing most antibodies against the donor blood cells and most ABO errors. The crossmatch, however, does not guarantee that no transfusion reaction will occur.

Transfusion products must be kept refrigerated at specific temperatures in order to avoid hemolysis. The actual transfusion is done through equipment that contains a filter that removes fibrin and other particulate matter. A venipuncture is performed with a 20 gauge or wider needle. If a narrower needle is used as it might be in children and infants, a pressure device or a pump may be used. Central venous lines should not be used for transfusion because the coldness of the components or the high concentration of potassium could cause arrhythmias, especially in neonates. The transfusion should be started only with normal saline, as both 5% dextrose in water and Ringer's lactate damage red cells. No medications should be added through the blood administration set. Confirmation of the identity of the recipient and the donor material is done again prior to administration.

Blood is warmed before administering only in cases of massive transfusions, rapid transfusions, exchange transfusions in infants, or in patients with cold agglutinins. This warming should be done only by a machine designed for this purpose.

Emergency transfusions are occasionally needed in life-threatening situations. There may not be time to complete the crossmatch, and the patient's physician must sign a release for the blood bank releasing the bank from responsibility. If time permits, about ten minutes is needed for ABO and rh typing so that group-specific blood can be provided. Type O negative blood may be given when such time is not available.

Whole blood should be reserved for cases of active bleeding and surgical procedures. In other situations, the patient should receive only the component in which they are deficient.

Red blood cells ("packed cells") are prepared by centrifugal or gravitational sedimentation of the RBCs in whole blood followed by the removal of the plasma. This is indicated when the patient requires more red cells but not an increase in intravascular volume.

Other blood components and derivatives available to treat patients include platelet concentrates, granulocyte concentrates, plasma, cryoprecipitate, albumin, and plasma protein fractions. Granulocyte transfusion requires pretransfusion compatibility testing although this is not needed in platelet concentrate transfusions. It should be remembered that both of these may transmit infectious diseases and may cause allergic and febrile reactions.

Transfusing plasma that was frozen shortly after collection will provide coagulation factors. Because of the risk of transmitting infection, plasma should not be used solely as a volume expander. Cryoprecipitate is a blood product containing high concentrations of fibrinogen and antihemophilic factor (Factor VIII). While both plasma and cryoprecipitate may transmit infectious agents, neither contains enough RBCs to require pretransfusion compatibility testing.

Albumin and plasma protein fraction, both derived from plasma, are usually given for rapid blood volume expansion. Stable at room temperature, these products do not transmit infectious diseases. Precompatibility testing is not required.

POSTPROCEDURE INFORMATION

The majority of transfusions are performed while the patient is in the hospital (figure 14–1). It is becoming more and more acceptable, however, to have outpatient undergoing transfusion for certain medical problems. If a patient receives a transfusion as an outpatient, family and/or friends should be advised to watch for complications such as rashes, fever, joint pains, malaise, and so on. These should be reported to the physician.

Transfusions are administered occasionally in the home by a visiting nurse. This requires careful attention to all details and good patient understanding of the procedure. Vital signs should be taken every 15 minutes during the first 30 minutes of the transfusion and every 30 minutes thereafter.

Hemolytic transfusion reactions can occur as long as 14 days after the transfusion, and infections such as hepatitis can develop from 2 weeks to 6 months later.

COMPLICATIONS

A multitude of potential complications may arise from the transfusion of blood products. Although these reactions are infrequent, blood transfusion should not be considered a procedure without risk. The transfusion should always be justified and close observation for a possible transfusion reaction is essential.

Transfusions should be discontinued if any event more serious than hives occurs during the procedure. The IV line should be kept open for supportive care and the blood bank should be notified immediately.

Complications of transfusions vary widely from mild chills and fever to severe fatal hemolysis. Febrile nonhemolytic reactions are usually mild episodes of chills and fever, rarely precipitating shock. This is thought to be caused by antibodies to leukocytes or platelets and may be pretreated with antipyretics. Future transfusions in these patients who have demonstrated this reaction should be of either leukocyte poor or frozen and thawed washed red cells.

Allergic reactions, often characterized by itching, urticaria, and, sometimes, headache, occur in 1% to 2% of all transfusions and are caused by hypersensitivity to an unknown agent in the donor blood. Previous history of transfusion allergies may suggest the need for pretreatment with antihistamines or steroids. Patients with antibodies to IgA may react more violently and with anaphylaxis. These individuals should receive extensively washed red cells or IgA-deficient donor blood.

Hemolytic transfusion reactions are the most severe. The severity will vary with the amount of blood given, the incompatibility, and the clinical condition of the patient. Often there is difficulty breathing, flushed face, and evidence of shock. Steps to maintain blood pressure and urine output should be taken imme-

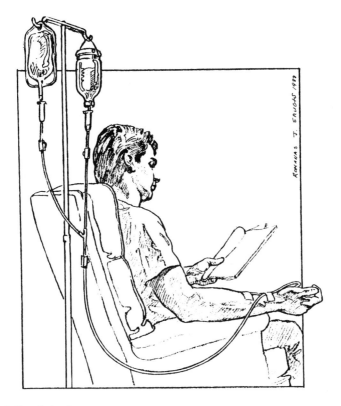

Figure 14–1. Transfusion in progress.

diately. If disseminated intravascular coagulation occurs, fresh frozen plasma and/or platelets may be administered.

Whole-blood transfusion may result in circulatory overload characterized by a rise in venous pressure, rapid pulse, pulmonary edema, and cyanosis.

The risk of disease transmission from donor to recipient includes blood borne organisms that cause malaria, syphilis, viral hepatitis, and AIDS. Delta hepatitis has been recognized recently as a cause of fulminant hepatitis in patients with concurrent hepatitis B infection. Since this infection appears to coexist with Hepatitis type B, screening for the latter antigen minimizes the risk of delta hepatitis. All donor blood is screened for the latter three illnesses, and malaria is avoided by careful screening of donors. None of the screening tests are 100% accurate.

Other less common complications of blood administration include pulmonary embolism secondary to a clot, foreign material, or air entering the bloodstream via the tubing, localized vasospasms caused by the administration of cold blood, and hyperkalemia caused by leakage of potassium from the stored red cells.

PATIENT QUESTIONS

How long does a transfusion take?

Whole blood and packed or frozen-thawed red cells are ordinarily administered within 2 to 3 hours per unit. Each unit administered should not require more than 4 hours. The longer the blood hangs, the warmer it becomes and the greater the dangers of bacterial proliferation and red cell hemolysis. Under certain circumstances, blood administration may need to be speeded up, and a unit of packed cells can be administered in as little as 5 to 10 minutes. Patients should be told what blood products they are receiving, how many "bags" will be hung, how long the procedure will take, and what they should watch for.

Will I get an infectious disease from the transfusion?   Will I get AIDS?

Blood transfusion is a potent vector for the transmission of a number of diseases. Much of this risk, however, is eliminated by the exclusion of commercial blood donors and screening blood donors both by obtaining appropriate historical information and by testing the blood for appropriate antibodies or antigens. The large majority of cases of posttransfusion hepatitis are of the non-A, non-B variety now that screening for hepatitis B has become standard. Rarely, cases of malaria, trypanosomiasis, and cytomegalovirus have been traced to blood transfusion.

Acquired immune deficiency syndrome (AIDS) remains a rare complication of blood transfusions. Prospective donors whose history shows them to be at high risk for contacting AIDS are not allowed to donate blood. As a further precaution, all blood donors are tested for antibodies to HIV virus. The possibility of a false negative antibody test during the early months of HIV infection is present. The precise risk of posttransfusion AIDS today is difficult to assess. Whether these measures will be successful in eliminating the risk of transmission of AIDS during blood transfusion remains to be determined.

Should I ask a relative to donate blood for my transfusion, or should I donate my own blood in advance in anticipation of a transfusion?

This is a complex question and depends on many factors. Most physicians in the United States feel that the blood supply is safe and the likelihood of disease transmission is small. The use of blood from a family member or autologous (patient's own blood) transfusions is becoming possible at many more medical institutions. The decision to do this depends on hospital and blood bank policies, the acuteness of need for transfusion, the medical reasons for the transfusion, the health of the relative, and the potential volume of blood that may be needed. Patients should discuss these issues with their physicians and family members.

How safe is transfusion of uncrossmatched blood and is its use preferable to using universal donor (type O negative) in the emergent situation?

Optimally, the 10 minutes needed for preparation of type-specific blood matching the ABO group and Rh type will be available. This type-specific transfusion eliminates the pathogenesis of hemolytic reactions to a large degree. This was done extensively during the Vietnam War with few adverse effects and is probably preferable to using universal donor blood that is relatively rare and is specifically indicated in many circumstances.

CONSENT

Although blood and blood-product transfusions are not specifically invasive procedures, it is wise to discuss the transfusion with the patient and obtain the patient's consent for transfusion. This consent should be informed, and should be obtained even if it is uncertain as to whether a transfusion will be needed in situations such as surgery when the patient will be unable to give consent.

When it is necessary to infuse uncrossmatched blood into a patient, an emergency release form must be completed on release of the blood. The form describes the nature of the emergency and identifies the product being used. The form also reminds the physician that uncrossmatched blood is being used. This required form is an "internal" form, but it is a good idea for the physician to inform the patient and/or family when uncrossmatched blood is being used. If possible, a special consent form for this procedure should be obtained. Verbal consent can be used if documented appropriately. If the transfusion is an emergency and no one is available to give consent, the procedure should be documented and done.

SELECTED BIBLIOGRAPHY

Bove JR: Transfusion associated hepatitis and AIDS. What is the risk? *N Eng J Med* 1987;Jul, 23:317:4:242.

Coffin CM: Current issues in transfusion therapy. *Postgrad Med* 1987;Jan 81:1:343.

Peterman TA: Transfusion associated acquired immunodeficiency syndrome. *World J Surg* 1987;Feb:111:37.

Renner SW, Howanitz JH, Fishkin BG: Toward meaningful blood usage review; comprehensive monitoring of physician practice. *QRB* 1987;Mar 13:3:76.

Shaikh BS: History and clinical practice of modern blood transfusion therapy: a review. *JPMA* 1987;Jan:37:1:13.

III
Anesthesia and Analgesia Procedures

15

Acupuncture

RICHARD SADOVSKY

Acupuncture is described as a system of medicine used to restore health as well as to prevent illness. The basic tenet, as practiced in China for thousands of years, is that treatment is directed at the cause of the problem rather than at the palliation of symptoms. Traditional acupuncture is based on the idea that "vital" energy travels in pathways or "meridians" in the body. Each meridian corresponds to one of the vital organs, and the insertion of needles into the points that lie along these meridians establishes a balance, or flow, of energy where there had previously been a blockage or imbalance.

More commonly, acupuncture is aimed at relieving a specific symptom. Painful acupuncture can have the generalized effect of increasing tolerance to pain throughout the body. In order to practice acupuncture in a less painful manner, the source of tenderness must be found. This is usually done by physical examination. If it is anatomically safe, the needle can be inserted relatively painlessly in the immediate proximity. There is much debate about the desirable approach to acupuncture methodology, point selection, and the methods of needle stimulation.

The use of acupuncture for anesthesia is beyond the scope of this chapter.

INDICATIONS

Currently, acupuncture is most commonly used in patients with chronic complaints including migraine, arthritis, phantom limb pain, cancer pain, depression, tinnitus, angina, asthma, drug or alcohol addiction, or other problems. Generally conventional medicine has not resolved their problems and the patients are desperate. There does appear to be a significant difference between the therapeutic effect of acupuncture versus placebo in the treatment of chronic pain, although this difference diminishes with time.

Acupuncture use in the treatment of chronic headache and back pain has been most thoroughly studied. Traditional acupuncture, which has its own method of classifying headaches, appears to have mixed results of patients with migraine and somewhat better results with tension headaches. The results of studies of patients with lower back pain also contain mixed results with some evidence of short-term beneficial effects from acupuncture.

ALTERNATIVES

Comparison of acupuncture with more conventional Western therapy for treatment of a variety of musculoskeletal problems has been performed with unclear results. The data suggest that a physical placebo results in 30% of the patients experiencing some pain relief; random needling giving a 50% relief response, and acupuncture decreasing pain symptoms in 50% to 80% of patients. Alternatives to acupuncture include analgesics, electrical stimulation, hypnosis, and other forms of drug therapy. Comparative studies have not clearly determined which treatment is best for which type of pain. No significant differences have emerged where acupuncture has been compared with transcutaneous electrical nerve stimulation (TENS), other forms of electrical nerve stimulation, or physiotherapy. Comparisons of acupuncture with drug therapy are few and often incomplete, but they imply a similar response rate.

POSSIBILITY OF FAILURE

Not all people improve with acupuncture. It is likely that a wide variety of physical and psychological factors such as extent of the pathology, presence of depression, and level of belief in the treatment may affect the patient's response to acupuncture. The proportion of patients helped over the short term appears to be in the 50% to 80% range. Those who tend to improve with acupuncture treatments when questioned postprocedurally are generally younger (under 40 years of age), had more treatments, had less chronic pain, and were less likely to have had surgery. At times, the main complaint is not improved, although a person may feel better in a more general way and may sleep better or feel more relaxed. Symptomatic relief is highest immediately following a course of treatment and tends to diminish with time. This may be caused by the development of tolerance following long periods of acupuncture stimulation.

CONTRAINDICATIONS

Patients who are depressed, passive, and have had a long duration of pain are poorer candidates for acupuncture and have less likelihood of pain relief following treatment. The presence of nonpain-related coexistent medical illness is more likely to be associated with failure.

Pain that has a clear neurophysiologic cause (e.g., sciatica) will probably not respond to acupuncture.

PREPROCEDURE PREPARATION

There is no preprocedure preparation for acupuncture.

PATIENT EDUCATION

For long-term relief, the most suitable cases for acupuncture are those patients who are well motivated and have minimal organic changes. Patients should understand that the first treatment may produce relief for only a few hours. The second treatment done several days later may produce a full day's relief, while the third treatment may provide longer relief. Usually at least 5 or 6 treatments are needed to obtain sustained relief.

Relief may be temporary with most studies concluding that the analgesic effect of acupuncture generally disappears within 6 months to a year following the course of therapy.

PROCEDURE

In traditional acupuncture therapy, the initial diagnosis involves considering the patient's current condition, medical history (including that of his family) and life pattern. This is combined with an examination and a "mapping out" of the meridians. This process may require several hours. The treatment sessions are generally short and done regularly with decreasing frequency over time.

After the selection of acupuncture points, the needle is inserted (figure 15–1) and stimulation may be applied using twirling by hand, heating the needle, or electrical stimulation. The treatment regimen may include massed or spaced treatment sessions.

R. SRUGIS '88

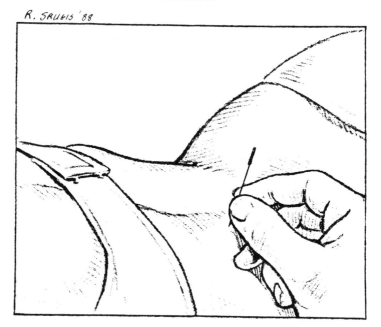

Figure 15–1. Acupuncture needle insertion.

POSTPROCEDURE INFORMAITON

There is no postprocedure information needed by the patient. If irritation occurs in the treated area, warm compresses can be applied and the acupuncturist should be informed.

COMPLICATIONS

Perhaps the most common side effect of acupuncture is the development of more pain within 48 hours of treatment. This is usually thought to be caused by the use of too many needles. This pain is usually self-limiting and rarely lasts more than a few days.

Other rare side effects have been hepatitis and local abscesses at the acupuncture site.

There are also reports of acupuncture relieving visceral pain. The practitioner must be careful not to mask pain that may be caused by significant visceral abnormalities.

PATIENT QUESTIONS

Will acupuncture make my pain disappear?

Acupuncture, like many analgesics, works for a limited period of time with an immediate success rate of 50% to 80%. Some studies report that, following completion of a full course of therapy, the analgesic effects disappear completely after 6 months, while others report longer relief periods. Long-term follow up of patients receiving courses of acupuncture has been difficult. It is clear, however, that the effect of acupuncture diminished with time, implying that the patient might have to seek further therapy directed at providing analgesia.

How do I know that the acupuncturist is competent?

Patients should be encouraged to go to acupuncture therapists who are known to the physician and who have had appropriate training and practical experience. At present, there are a number of societies for acupuncturists and it is difficult to check credentials thoroughly. The question as to which acupuncture points (whether classical points, trigger points, motor points, or others) are most thera- peutic when stimulated is not answerable at present.

CONSENT

It is wise to obtain informed consent prior to acupuncture therapy.

SELECTED BIBLIOGRAPHY

Vincent CA, Richardson PH: Acupuncture for some common disorders: a review of evaluative research. *J R Coll Gen Pract* 1987;Feb:37:395:77.

Richardson PH, Vincent CA: Acupuncture for the treatment of pain: a review of evaluative research. *Pain* 1986;Jan 24:1:15.

Laborde JM: Acupuncture treatment: a perspective. *J Pain Symptom Manag* 1986;Fall:1:4:232.

Fan SG: Acupuncture analgesia. *Acta Neurocir* 1987;Suppl 38:82.

Mayer DK: Non-pharmacologic management of pain in the person with cancer. *J Adv Nurs* 1985;10:325.

16

Electrical Stimulation Therapy

RICHARD SADOVSKY

As recognized medical practice, electrical stimulation has been used most frequently to diminish both acute and chronic pain. The selective stimulation of primary afferent nerve fibers has been reported to decrease acute pain in 50% to 60% of patients and to control chronic pain for prolonged periods in approximately 30% of patients. Peripheral nerve stimulation is applied most commonly to the skin surface (transcutaneous electrical nerve stimulation, TENS) (figure 16–1) or by implanted electrodes.

Peripheral nerve stimulation utilizes large, myelinated, afferent nerve fibers to initiate local inhibitory circuits within the dorsal horn of the spine cell (the "gate control" theory). Transmission through the spinal cord is then decreased in a segmental distribution. Higher levels of stimulation can be used to activate polysegmental inhibitory circuits. Most frequently, the segmental approach is used to treat pain by the production of nonpainful paresthesia in the region of the body where the pain is located. This differs from acupuncture techniques, which are extra-segmental and often use painful stimuli.

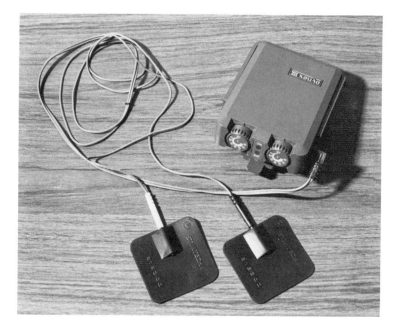

Figure 16–1. Transepidermal nerve stimulation unit.

Deep-brain and spinal-cord electrical stimulation have documented roles in chronic pain relief, but these therapies are too complex to discuss here.

Electrical stimulation has been used to promote healing in certain orthopedic problems such as fractures. Electrodes are used either internally or externally and the treatment generally requires several months. Good randomized studies have not yet documented clearly the efficacy of this use of electrical stimulation.

INDICATIONS

The indications for pain therapy must be considered with effectiveness of therapy and evaluation of side-effects. Any localized pain of somatic or neurogenic origin is an indication for electrical stimulation therapy provided that paresthesia can be obtained in the region of pain. Acute pain that is most responsive to TENS includes traumatic pain, postoperative pain, and post-herpetic neuralgia. Minor trauma produces transient pain that may or may not require TENS, while major trauma usually requires systemic analgesics for multiple injuries. TENS is often ineffective in these latter cases but can often be helpful in unique situations such as rib fractures. Postoperative pain is treated with TENS more frequently. Sterilized electrodes can be places next to the incision by the surgeon at the conclusion of the procedure. This has been done following abdominal and thoracic surgery, total hip replacements, and lumbar-spine operations. Pain secondary to post-herpetic neuralgia responds well, especially if the patient has not already been exposed to some other type of pain management regimen. Two other acute pain states for which TENS has been used include childbirth and acute orofacial pain caused by periodontal infections and routine dental procedures.

Chronic pain is a greater clinical problem and, when the pain is neurogenic such as peripheral nerve injury, postherpetic neuralgia, and intercostal neuritis, TENS is particularly helpful. Chronic back pain, radiculopathies, and compression syndromes are also suitable to this technique. Chronic pain states not suitable for this treatment are those that are widespread and poorly localized, including visceral pain, and psychogenic pain.

The indications for implanted electrodes are less well known because this more complex procedure is used less than the transcutaneous method. Criteria must be rigorous and include the existence of severe, unremitting pain. The most suitable patients appear to be those with peripheral nerve injury. In general, an adequate trial of TENS should be attempted before using more invasive procedures.

Electrical stimulation therapy for nonunion (i.e., failure of a fracture to heal after 6 to 9 months) may relieve patients from permanent disability by promoting healing. This application is presently under study.

ALTERNATIVES

Conventional forms of pain therapy, which include medication, physical modalities such as immobilization and strapping, and intercostal blocks are associated with complications. Prostaglandin synthetase inhibitors such as anti-inflammatory agents can cause gastric erosion in stressed patients. Narcotic agents decrease the respiratory drive. Immobilization may predispose the patient to emboli while strapping (in the case of rib fractures) diminishes ventilatory excursion. Intercostal blocks may require repeated injections.

The main advantage of TENS over narcotic analgesia is that pain relief is continuous. Narcotic requirements of patients who use TENS postoperatively are substantially decreased. In addition, there is no respiratory depression and no alteration of bowel motility. (The use of acupuncture is discussed in chapter 15.)

Surgical treatment of pain includes ablation of the nerve. This procedure has all the risks that accompany surgery, but it has the advantage of not requiring the necessary discipline on the part of the patient when using nerve stimulation.

The alternatives to electrical stimulation therapy for bone nonunion include additional conservative management or surgical fixation and repair.

POSSIBILITY OF FAILURE

The efficacy of treatment of pain with electrical stimulation therapy often decreases with time. With treatment of chronic pain, only around 20% to 35% of patients will report relief after using TENS for more than 1 year. This contrasts with the 60% to 80% relief rate of chronic pain in the early stages of the use of TENS, perhaps due to a decrease in placebo effect occurring with time.

Success rates of electrical stimulation therapy for nonunion vary depending on the type, location, and complexity of the fracture, the nature of additional bone grafting, and the use of any fixation devices. Success rates as high as 80% to 90% have been reported.

CONTRAINDICATIONS

The only absolute contraindication for TENS is in patients with pacemakers or other implanted electrical devices. These may be affected by the electrical field produced by the generator. It is also probably best not to use TENS in patients who cannot understand the controls since a sudden increase in amplitude can cause a highly painful muscle contraction.

The safety of nerve stimulation over the carotid sinus or during pregnancy is uncertain. Nerve stimulation for pain relief is also inappropriate in progressive pathologic disorders in which it is necessary to accurately follow the progression of pain.

Electrical stimulation therapy for nonunion of bone is contraindicated in the presence of any inflammatory process including systemic infections, osteomyelitis, or bone tumors. Neither can congenital or developmental conditions be managed by this treatment.

PREPROCEDURE PREPARATION

Prior to electrical stimulation therapy for pain relief, a complete evaluation of the patient's pain symptom complex is essential, including a description of prior efforts to eliminate the pain, if any. A prior or current history of narcotics addiction may indicate a patient who is less likely to respond to stimulation therapy. It is also helpful to know whether the patient is involved in litigation or receiving financial compensation for the pain.

Clear descriptions of the locus of pain should be obtained to facilitate electrode placement. This, along with the physical examination evaluating any functional losses caused by the pain, will help to evaluate the results of pain relief therapy.

No specific preparation is needed for use of electrical stimulation therapy for resolution of bone nonunion.

PATIENT EDUCATION

Patients need to understand thoroughly the procedure and its indications. The patient's motivation, education, and cultural background may affect the efficacy of electrical stimulation therapy for pain. Family education should be included in the teaching program.

If electrical stimulation therapy is being used for nonunion of bones, the patient must cooperate with the treatments and avoid weight bearing on the affected area.

DESCRIBE PROCEDURE

Multiple techniques can be used to produce nonpainful parasthesias. These include (1) transcutaneous electrical nerve stimulation (TENS) using superficial electrodes placed on the skin; (2) peripheral nerve stimulation through subcutaneously implanted electrodes; (3) peripheral nerve activation using electrodes directly implanted at the nerve; and (4) activation of collaterals by direct stimulation of the dorsal columns or through the dura.

Electrical stimulation requires a pulse generator, an amplifier, and a system of electrodes. The pulses can be continuous or intermittent with varying frequencies. The amplifier intensifies the signal in order to deliver adequate current to the electrode.

The threshold for stimulation of peripheral nerves can be variable because of the heterogeneity of the body's impedance and the nonpassive characteristics of peripheral nerves. The larger the individual nerve fibers, the lower the threshold. Fibers on the surface of the nerve will be stimulated before the deeper ones. Younger patients do well with a unit that offers a variety of modes of stimulation while an elderly patient may achieve good results with a unit that has present parameters and can be used with minimal adjustment. For practical purposes, the goal is to activate large sensory muscle fibers without causing muscle contractions, dysthesia, or pain.

Positioning of the electrodes should be as close as possible to the course of the peripheral nerve innervating the site of the pain. It is best to stimulate close to the pain, but this is not essential. Electrical stimulation of specific points, such as trigger, motor, or acupuncture points, has been reported to be effective in reducing pain. The site of most effective stimulation can often be predicted by trial stimulations, especially in the case of the transcutaneous electrode units. Bilateral stimulation can be extremely helpful and is often used for unilateral pain conditions. There can be a contralateral transmission from afferent nerves activated unilaterally by the TENS device. For some patients, this may require admission to a hospital to ensure adequate trial. Areas of insensitivity and hyperesthesia should be avoided in electrode placement. Placement over bony prominences and haircovered areas is not recommended because of the decrease in skin contact.

With transcutaneous electrodes, it is necessary to stimulate the afferent nerves without damaging the skin. Many types of electrodes have been used, all requiring attachment to the skin with adhesive tape or with self-adhesive methods. The electrodes should be at least 2 cm in diameter to prevent skin irritation from too high a current density. Impedance is minimized by applying electrolyte gel that prevents skin irritation. The vast majority of patients prefer frequencies between 40 and 70 Hz with pulse widths of 0.1 to 0.5 msec.

Implanted electrodes can be used subdermally to treat acute or chronic pain. This requires implantation under local anesthesia with suturing in such a way that maximal parasthesias realized with minimal muscle contraction.

Electrical stimulation used to resolve nonunion of bones may utilize a noninvasive coil system, a semi-invasive percutaneous stimulator, or a fully implantable direct current stimulator. Treatment generally lasts 3 to 6 months and requires good patient cooperation.

POSTPROCEDURE INFORMATION

The family should understand the mechanism of electrical stimulation therapy and be supportive of the patient's use of this mode of therapy. Instructions need to be taught to persons other than the patient so that guidance and monitoring can be done by appropriate family members.

COMPLICATIONS

TENS is a safe procedure with remarkably few side effects. Occasional pain occurs when impedance between the electrode and the skin is lowered because of perspiration or inadequate use of the electrolyte gel. An allergic dermatitis caused by the tape used to attach the electrode to the skin may occur.

Implanted electrodes require much less current than surface electrodes, but the risk of damage to tissues by electrochemical changes at the interface of the electrode and the tissue.

In treatment of nonunion, local skin irritation can occur around the cathode pin sites causing swelling, pain, and redness. Implanted cathode pins have been known to break, but this does not appear to increase morbidity.

PATIENT QUESTIONS

Will I have pain when using the TENS unit?

TENS is a painless technique when done properly, requiring the appropriate amount of current for stimulation and the use of electrolyte gel between the skin and the electrodes. Absence of gel may cause a sudden pricking pain due to thermal damage of the external layer of the skin. A localized area of low impedance may be caused by perspiration, emphasizing the need for the gel.

How long does it take for TENS to be effective?

The effective induction time for TENS varies from an instant to several hours with the average time being about 20 minutes. Patients with chronic pain often have a cumulative effect with the extent of pain relief increasing over several weeks. Perseverance is required to obtain maximal benefit and patients need training and encouragement. The amount of post-stimulation relief varies with some patients finding considerable periods of relief. The reasons for these variations are not clear and probably reflect many factors.

Can I use nerve stimulation to decrease pain as often as I want?

The patient should be instructed to use the nerve stimulation device daily for a specified amount of time rather than whenever needed. The longer one uses nerve stimulation, the less effective the treatment seems to be. Several hours per day is probably the maximum amount of time for the use of these devices.

Will electrical stimulation treatment of my unhealed fracture be painful?

No discomfort is felt by patients using electrical stimulation therapy for nonunion of a fracture. Local pain, when present, indicates superficial irritation and should be reported to the surgeon.

CONSENT

Consent should be obtained for any invasive form of electrical stimulation therapy. Consent is generally not obtained when a TENS unit is used.

SELECTED BIBLIOGRAPHY

Geier KA, Hesser K: Electrical bone stimulation for treatment of nonunion. *Orth Nurs* 1985;Mar/Apr:4:2:41.

Gybels J, Kupers R: Central and peripheral electrical stimulation of the nervous system in the treatment of chronic pain. *Acta Neurochir* 1987;Suppl 38:64.

Jensen JE, Etheridge GL, Hazelrigg G: Effectiveness of transcutaneous electrical neural stimulation in the treatment of pain. *Sports Med* 1986;Mar–Apr:3:2:79.

Latham J: Transcutaneous nerve stimulation. *Prof Nurse* 1987;Feb 2:5:133.

Lehmann TR: Efficacy of electroacupuncture and TENS in the rehabilitation of chronic low back pain patients. *Pain* 1986;Sept 26:3:277.

Moore DE, Blacker HM: How effective is TENS for chronic pain? *Am J Nurs* 1983;Aug 83:8:1175.

17

General Anesthesia

JEFFREY SCHWARTZ

General anesthesia refers to a reversible state of unconsciousness and analgesia. In clinical practice the anesthetist not only induces and maintains the anesthetic state but also supports and monitors vital functions such as ventilation and circulation. To this end, the anesthetist is responsible for everything from establishing intravenous access and proper positioning of the patient on the operating table to administering of fluids and blood and transporting the patient to a recovery facility (figure 17–1).

General anesthesia is based on the observation, first made in the mid 1800s, that inhaling certain gases could safely and reversibly produce unconsciousness. The original inhaled anesthetics were ether and chloroform. These were supplanted by various agents over the years because of concerns of toxicity and flammability. Today, in the United States, the most commonly administered inhalation anesthetic is nitrous oxide. More potent gases, such as halothane, enflurane, and isoflurane may be administered, as well. The anesthetist also supplements with intravenous drugs such as narcotics, barbiturates, benzodiazepines, and neuromuscular blocking agents.

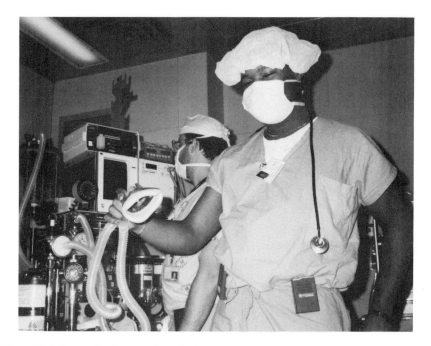

Figure 17–1. Preparation for general anesthesia.

It is curious that though a great deal is known about the pharmacology and effects of these agents, the mechanism of general anesthesia is poorly understood.

INDICATIONS

General anesthesia can be considered for patients of any age, in any state of health, and for any surgical procedure. Certain peripheral procedures with limited invasiveness and blood loss are best done under regional anesthesia, thereby avoiding the risk of general anesthesia. These would include, for example, colonoscopy, endoscopy, cataract removal, small skin or nail excisions, many kinds of biopsies, and many dental and plastic surgery procedures. Any operation of greater invasiveness, that enters a body cavity, that involves significant blood loss or fluid shifts, or that requires immobility or uncomfortable positioning for adequate surgical maneuvers should be especially considered for general anesthesia.

ALTERNATIVES

For certain operations, many patients may be suitable for regional anesthesia or local anesthesia. Issues that enter into the decision as to which method is to be chosen include patient's preference, location and duration of the surgery, general medical condition and position that the patient will be in during the operation. It is up to the anesthetist, in consultation with the surgeon if necessary, to decide which type of anesthesia is best for a particular patient. It must be remembered that regional anesthesia has a small but definite failure rate, therefore an operation that is to be performed under regional anesthesia may require general anesthesia.

It is a misconception that regional anesthesia is inherently less risky than general anesthesia. On the contrary, a patient who has overdosed is probably managed better under general anesthesia in order to protect the patient from aspiration. The patient with poor pulmonary function might do better with a regional anesthetic, but many do better with a general anesthetic because of increased control of the airway, and the ability to suction the trachea. Patients with severe chronic obstructive pulmonary disorder (COPD) or congestive heart failure (CHF) often cannot lie awake and supine for long periods of time. Patients with significant aortic stenosis usually do better with a general anesthetic. The important principle is that all these considerations must be weighed by the anesthetist in formulating the anesthetic plan.

POSSIBILITY OF FAILURE

Very rarely, certain problems may arise after induction of general anesthesia, that is, after the patient is asleep. These include the inability to intubate the trachea, occurrence of abnormal heart rhythms, evidence of myocardial ischemia, and sudden rise in body temperature. The decision may be made that it would be best to postpone the surgery and wake the patient up. After the patient's condition is improved, a decision can be made on how to better prepare him preoperatively and/or to alter the anesthetic technique.

CONTRAINDICATIONS

There are no absolute contraindications to general anesthesia. However there are certain situations in which general anesthesia is relatively contraindicated and regional anesthesia may be preferable. These include a history of asthma (especially if there is active wheezing), recent food ingestion, severe cardiopulmonary compromise as evidenced by poor pulmonary function tests or poor ejection fraction, and anticipated difficulty in maintaining a patient's airway. The risks and benefits of each approach have to be weighed in each particular situation. It must be emphasized that a regional anesthetic may, at any time, have to be converted to a general anesthetic because of either inadequate anesthesia or unanticipated surgical problems.

PREPROCEDURE PREPARATION

Before the surgery, the anesthetist will see the patient in the preoperative interview. At that time he/she will take a history, do a physical examination, and review laboratory data to help decide on the safest anesthetic. Tests such as complete blood count (CBC), blood chemistries, chest roentenogram and electrocardiogram (ECG) may be necessary before the anesthetic. Selected patients may require further evaluation such as pulmonary function tests or echocardiogram. It is common for a medical specialist to be asked to evaluate a patient and optimize the patient's preoperative condition.

In addition, the patient will be told to take nothing by mouth, except medications, after midnight preceding surgery. A premedication may be ordered and the patient may expect a pill or injection before coming to the operating room.

PATIENT EDUCATION

The importance of taking nothing by mouth before the operation is emphasized. All removable dental fixtures should be taken out before patients leave their rooms. They should be assured that they will be asleep for the surgery and that an anesthetist will be in attendance the entire time monitoring their vital functions.

Patients can decrease the incidence and severity of complications by being in the best physical condition possible before the operation. Patients should stop smoking. Even 24 hours of no smoking has been shown to decrease carbon monoxide levels in the blood and improve ciliary clearance. Overweight patients should lose weight. Lung function is inevitably compromised to some degree, and obesity can worsen the dysfunction. Patients on chronic medications should comply with their prescriptions.

PROCEDURE

The sequence of events leading to the induction of general anesthesia is variable and depends on the age of the patient, underlying medical problems, the nature of the surgery, and the preference of the anesthetist.

A healthy adult would typically be given a sedative, either orally or intramuscularly, before transport to the operating room. An intravenous cannula is inserted after local skin infiltration. Routine monitors, such as a blood pressure cuff and ECG leads are applied. The patient is asked to breathe oxygen through a face mask while anesthesia is induced intravenously. Typically, an endotracheal tube is inserted once the patient is asleep but this may not be necessary for short procedures. Anesthesia is maintained with a combination of intravenous and inhalation agents. Vital signs are monitored constantly and the anesthetic effect is carefully titrated. When the surgery is completed the patient is awakened by discontinuation of the anesthetic, the trachea is extubated and the patient brought to the recovery room. The patient remains in the recovery room until all vital signs are stable and the patient is awake and alert.

Certain patients may need arterial or central venous catheters placed before induction of anesthesia. For young children, anesthesia may be induced with drugs administered rectally, intramuscularly, intravenously or by breathing anesthetic gases. Parents are frequently allowed to accompany the child into the operating room.

Certain patients, due either to their poor health or to the extensive nature of their surgery, will require postoperative mechanical ventilation. These patients will be told preoperatively that they will not wake up immediately after the operation but will wake up in an intensive care setting. There will be an endotracheal tube in their throat preventing them from speaking. They will be made comfortable with sedatives and analgesics until their condition is stable enough to warrant extubation.

POSTPROCEDURE INFORMATION

After routine inpatient surgery family members should expect patients to be drowsy for most of the day. They may eat, if there is no surgical ileus, as soon as they are awake and hungry. In the hospital, patients are often given incentive spirometers and encouraged to breath deeply and cough. Outpatient surgery is becoming increasingly common. Once awake and stable, patients are discharged home with a responsible person. If dizziness, pallor, labored breathing, excessive pain or bleeding, fever, inability to void, inability to take liquids, or excessive vomiting develop they should call the hospital immediately. Following anesthesia, a patient should not operate heavy machinery or make important decisions for at least one day.

COMPLICATIONS

Common and self-limiting complications after general anesthesia include hoarseness, sore throat, nausea and vomiting and back pain. Patients with a history of prolonged nausea or vomiting postoperatively can be treated with antiemetics before awakening that will decrease the incidence and severity.

Less common complications include dental injury, peripheral nerve injury, and anaphylactic reactions.

Rare but more serious complications include myocardial infarction, stroke, brain damage, kidney failure, congestive heart failure, aspiration, and pneumonia.

Many times serious morbidity can be avoided or lessened by more invasive monitoring such as a pulmonary artery catheter. Good postoperative care in an appropriate setting is also an important factor in avoiding complications. The most important factor in decreasing morbidity is a careful and thoughtful anesthetic technique.

The mortality after general anesthesia is estimated at $1/10,000$ to $3/10,000$. It is difficult to separate the role of anesthesia from that of surgery, the patient's disease, and the underlying medical condition when reviewing the mortality rates following administration of general anesthesia.

PATIENT QUESTIONS

Will it hurt?

During the surgery itself the patient will be unconscious and not feeling any pain. Before anesthesia is induced, procedures such as inserting an intravenous or intraarterial catheter may briefly cause some pain. This is done under local infiltration and often some sedation. After anesthesia is terminated, the patient may feel incisional pain from the operative site. This will be treated with narcotics in the recovery room.

When will I wake up?

Generally, anesthesia is terminated at the completion of the surgery and the patient awakened shortly thereafter. It is common, however, to have no memory of awakening in the operating room. Certain critically ill patients, after open heart surgery for instance, may be left anesthetized and on a ventilator until their condition stabilizes. These patients can expect to wake up some number of hours to a day after the surgery.

Will I have to breathe gas from a mask?

Many patients have a bad memory of an ether induction by mask from twenty or more years ago. This was an unpleasant experience, associated with much anxiety, nausea, and discomfort. Today, in any patient old enough to accept an intravenous cannula, anesthesia is induced with intravenous drugs. This is very fast and pleasant. Thiapental (Pentothal®) is the prototype drug. It is advisable for patients to breathe oxygen, which is odorless, through a mask before induction.

Do I have to go to sleep for the operation?

Many operations can be done under regional or local anesthesia. The anesthetist will discuss with the patient whether it is possible or advisable to utilize a regional technique.

Will I wake up during the operation?

Awareness during anesthesia is a very rare phenomenon. The anesthetist is constantly alert to signs of light anesthesia such as a rise in blood pressure and pulse rate. If this occurs, the anesthetist will deepen the anesthesia with additional drugs before the patient is conscious.

Will I be nauseated after the operation?

Postoperative nausea and vomiting are very common with an incidence of about 30%. It occurs more frequently in women, obese patients, children and adolescents, and after intraabdominal surgery. It is generally self-limiting and may be treated with antiemetic drugs.

CONSENT

Signed informed consent is obtained before administering general anesthesia. Only in an emergency situation in which the patient is not competent to sign the consent form and no family member can be contacted is the informed consent waived.

SELECTED BIBLIOGRAPHY

Burns K: Postoperative care and review of complications. In Woo SW, ed: *Ambulatory Anesthesia Care.* Boston: Little, Brown & Company, 1982;27–34.

Goldman L, Caldera DL, Nussbaum SR: Multifactorial index of cardiac risk in noncardiac surgical procedures. *N Engl J Med* 1977;297:845.

Harrison GG: Death attributable to anaesthesia. *Br J Anaesth* 1978;50:1041.

Vacanti CJ, VanHouten RJ, Hill RC: A statistical analysis of the relationship of physical status to postoperative mortality in 68,388 cases. *Anesth Analog* 1970;49:564.

18

Postoperative Pain Management: Spinal and Epidural Narcotics and Patient-Controlled Analgesia

JUSTIN McKENDRY AND MATHEW LEFKOWITZ

Pain management is a multidisciplinary specialty involving the primary care physician, anesthesiologist, psychologist, neurologist, and physical therapist. Pain specialists treat acute and chronic pain with analgesics, nerve blocks, psychotherapy, transcutaneous electrical nerve stimulation (TENS), acupuncture, spinal opioids, and patient-controlled analgesia. This chapter will discuss spinal opioids and patient-controlled analgesia.

Narcotics can be injected intrathecally or into the epidural space. Spinally administered opioids act by blocking painful afferent impulses at endogenous opioid receptors in laminae I through V of the dorsal horn of the spinal cord. These endogenous opioid receptors together with descending supraspinal pathways function to modify incoming pain information before it is transmitted to supraspinal levels. The blockade is selective, sparing somatic, sensory, motor, and sympathetic function. The technique avoids the sedation and mood changes of systemically administered narcotics. The most serious complication is delayed respiratory depression.

Patient-controlled analgesia is the use of a patient-controlled intravenous narcotic infusion pump for postoperative pain control. The machine is activated by the patient by means of a hand-held button that is connected to the machine. It infuses a preset amount of narcotic and has determined intervals during which time the machine cannot be activated.

INDICATIONS

Spinal opioids are typically used for postoperative pain relief, cancer pain, chronic pain disorders, and have been reported useful in painful sickle cell crises. Spinal opioids are effective in relieving the pain of thoracic, abdominal, pelvic, and lower extremity surgery. Specifically, spinal opioids relieve the pain of sternotomies, thoracotomies, rib excisions, cholecystectomies, colectomies, nephrectomies, prostatectomies, hysterectomies, caesarean sections, and lower extremity amputations. Most postoperative pain, excluding head and neck surgery, can be effectively controlled by spinal narcotics.

The indication for patient-controlled analgesia is postoperative pain requiring narcotic analgesics. Patient-controlled analgesia may be used also in the home for the terminally ill.

ALTERNATIVES

Pain treated with spinal narcotics can be treated alternatively with intravenous, intramuscular, or oral narcotics. These forms of analgesia, however, result in greater sedation, mood changes, and more variable pain relief than spinal narcotics. The greater sedation and mood changes result from the increased concentration of systemically administered narcotics reaching supraspinal structures. The less predictable pain relief results from the more variable absorption, particularly when the narcotic is administered intramuscularly or orally.

When administered to relieve pain but to avoid sedation, intravenously administered narcotics with patient-controlled analgesia results in a more stable, therapeutic serum drug level than traditionally administered intramuscular narcotics. The more consistent narcotic blood levels result in less pain, less sedation, increased cooperation with physical therapy, improved pulmonary function, and earlier postoperative mobilization. Perhaps the most important aspect of patient-controlled analgesia is that it enables the patient alone to treat the pain himself or herself.

CONTRAINDICATIONS

Absolute contraindications to intrathecal and epidural narcotics include infection at the site of injection, sepsis, bleeding disorders, allergies to injected narcotics, increased intracranial pressure, and inadequate facilities for postoperative monitoring of patient respirations. Sepsis and infection at the site of injection expose the central nervous system to the infectious agent. Bleeding disorders risk epidural and subdural hematomas. Dural puncture with increased intracranial pressure result in brain stem herniation. Spinal opioids without adequate monitoring expose the patient to unnecessary risk of undetected respiratory depression.

Relative contraindications to spinal narcotics are severe cardiac or pulmonary disease, previous laminectomy, and an abnormal neurological examination. Severe cardiac or pulmonary disease results in a smaller margin of safety if respiratory depression should occur. A previous laminectomy distorts the anatomy making epidural and spinal placement more difficult. An abnormal neurological examination may contribute to confusion between previous illness and postoperative analgesia complications.

Patient-controlled analgesia is contraindicated in confused, debilitated patients because of their inability to cooperate. The system cannot be used when intravenous access is unobtainable.

PREPROCEDURE PREPARATION

Communication between the surgeon, anesthesiologist, and nursing staff regarding postoperative patient care must precede the decision to use spinal narcotics. The anesthesiologist examines the patient, obtains a medical history, reviews the pertinent lab data, and explains the risks and benefits of the procedure to the patient. The coagulation profile should be checked and a careful neurological examination, including an evaluation of cerebral spinal fluid pressure, is essential.

PATIENT EDUCATION

Education for patient-controlled analgesia involves a patient-anesthesiologist interview, maintenance of an intravenous line, a nursing staff educated in the system, and a pharmacy that can maintain and fill the pumps. (figure 18–1).

The patient should be informed of the risks and benefits of spinal opioids. The risks include respiratory depression, urinary retention, pruritus, nausea, vomiting, and headache. The necessity of respiratory monitoring via nasal canula attached to an apnea monitor should also be explained to the patient. The patient should be assured that spinal and epidural catheter placement is safe and accompanied by minimal discomfort.

The patient-controlled analgesia device and strategy should be explained to the patient. The patent is taught to use the device prophylactically prior to physical therapy, ambulation, and dressing changes. The patient is taught to minimize the bolus during waking hours to avoid sedation, while maximizing the bolus before sleeping to extend the dosing interval. The patient should aim at avoiding *distressing* pain rather than eliminating all pain.

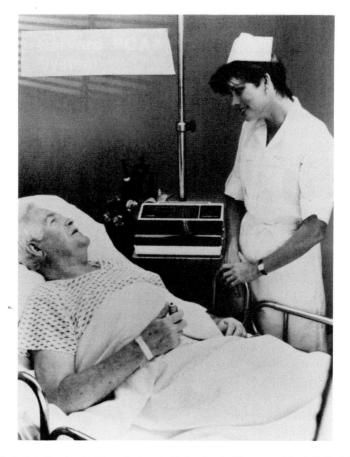

Figure 18–1. Orienting a patient to patient-controlled analgesia (Courtesy of Bard Medical Systems).

PROCEDURE

Intrathecal narcotics are injected into the cerebrospinal fluid (CSF) through a spinal needle in a lumbar space after free flow of CSF has been established. Any lumbar space beneath L2, where the spinal cord usually ends, is chosen for needle placement. The narcotic dose usually accompanies the local anesthetic providing regional anesthesia for the surgery. Intrathecal narcotic results in 12 to 24 hours of analgesia. Repeated doses of intrathecal narcotic require repeated spinal taps.

Epidural catheters can be placed at any level of the spinal cord. The advantage of epidural narcotics over spinal narcotics is that repeated doses can be given through the indwelling epidural catheter. The technique of epidural catheter placement is as follows: the epidural needle attached to a syringe is moved slowly through the supraspinous and interspinous ligaments as well as the ligamentum flavum. A loss of resistance in the syringe plunger occurs when the epidural space has been entered. The syringe is removed and a catheter is threaded through the needle. The needle is then removed. The catheter is checked for CSF or blood return. Placement is checked with a test dose of local anesthetic with epinephrine. The catheter is then taped in place and ready for narcotic injection.

The usual narcotics chosen for either intrathecal or epidural use are morphine or fentanyl. Morphine is a water-soluble narcotic with a 12 to 24 hour duration of action when used by these routes. Its high-water solubility allows its slow passage through the CSF to the respiratory center in the brainstem. This accounts for the uncommon occurrence of respiratory depression. The usual intrathecal dose of morphine is 0.4 to 0.5 mg. The usual epidural dose is 6 to 8 mg.

Fentanyl is a highly lipid soluble, short-acting narcotic with a 4 to 6 hour duration of action when used intrathecally or epidurally. Its lipid solubility results in its rapid movement through the spinal tissue to opiate receptors in the spinal cord. This rapid absorption explains the more localized analgesic effect of fentanyl when compared with morphine. Fentanyl's poor water solubility results in very rare respiratory depression because of limited transport of the narcotic to the respiratory center in the brainstem. The usual epidural dose of fentanyl is 50 to 100 mcg. The usual intrathecal dose is 5 to 10 mcg. The choice between morphine and fentanyl generally depends on the desired duration of action.

The patient-controlled analgesia pump is connected to the patient's intravenous line. A bolus dose is chosen that relives pain but avoids sedation. A typically interval dose might be 1 mg of morphine. This dose is increased by 50% if analgesia is not achieved and decreased by 50% if sedation occurs. A dosing interval is chosen that is just longer than the time to peak effect of the intravenous narcotic analgesic. Typically this would be 5 to 10 minutes for morphine. Adjustments in dose and dosing interval are made on the basis of twice daily interviews with the patient by the anesthesiologist.

POSTPROCEDURE INFORMATION

Patients can receive epidural narcotics for extended periods of time in outpatient settings. These long-term epidural catheters are placed in the usual manner with the end tunneled into a subcutaneously placed narcotic reservoir or pump. The reservoir is refilled by a percutanous injection. The pump rate can be adjusted by a remote control device held over the pump. Patients families can be taught to recognize over-sedation and respiratory depression. These symptoms, however, are exceedingly rare in chronic narcotic administration.

Patient-controlled analgesia can be employed outside the hospital when oral narcotics are unable to control the patient's pain. Intravenous access must be available (figure 18-2). In this situation, the family is also taught to recognize over-sedation and respiratory depression, uncommon complications with chronic narcotic administration.

COMPLICATIONS

Side effects of spinal narcotics are respiratory depression, pruritus, nausea, vomiting, urinary retention, and headaches. Respiratory depression is the most serious and the least common complication. In a series of over 1,000 patients treated with epidural narcotics for postoperative pain relief, approximately 10 experienced depressed respirations. The depressed respirations were gradual in onset, easily detected, and successfully treated with intravenous naloxone without pain breakthrough.

Pruritus occurs in approximately 11% of patients receiving spinal opioids. The pruritus is treated with intravenous naloxone without pain breakthrough. Nausea, vomiting, and urinery retention occur with equal frequency following spinal or intramuscular narcotics. The nausea and vomiting can be treated with prochlorperazine as well as naloxone. The urinary retention is relieved with a Foley catheter. Headaches usually occur from inadvertent dural puncture during epidural catheter placement. They are treated with bedrest, hydration, and analgesics.

Patient-controlled analgesia morbidity is secondary to the narcotic administered. Urine retention, nausea and vomiting, tolerance to prolonged narcotic administration, and respiratory depression have all been reported. Respiratory depression is rare when the lock out interval is longer than the time to peak action of the narcotic.

PATIENT QUESTIONS

Will the epidural catheter injure my spinal cord?

Epidural catheters are not in contact with the spinal cord. Autopsies performed on cancer patients who had received long-term epidural narcotics showed no pathological changes in the cord or the dura from the catheter or administered drug.

Will I be able to lie on my back or walk with the epidural?

Epidural catheters are made of flexible plastic that allows complete freedom of movement. After the catheter has been properly secured with benzoin and tape,

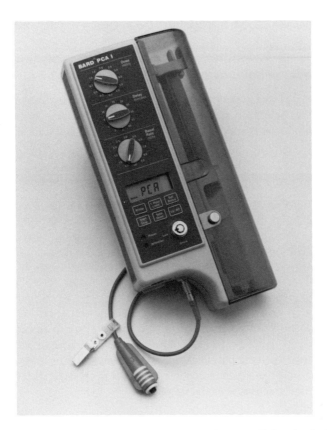

Figure 18–2. Portable pump mechanism for intravenous patient-controlled analgesia (Courtesy of Bard Medical Systems).

the patient can move about in the bed, the chair, or on the floor without catheter's kinking or dislodging. Because of the catheter's narrow diameter, the patient can lie on his or her back without discomfort. The patient who has a subcutaneously placed catheter and pump may also engage in normal daily activities including showering or bathing without damage to the catheter. More vigorous athletic activity, which is rarely possible for these terminally ill patients, will probably not dislodge the catheter.

Is this experimental? Why haven't I heard of it?

Epidural and spinal narcotics have been used for more than 10 years with proven efficacy and safety. Most anesthesia departments now offer epidural and spinal narcotics for postoperative pain. Because all anesthesiologists now in training learn the techniques of pain management, the frequency of these procedures will increase.

How long will the epidural catheter remain in place?

Subcutaneously placed catheters for chronic pain have remained in place for months. The catheters do not need to be replaced as long as they function properly. Epidural catheters for postoperative pain are usually left in place for 2 to 3 days.

Will patient-controlled analgesia relieve all of my pain?

Patient-controlled analgesia results in more complete pain relief than the traditional intramuscular or intravenous injection of narcotic. The pain relief is not 100%. Narcotics are best at relieving dull, aching visceral pain. Discomfort from nasogastric (stomach) tubes and Foley urinary catheters, transmitted by somatic pain fibers, may persist.

Will I become addicted to narcotics?

Short term, post-operative use of narcotics does not result in addiction. Studies show that patients using the patient-controlled analgesia actually use fewer narcotics than those receiving physician-ordered intramuscular or intravenous injections. A more stable analgesic narcotic blood level is obtained with the frequent, small-dose, patient-activated analgesic pumps.

How long will I use the pump?

Patient-controlled analgesia for postoperative pain is discontinued when the patient would normally be switched to an oral analgesic. The oral analgesic may be a narcotic or a nonsteroidal depending on the severity of pain. Patient-controlled analgesia for chronic cancer pain may be used as long as intravenous access is available and the patient is able to manage the process.

Consent

Informed consent is required for epidural and intrathecal narcotics, as well as for patient-controlled analgesia.

SELECTED BIBLIOGRAPHY

Behar, M. et al: Epidural Morphine in Treatment of Pain. *Lancet* 1979;1:527–529

Bennet R, Griffen W: Patient-controlled Analgesia. *Contemp Surg* 1983; April: Vol 23: 27–33.

Cousins MJ, Mather LE: Intrathecal and epidural administration of opioids. *Anesthesiol* 1984;6:276.

Graves D et al: Patient-controlled analgesia. *Ann Intern Med* 1983;99:360–366.

Slater E: Experience with epidural morphine for postsurgical pain in a community setting. *Anesthesiol Re* 1985;May/June:12:3:37.

White, P: Patient-controlled analgesia: a new approach to the management of postoperative pain. *Semin Anesth* 1985; Vol IV:3:255–266.

Yaksh, T: Spinal opiate analgesia: characteristics and principles of action. *Pain* 1981;11:293–346.

19

Regional Anesthesia

HOWELL R. GOLDFARB AND JOEL MANN YARMUSH

Regional anesthesia enables surgery to be performed without the loss of consciousness. It began about 40 years after general anesthesia with the introduction of local anesthetics that could be used to reduce or eliminate multiple sensations, including pain, in a discrete part of the body. This can affect an area as small as a patch of skin during a local anesthetic or as large as the area from the chest to the toes during a spinal anesthetic. Local anesthetics are injected near the appropriate nerves that block conduction of sensory, motor, and autonomic impulses. The type of impulses and in what proportion they are blocked depends on several factors that include the specific drug used (e.g., lidocaine versus bupivacaine), the amount used (i.e., concentration and volume), and the local conditions at the injection site.

INDICATIONS

The need for pain relief during surgical manipulation is an indication for anesthesia. While regional anesthesia may be preferred in some situations, there is no absolute indication for regional anesthesia as opposed to general anesthesia.

However, there are a number of relative indications. These include patient and physician preference, and certain operative procedures (i.e., transurethral prostatectomies, hip surgery).

Patients often prefer regional anesthesia because there is usually little postanesthetic nausea and vomiting. It is favored in the patient who dislikes lack of control associated with losing consciousness under general anesthesia. It is also chosen because of potential excellent postoperative pain relief. Physicians often prefer regional anesthesia because some operative procedures can be easily performed in the office under local infiltration.

Complications in certain procedures can be minimized using regional anesthesia. In a transurethral prostatectomy, hyponatremia and bladder perforation can be discovered and dealt with earlier in the awake patient. In hip surgery, blood loss and thromboembolic phenomena can be decreased using regional anesthesia.

In the elderly, regional anesthesia has been shown to lessen or prevent postanesthetic confusion. In obstetrical patients, regional anesthesia allows early mother-child bonding and obviates the risks of using general anesthesia in the parturient. In asthmatics, regional anesthesia avoids manipulation of the airway, which can initiate an attack.

Regional anesthesia leaves the airway reflexes intact thereby reducing the chance of vomiting and aspiration in the patient with a full stomach. It also reduces the chance of potential catastrophic complications in the patient with a difficult airway.

ALTERNATIVES

Although general anesthesia is not practical for minor procedures (i.e., superficial laceration repair, splinter removal, and so on), it is always an acceptable alternative to regional anesthesia. Also, different types of regional anesthesia can be utilized for the same surgical procedure. For example, anesthesia for an uncomplicated inguinal hernia repair in an otherwise healthy young man can proceed using local (infiltrative), major regional (spinal or epidural), general, or even a combination of local and "light" general anesthesia.

Local anesthesia is easy to administer and offers good, but short, postoperative pain relief. Normal activities usually resume soon after the operation.

Major regional anesthesia requires more technical expertise and experience, and can offer excellent postoperative pain relief. The patient can usually resume normal activities several hours after the operation.

General anesthesia requires technical expertise and offers variable postoperative pain relief. It may be necessary in the event of unsuccessful regional anesthesia. Normal activities resume at variable times depending on patient response to the anesthesia.

Combination local and light general anesthetic requires technical expertise and can offer good postoperative pain relief. Normal activities can resume soon after surgery.

All four alternatives discussed above offer acceptable anesthesia. The choice will depend upon the preferences of the surgeon and anesthesiologist after discussion with the patient.

POSSIBILITY OF FAILURE

While regional anesthesia is usually successful and a good experience for all, there are times when it will be unsuccessful. The reasons include technical difficulty, anatomic variability, and patient discomfort. Some regional anesthetics are technically difficult and often carry a significant failure rate. This is the case with an axillary block used to anesthetize the brachial plexus. After positioning and preparation, a needle is inserted into the axilla in search of the brachial plexus. Proper placement is usually confirmed by parasthesias, arterial puncture, or muscle stimulation. Despite deemingly correct needle placement the incidence of an unsuccessful or partially successful block can be as high as 5% to 10% depending on the skills of the anesthesiologist.

Regional anesthetics can fail because of anatomic variability. An epidural block may be very difficult in the elderly patient with osteosclerosis or the young patient with scoliosis. The incidence of failure of a caudal block may be as high as 5% to 15%. Anatomic reasons are commonly thought to be the cause of failure.

Patient discomfort can also be a cause of regional anesthetic failure. This is true even if the block is technically successful and anesthesia adequate for the procedure. It is usually seen in an ill-prepared patient who becomes overly anxious and uncooperative. For example, under regional anesthesia, a patient may still experience nonpainful pressure sensations. These may be unpleasant if not anticipated. Other bothersome possibilities are the operating room noises (such as drills) or even a backache from lying in one position for an extended period of time.

When regional anesthesia is not successful there are several alternatives. An unsuccessful ankle block can be repeated. A partially successfully axillary block can be supplemented by distally blocking the particular nerve that was missed. A failed epidural block can often be converted to a spinal block. An anxious patient anesthetized with regional anesthesia can be accommodated with anxiolytics, allaying fears, and decreasing awareness.

Since general anesthesia is always an alternative to unsuccessful regional anesthesia in the operating room setting, all patients receiving regional anesthesia need also be prepared for general anesthesia.

CONTRAINDICATIONS

Absolute contraindications include patient refusal and skin infection at the site of injection. Most contraindications for regional anesthesia are relative, and only discussion with the patient, surgeon, and anesthesiologist about the risks and benefits can determine if regional anesthesia should proceed. Relative contraindications are (1) lack of technical skill of the anesthesiologist, (2) previous allergy to local anesthetic, (3) septicemia, (4) uncooperative patient, (5) neurologic disease (increased intracranial pressure, spinal cord pathology, multiple sclerosis, or peripheral nerve disease), (6) hypovolemia, and (7) bleeding tendencies.

PREPROCEDURE PREPARATION

The patient is prepared for surgery in the usual manner (i.e., shave, prep, lab tests). Nothing can be taken by mouth (other than ordered medications with a sip of water) after midnight on the night prior to surgery. An anesthesiologist will make a preoperative visit and take a history and physical examination. He or she will describe what will occur before, during, and after the operation.

PATIENT EDUCATION

The patient should know that the procedure itself may involve minor discomfort. To position a needle for some peripheral blocks the involved nerves need to be contacted. This will cause parasthesias in the nerves' distribution, which will confirm proper needle placement. The patient is encouraged to remain still despite these possibly unpleasant sensations. The paresthesias cease after injection of local anesthetics near the nerves, further confirming a successful block.

The patient should also know that other nonpainful sensations such as pressure may remain intact. It is hoped that the patient will then be less likely to become anxious and misinterpret these sensation as incomplete anesthesia. Anxiolytics can be given as needed.

PROCEDURE

After arrival in the operating room waiting area, an intravenous catheter is placed. The patient is then brought into the operating room where appropriate monitoring equipment (i.e., ECG, blood pressure cuff, pulse oximeter) is applied. The patient is positioned accordingly and the involved area is sterilely cleaned and prepped. A small (25 to 26 gauge) needle is used to anesthetize the skin and subcutaneous tissue with local anesthetic. A larger gauge needle is then introduced through the anesthetized area. After proper needle placement, more local anesthetic is injected blocking the involved nerves (figure 19-1). The type and amount of local anesthetic used will not be discussed here as it is beyond the scope of this chapter.

There are numerous regional nerve blocks. Some of the more common ones are spinal, epidural, axillary, retrobulbar, and ilioiguinal nerve blocks.

Spinal anesthesia is usually performed in the lateral decubitus or sitting position. A long, 22 or 25 gauge spinal needle is introduced at the L3–L4 or L4–L5 intervertebral space well below the level (L1–L2) of the spinal cord in adults. Proper placement in the subarachnoid space is usually readily achieved and confirmed with free flow of cerebrospinal fluid.

Epidural anesthesia is performed by introducing a large, blunt (16- or 17-gauge) needle into the epidural space. This is a potential space immediately outside the dura mater and subarachnoid space. It is usually performed in the lateral decubitus or sitting position at the same vertebral level as the spinal block. Other vertebral levels (i.e., cervical, thoracic, and sacral) can also be used. The epidural needle is slowly advanced until loss of resistance is encountered. This signals entrance into the epidural space. A flexible catheter is passed through the needle and secured in the epidural space. After removal of the needle, injection of local anesthetics is possible for as long and as often as an epidural block is needed.

An axillary block is performed with the patient in the supine position. The arm is abducted, the elbow flexed 90°, and the axillary artery is palpated. A blunt, 22-gauge needle is introduced into the axilla until proper placement is assured. This may be achieved using one of several techniques (i.e., paresthesias, arterial puncture, muscle stimulation) depending on the expertise and preference of the anesthesiologist. Local anesthetic is then injected into the axillary sheath that surrounds the brachial pluxus.

A retrobulbar block is the most common block for cataract extraction. It is performed in the supine position with the patient keeping still and looking upward and inward. As injection underneath and behind the eye can be a somewhat frightening experience, continued reassurance is necessary.

Regional anesthesia is very common for inguinal hernia repair. A nerve block is usually performed by the surgeon. It involves infiltration of the skin and subcutaneous tissue with local anesthetic followed by injection near the ilioiguinal and iliohypogastric nerves. As the operation progresses more local anesthetic can be given by the surgeon as needed.

POSTPROCEDURE INFORMATION

In the postoperative period the patient may have somewhat decreased sensations in the previously anesthetized area. During this time, motor function may also be diminished. This should resolve completely once the local anesthetics have

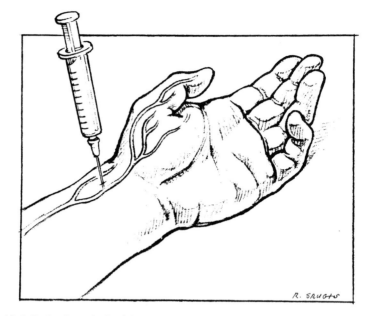

Figure 19–1. Regional anesthesia of the radial nerve.

worn off. Pain management therapy can then be initiated and normal activities resumed.

Any persistent difficulties (e.g., headaches, muscle spasms, tingling) should be related to the involved physician for recommendations on appropriate management.

COMPLICATIONS

Regional anesthesia is thought to have the same overall mortality as general anesthesia. However, in certain cases, studies have shown that morbidity might be decreased. For example, regional anesthesia for hip surgery in the elderly decreases morbidity including that from thromboembolic events or postoperative confusion.

The incidence of complications in regional anesthesia is dependent on the skills and experience of the anesthesiologist. Most of the complications are easily treated. They include hypotension from spinal or epidural block, infection, nausea and vomiting, backache, postdural puncture headache, intravascular injection, hematoma, and nerve damage.

Hypotension with major regional block is usually secondary to decreased peripheral vascular resistance from sympathetic blockade. Hydration and, occasionally, vasoconstricters are used to prevent or minimize this hypotension.

Infection is very rare in regional anesthesia utilizing standard sterile technique and is contraindicated if an infected site exists.

Nausea and vomiting are thought to occur less often with regional anesthesia than with general anesthesia. The incidence is unknown. It can also be an early sign of hypotension and is relieved with correction of the hypotension. In all cases, antiemetics can be given as needed.

Backache in regional anesthesia is no more prevalent than in general anesthesia. This lends credence to the assumption that the majority of postoperative backaches are due to the position of the patent and length of the procedure. The incidence of postoperative backaches is as high as 15%. They are usually transient.

One of the most annoying complications of major regional anesthesia is the postdural puncture headache. It is caused by cerebrospinal fluid leakage through the dura mater and its incidence varies inversely with the age of the patient and gauge of the needle used. In obstetrical populations recent studies have shown an incidence as high as 25%. The headache is postural: often severe when standing and relieved when supine. Although the headache can be quite distressing, it usually resolves in a couple of days. Conservative treatment includes hydration, bed rest, and analgesics. For more severe headaches, an autologous epidural blood patch can be used, which usually provides good relief.

Intravascular injection can be minimized by frequent aspiration. Complications associated with intravascular injection include central nervous system (CNS) toxicity and cardiovascular instability.

Hematomas are usually of little consequence but can be catastrophic if they occur in the subarachnoid or epidural spaces. Their incidence can be reduced by avoiding, when possible, major regional anesthesia in those patients on anticoagulative therapy or those with bleeding problems. Bleeding times can be performed on those patients taking aspirin or other drugs affecting platelet function.

Peripheral nerve trauma is seen most frequently in techniques where parasthesias are sought. The incidence can be as high as 3%. The injury is transient and usually does not last for more than several weeks or in the most severe cases, months.

PATIENT QUESTIONS

Will I experience pain?

Patients may experience some pain or discomfort during the anesthetic procedure as explained above. This should be minimal and, if expected, not very bothersome. During the operation itself patients should not experience pain but may have other sensations such as pressure. Again, if expected, this should not be bothersome. If pain is not completely abolished the regional anesthetic can be repeated, supplemented, or converted to general anesthesia.

Will I be awake or remember the operation?

Following regional anesthesia, level of consciousness varies with the status of the patient and the nature of the operation. During, and consequently after, a transurethral prostatectomy, patients are kept awake so that CNS function can be readily assessed. In other operations, patients may prefer to be heavily sedated with no recall of operating room events. Thus, the anesthesiologist will control the level of awareness taking into consideration the patient's needs and wishes.

Will I be paralyzed by either spinal or epidural anesthesia?

Extensive studies have been completed that have shown no episodes of paralysis with major regional anesthesia. This indicates that the incidence of paralysis is extremely small. Neurological deficits are usually the result of hematomas that can be minimized by avoiding the use of this technique on patients who are taking anticoagulants or who have bleeding problems.

Why shouldn't I use general anesthesia and be asleep during the procedure?

Regional anesthesia is the preferred anesthetic in certain situations, especially during minor surgical procedures that are performed in the physician's office. General anesthesia does have a risk of morbidity and mortality and should be reserved for situations in which regional anesthesia is impractical or cannot be performed.

CONSENT

The patient should sign a written consent for surgery and anesthesia. They need not be separate forms. Consent should indicate an awareness of the anesthetic procedure, alternatives, restrictions (if any), and side effects. This should be further confirmed in the anesthesiologists preoperative note.

SELECTED BIBLIOGRAPHY

Chung F, Meier R: General or spinal anesthesia: which is better in the elderly? *Anesth* 1987;67:422.

Harrison RT, Roberts MT, Thadaka R: Prospective, multi-centre trial of mortality following general or spinal anesthesia for hip fracture surgery in the elderly. *Brit J Anaesth* 1987;59:1080.

Job CA, Fernandez MA: Inguinal hernia repair: comparison of local, epidural and general anesthesia. *N Y S J Med* 1979;79:1730.

Modig J. Borg T: Thromboembolism after total hip replacement: role of epidural and general anesthesia. *Anesth Analg* 1983;62:174.

Phillip BK: Supplemental medication for ambulatory procedures under regional anesthesia. *Anesth Analges* 1977;32:63.

IV
Pulmonary and Chest Cavity Procedures

20

Bronchoscopy

P. SMITH AND R. SADOVSKY

Bronchoscopy or direct visualization of the tracheobronchial tree may be performed with the fiberoptic (flexible) bronchoscope or the rigid bronchoscope. Rigid bronchoscopy was introduced around the turn of the century by Killian and was modified by Jackson to the basic design that remains in use today. The standard Jackson bronchoscope is a hollow tube 40 cm long with a 7 mm lumen. A light carrier provides illumination at the distal end. There are a variety of lenses for magnification and right angle-viewing and retroverted telescopes for visualization of upper-lobe lesions.

In 1967, the flexible fiberoptic bronchoscope developed by Ikeda became commercially available. Because of its ease of insertion, better acceptance by patients, and smaller diameter permitting visualization of more distal bronchi, the flexible scope has supplanted the rigid bronchoscope for most clinical purposes. Fiberoptic bronchoscopes most frequently used today are 5 mm or less in diameter. They are composed of thin glass fibers that transmit light. Within the scope one bundle of fibers transmits illumination from an external light source and another bundle transmits the image back to the operator. There is a channel for suction and the passage of biopsy instruments. Angulation of the distal tip of the scope is controlled by a lever at the operator's end allowing the scope to be directed into the various bronchial orifices. Still photography can be performed, and the scopes can be fitted with a video camera to permit viewing on a monitor and recording on video tape.

INDICATIONS

The most frequent diagnostic indications for fiberoptic bronchoscopy are (1) suspicion of lung cancer, (2) diagnosis of diffuse lung disease, (3) diagnosis of pneumonia in the immunocompromised host, and (4) hemoptysis.

Bronchogenic carcinoma might be suspected because of radiographic abnormalities showing a mass or nodule, hilar or mediastinal adenopathy, atelectasis, or unresolved pneumonia. Symptoms and signs such as chronic cough, hemoptysis, localized wheezing, or recurrent laryngeal nerve paralysis may also be due to lung cancer and indicate the need for bronchoscopy.

The fiberoptic bronchoscope permits examination of the airways to the subsegmental level. Areas appearing abnormal are sampled by brushing and biopsy. Brushes are introduced within a plastic sheath through the suction channel of the scope. Samples obtained are smeared on microscope slides and fixed and stained for cytologic examination. Secretions aspirated through the bronchoscope and washings of the abnormal areas using normal saline are also submitted for cytology. A variety of biopsy forceps provide small (up to several mm) but satisfactory specimens for histological examination. The diagnostic yield on biopsy of carcinomas visible within the tracheobronchial tree is greater than 90%.

Lesions that are too peripheral to be directly visualized with the bronchoscope can still be brushed or biopsied using fluoroscopy to guide the sampling instrument. Using a combination of techniques (transbronchial brushing and biopsy) diagnostic yields of 60% to 75% have been reported for peripheral cancers.

Bronchoscopy is also an important tool for staging bronchogenic carcinoma and determining resectability. In general, tumors extending to within 2 cm of the main carina are not resectable. In addition, mediastinal lymph nodes may be aspirated for cytological examination using a needle within a plastic sheath (transbronchial needle). The main carina, trachea, or mainstream bronchus is pierced with the needle, which then samples the subjacent nodes in these regions. Metastatic involvement in subcarinal nodes or nodes contralateral to the primary lesion preclude surgical resection.

In the diagnosis of diffuse lung disease, fiberoptic bronchoscopy with transbronchial lung biopsy provides good diagnostic yields in some conditions. Sarcoidosis, for example, even with only hilar and mediastinal adenopathy and no radiographically apparent lung involvement can be diagnosed by transbron-

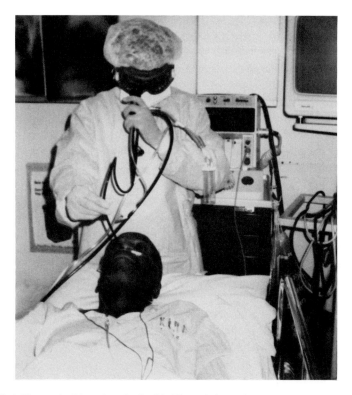

Figure 20–1. Nasotracheal insertion of a flexible fiberoptic bronschoscope.

chial biopsy in up to 60% of cases. The yield is 90% or greater when pulmonary parenchymal involvement is seen on chest roentgenogram.

Bronchoalveolar lavage is a technique that has increased the diagnostic capabilities of the fiberoptic bronchoscope in diffuse pulmonary disease. Lavage is performed by wedging the scope in a subsegmental orifice and sequentially instilling and aspirating 20 to 50 cc aliquots of normal saline. The recovered fluid can be analyzed in a variety of ways. Cytological studies and smears and cultures for microorganisms are routinely done. Special stains, or the use of electron microscopy, may allow diagnosis of such entities as pulmonary hemorrhage, alveolar proteinosis, and histiocytosis-X.

Research applications of bronchoalveolar lavage have added significantly to understanding the pathogenesis of some diffuse lung diseases such as sarcoidosis and idiopathic pulmonary fibrosis. More recently, bronchoalveolar lavage has provided important insights into the routine of airway inflammation in the pathogenesis of asthma.

In immunosuppressed patients, transbronchial biopsy and bronchoalveolar lavage have proven extremely valuable for diagnosing opportunistic pulmonary infections. *Pneumocystis carinii* pneumonia in patients with the acquired immunodeficiency syndrome can be diagnosed by lavage alone in more than 90% of cases. Growing experience with this technique suggests that other opportunistic pulmonary infections such as those caused by cytomegalovirus, cryptococcus, and mycobacteria may be accurately diagnosed as well.

Bacterial cultures of aspirated secretions, washings, and lavage may not accurately identify lower respiratory flora and, therefore, miss the true cause of a bacterial pneumonia. This is because the bronchoscope and suction channel are contaminated with bacteria from the nose, mouth, and pharynx during the passage of the scope. However, using a special microbiologic brush system, accurate cultures of the lower respiratory flora are possible. The brush is enclosed in a double-sheathed plastic catheter, sealed at the distal end with a plug that dissolves when extruded into the airway. The brush is extended in to the desired area to obtain a culture.

In the evaluation of hemoptysis, bronchoscopy has two major purposes: localization of the site of bleeding and diagnosis of the underlying condition. Localization of bleeding is crucial should surgical resection be required for hemorrhage that increases and becomes life-threatening. Bronchoscopy is also helpful to identify the site of bleeding prior to bronchial artery embolization, an alternative approach for control of massive hemoptysis.

Therapeutic fiberoptic bronchoscopy is indicated in three major situations: (1) endobronchial suctioning to relieve atelectasis, (2) foreign-body removal, and (3) laser therapy. In acute collapse of a pulmonary segment, lobe, or an entire lung, bronchoscopy with vigorous suctioning and instillation of aliquots of saline can improve removal of retained or inspissated secretions when a trial of vigorous bronchial hygiene fails. The latter should always be attempted before resorting to bronchoscopy and should include suctioning, chest percussion, bronchodilators, and encouragement to cough.

Foreign-body removal may be done with the fiberoptic bronchoscope using a variety of grasping forceps and baskets. Usually, endotracheal intubation is indicated to prevent unintentional release of the object during passage through the glottis or loss in the pharynx or nose as the scope, grasping instrument, and foreign body are withdrawn.

Laser therapy via the fiberoptic bronchoscope has been shown effective in relieving obstructions in the trachea and main bronchi due to tumor. In general, laser therapy has been reserved for patients in whom radiation and surgical therapy have failed or are not appropriate. Excellent short-term results have been reported with relief of symptoms and improvement in function. Lasers have also been used successfully for control of bleeding from endobronchial tumors. Most procedures are now done using the Neodymium:YAG laser. Obstructions due to benign processes such as granulation tissue causing tracheal stenosis are also amenable to laser therapy. In addition, experience is accumulating in the use of lasers to treat more distal obstructions (in lobar or segmental bronchi) and to treat early malignant lesions.

Rigid Bronchoscopy

The use of rigid bronchoscopy had declined with the advent of fiberoptic bronchoscopy. There are, however, several circumstances where the rigid scope is indicated. Foreign-body removal is often more easily done through the rigid scope. Extensive bleeding or copious bronchial secretions also require the rigid bronchoscope and its greater capacity for suction. Similarly, it is indicated in patients with large pyogenic abscesses, since manipulation may lead to flooding the airways with purulent material. Finally, the rigid scope is preferred by some for laser therapy because of better control of bleeding and removal of necrotic tumor debris.

ALTERNATIVES

Alternatives to fiberoptic bronchoscopy for diagnostic purposes include transthoracic fine-needle aspiration and open lung biopsy. Fine-needle aspiration is performed with fluoroscopic of CT guidance and can provide material for cytological and microbiological studies. The diagnostic yields are high for solitary or multiple malignant lung nodules. Hilar or mediastinal masses and diffuse lung infiltrates may also be diagnosed by fine-needle aspiration. Pneumothorax and hemoptysis are the possible complications of this procedure. Candidates for fine-needle aspiration in preference to bronchoscopy would include some patients with coronary artery disease since bronchoscopy is more likely to result in increased myocardial work and ischemia. It may also be preferred in patients with peripheral or pleural-based lesions that are easily sampled with this technique.

Open lung biopsy is an appropriate alternative to bronchoscopy in the immunocompromised patient with respiratory failure and suspected opportunistic infection who is either too unstable to permit bronchoalveolar lavage or in whom the need to rapidly establish a diagnosis warrants an open biopsy with its higher diagnostic yield. Open lung biopsy is also indicated in patients with uncorrectable coagulopathies to provide adequate hemostasis.

POSSIBILITY OF FAILURE

Bronchoscopy, like all diagnostic procedures, may occasionally fail to provide adequate diagnostic information. The frequency of false negative results depends on several factors, including the type of pathology, the operator's experience, and the patient's cooperation. For example, peripheral lung nodules that are small (especially when less than 1 cm) are often difficult to biopsy using transbronchial biopsy guided by fluoroscopy. Transthoracic needle aspiration may be more appropriate in some of these cases. Transbronchial lung biopsy may also fail with certain diffuse lung diseases where the pathology will not be adequately reflected by the small biopsies that are obtained. A good example is idiopathic pulmonary fibrosis (IPF). When the results of transbronchial biopsy are nondiagnostic and IPF is being considered, open lung biopsy should be done.

Bronchoscopy may also fail when the patient will not, or cannot, cooperate fully to allow an adequate examination. This may occur during bronchoscopies done under topical anesthesia with patients who are very anxious or very ill and unable to tolerate the procedure for a long enough time to obtain adequate specimens.

CONTRAINDICATIONS

There are few absolute contraindications to fiberoptic bronchoscopy. These include (1) lack of patient consent, (2) inadequately trained personnel to perform the procedure, and (3) inadequate facilities or experience to manage the potential complications. Relative contraindications include recent myocardial infarction or unstable angina, serious cardiac arrhythmia, unstable asthma, and respiratory failure with hypercapnia or severe hypoxemia. Uncorrected coagulation defects and platelet dysfunction associated with renal failure militates against biopsy.

PREPROCEDURE PREPARATION

Patients should be screened for any problems that might be contraindications to bronchoscopy. The usual preprocedure workup includes complete blood count, platelet count, coagulation profile, SMA-6, chest roentgenogram, arterial blood gases, and eletrocardiogram.

Optimally, patients should take nothing by mouth for 6 to 8 hours prior to the procedure and should avoid smoking for as long as possible.

Premedication frequently consists of intramuscular injections of an anticholinergic agent and a narcotic and/or sedative 30 to 60 minutes before the procedure. An intravenous line is started to allow additional sedative medications to be given and for emergency drug administration.

PATIENT EDUCATION

The patient should understand the procedure and be reassured that breathing will not be impaired during bronchoscopy. If a biopsy is being considered, the patient should be aware of this possibility and the additional risks. Someone should accompany the patient if the procedure is being performed on an ambulatory basis.

PROCEDURE

Fiberoptic bronchoscopy may be done in the operating room, specially designed endoscopy suites, or at the bedside. In stable patients, fiberoptic bronchoscopy may be performed on an ambulatory basis. Several hours of observation are required after the procedure to identify any untoward reactions and to allow sedative and narcotic medications to wear off before the patient is sent home. The fiberoptic scope is usually inserted via the nose but can also be passed orally or via an endotracheal tube or tracheostomy.

Topical anesthesia is applied to the pharynx by gargling or via a spray or nebulizer. For transnasal passage of the fiberoptic bronchoscope, an anesthetic lubricant such as viscous lidocaine is instilled into the nostril. Oxygen is administered via nasal cannula or mask, and electrocardiographic leads are placed for continuous monitoring. After passage of the scope to the level of the hypopharynx, additional anesthetic is sprayed under direct visualization on the larynx and vocal cords through the suction channel. When the cords are adequately anesthetized, the scope is passed through the glottis and into the trachea. The trachea, main stem bronchi, and more distal airways are anesthetized as needed to minimize coughing.

The tracheobronchial tree is examined in a sequential manner, usually beginning on the side contralateral to the known or suspected pathology. After inspection, bronchoalveolar lavage, brushings, biopsies, and washings are done as indicated.

Rigid bronchoscopy is considerably more uncomfortable and frequently requires general anesthesia. The rigid scope is introduced transorally, and the procedure is generally performed in the operating room.

POSTPROCEDURE INFORMATION

After bronchoscopy, the patient should remain in bed and have frequent monitoring of vital signs over the next three hours. The intravenous line is maintained, and nothing is given by mouth during this period. Blood-streaked sputum and minor degrees of hemoptysis are frequent after biopsy. Greater degrees of bleeding require investigation.

Patients with significant hypoxemia (PaO_2 less than 60 mm Hg breathing room air) should receive supplemental oxygen and monitoring with arterial blood gases or oximetry. Oxygen is often given routinely for several hours after bronchoalveolar lavage since hypoxemia is frequent after this procedure. Those undergoing transbronchial biopsy should have a chest radiograph to rule out pneumothorax.

The patient should be reassured concerning sore throat, hoarseness, or loss of voice that are temporary and usually last less than 24 hours. Lozenges or a soothing gargle can be used to ease discomfort when the gag reflex returns (usually with 2 hours of the completion of the procedure). Fever may occur following bronchoscopy, but it is almost always transient and usually not clinically important.

Coughing often persists for at least several hours after bronchoscopy but usually requires no specific treatment. Postprocedure sputum specimens are collected for cytological examination and appropriate cultures as indicated by the particular clinical situation.

COMPLICATIONS

In experienced hands, fiberoptic bronchoscopy is well tolerated, and major complications are unusual. Even in critically ill patients, for example, those with respiratory failure due to opportunistic pulmonary infections, fiberoptic bronchoscopy may be safely done with appropriate preparation and monitoring. Moreover, diagnostic information may be provided that would otherwise be obtained only by more invasive procedures such as open lung biopsy.

Complications may be caused by premedication, topical anesthesia, general anesthesia (if used), bronchoscopy itself, or the biopsy and brushing procedure. Premedication and topical anesthesia are the causes of at least half of the reported complications. Since some patients are comfortable with minimal or no preoperative sedative or narcotic agents, the doses of such drugs should be based on an individual patient's needs and underlying medical conditions. Complications related to topical anesthesia include laryngospasm, bronchospasm, and seizures. Significant absorption of these agents occurs via transbronchial mucosa. Lidocaine is probably the most frequently used, and is well tolerated with a low risk of toxicity.

Potential complications of the bronchoscopic procedure itself include laryngospasm, bronchospasm, hypoxemia, cardiac arrhythmias, cardiac ischemia, myocardial infarction, and cardiac arrest. Hypoxemia and sympathetic stimulation due to manipulation at the level of the larynx and in the tracheobronchial tree are key factors that may precipitate adverse cardiac events in patients with ischemic heart disease.

The overall morbidity from fiberoptic bronchoscopy has been estimated to be .08% to .15%. The mortality rate is .02% to .04%. With the addition of transbronchial biopsy, the rates are 2% and 0.2%, respectively.

Fever is not unusual following bronchoscopy and has been reported in up to 16% of patients. It is usually transient and requires no specific treatment. Pneumonia and bacteremia are rare occurrences.

Biopsy and brush procedures may result in bleeding. Significant bleeding (greater than 50 cc) has been reported in up to 4% of patients undergoing transbronchial biopsy. The risk is greater in some patients, particularly in the presence of uremia or immunosuppression. Pneumothorax occurs in approximately 5% of patients undergoing transbronchial biopsy and necessitates a chest tube in about half of these.

Laser therapy has its own set of complications in addition to those encountered with bronchoscopy alone. Many patients requiring laser treatment are at increased risk because they are seriously ill with advanced malignancies. Most reported major complications are caused by cardiovascular decompensation. Massive bleeding may occur when treating tumors that are in proximity to major vessels or invade vascular structures. Other potential complications are penetration of the tracheal wall and fires due to ignition of the fiberoptic scope of endotracheal tube.

PATIENT QUESTIONS

Will the procedure hurt?

Rigid bronchoscopy is quite uncomfortable and is usually done under general anesthesia. Flexible bronchoscopy, on the other hand, is only mildly uncomfortable. Cough is the main discomfort in most patients. It is usually controllable with adequate topical anesthesia, Narcotic and sedative medications given before or during the procedure also help relieve discomfort and reduce anxiety.

The tracheobronchial tree and pulmonary parenchyma do not contain pain fibers, and no pain is caused by procedures performed on these tissues. The numbness of the throat due to the local anesthetic resolves quickly. Patients are generally able to resume oral intake after three hours.

How will topical anesthesia be administered?

Topical anesthesia for the oropharynx and the hypopharynx is administered either by gargling or by inhalation via a nebulizer. Nebulization also provides some anesthesia to the larynx and the tracheobronchial tree. Additional anesthesia is given through the bronchoscope. An anesthetic lubricant is applied to the nose when the transnasal approach is used.

Should I have general or topical anesthesia?

The most common risks to the patient posed by bronchoscopy are related largely to the anesthetic employed rather than to the bronchoscopic procedure itself. Topical anesthesia is undoubtedly safer than general anesthesia, although the latter is more comfortable for the patient and appropriate in some cases, especially for rigid bronchoscopy.

Will I be able to breathe during the procedure?

The fiberoptic bronchoscope occupies a relatively small area within the airways and will not obstruct breathing. Although the rigid scope is larger, it is hollow, allowing spontaneous breathing or mechanical ventilation if general anesthesia is employed.

CONSENT

A fully informed, written consent is required.

SELECTED BIBLIOGRAPHY

Fitzpatrick SB, March B, Stokes D, Wang KP: Indications for flexible fiberoptic bronchoscopy in pediatric patients. *Am J Dis Child* 1983;6:595.

Fulkerson WJ: Fiberoptic bronchoscopy. *N. Eng J. Med.* 1984;311:511.

Sackner MA: Bronchofiberoscopy. *Am Rev Resp Dis* 1975;111:62.

Shure D: Fiberoptic bronchoscopy—diagnostic applications. *Clin Chest Med* 1987;8:1.

Van Gundy K, Boylen CT: Fiberoptic bronchoscopy. *Postgrad Med* 1988;1:289.

21

Chest Tube Insertion

RICHARD M. STILLMAN

The space between the visceral pleura and the parietal pleura of the lung forms a sac that extends into the neck, costophrenic sinuses, interlobar fissures, and retrosternal area. The right and left pleural spaces are separate and do not communicate. Normally, there is a thin layer of viscous fluid that acts as a lubricant within the pleural space. The entry of air, fluid, blood, or pus into this cavity can result from a variety of pathologic processes and can cause respiratory distress. Removal of the offending material can be performed by placement of a chest tube.

INDICATIONS

A chest tube is used to allow drainage of air, fluid, or blood from the pleural cavity. This allows the lungs to function with normal pressures preventing compression of the trachea and mediastinum toward the unaffected side and preventing infection in the pleural space. When the pleural space becomes filled with blood, fluid, or air, collapse of the lung occurs with resulting symptoms of chest pain and dyspnea and a possible shift of the mediastinum and the trachea to the opposite side. This latter problem can be life threatening because it may interfere with the venous return to the heart and result in shock and death. Patients with slow accumulation of pleural fluid may have minimal or no symptoms until a large amount of fluid has compromised ventilation. Emergency cases may require immediate placement of a chest tube while subacute cases may permit pleural tap or needle aspiration as well as other examinations to confirm the diagnosis. Medical problems requiring placement of the chest tube can be broadly classified as traumatic, iatrogenic, or nontraumatic. Traumatic causes include hemothorax, hemopneumothorax, open pneumothorax, pneumothorax, and tension pneumothorax. Iatrogenic causes include complications of bronchoscopy, central venous access, intercostal nerve block, pleural biopsy, positive pressure ventilation, postoperative, and thoracentesis procedures that lead to pneumothorax or hemothorax as complications.

Nontraumatic causes include chylothorax, empyema, hemothorax, recurrent pleural effusion, spontaneous pneumothorax, and tension pneumothorax.

Because chest-tube insertion will be accomplished with local anesthesia and minimal blood loss, any patient with pneumothorax, hemothorax, or fluid collection in the fluid cavity that interferes with lung function requires evacuation of the offending agent.

Refractory spontaneous pneumothorax and malignant effusions are often treated by sclerosing solutions injected through the tube.

ALTERNATIVES

In emergency circumstances, needle, trocar, or catheter thoracentesis might be appropriate when needed equipment or trained personnel are not available.

POSSIBILITY OF FAILURE

Very rarely, a second chest tube will be required to drain a loculated cavity (e.g., abscess) that does not communicate with the first chest tube.

CONTRAINDICATIONS

Under ordinary circumstances in the hospital there are no contraindications to chest tube insertion. If an underwater drainage system is not available or cannot be improvised from available equipment, a chest tube should not be inserted unless the pathology is life threatening. The presence of any abnormal bleeding state requires caution and possibly infusion of the needed components.

PREPROCEDURE PREPARATION

The majority of chest tube insertions are performed in emergency circumstances and no preparation is required. When practical, a chest radiograph is advisable as are tests of bleeding function. When chest tube insertion is performed for drainage of chronic progressive fluid collections, an antiseptic soap scrub is applied to the chest wall.

PATIENT EDUCATION

The patient should be advised of the indication for placement of the chest tube and about the use of local anesthesia. There will be some pain as the chest tube literally pops into the pleural cavity. This pain will last only a few seconds, but the presence of the tube itself may be uncomfortable and analgesia may be required. Patients who have a symptomatic pneumothorax should be advised that the symptoms themselves will disappear almost immediately upon insertion of the chest tube. The patient should be aware that the tube will remain in place for several days and, during this period, it must remain constantly attached to the underwater drainage system.

PROCEDURE

Following the antiseptic preparation of the chest wall, the patient is placed in a supine position with the affected side slightly elevated. The fifth or sixth intercostal space at the midaxillary line is identified for placement of chest tubes meant to evacuate air and fluid or blood and fluid alone. When a pneumothorax alone is being evacuated, the chest tube may be placed in the mid-clavicular line anteriorly to the second intercostal space. Iodine solution is widely applied to the skin and superficial anesthesia is affected by use of injection of a topical agent. The injection of anesthetic is administered into the subcutaneous tissue and the periosteum of adjacent ribs. Sterile drape sheets are positioned.

A transverse incision about 2 to 5 cm is made over the premarked interspace. The incision is carried through subcutaneous tissue to the periosteum of the rib and a blunt clamp is popped through the intercostal membrane just above the lower rib. Upon entry into the pleural space there will be an immediate rush of air or an outflow of fluid. A soft plastic chest tube ranging in size from 12 to 40 mm in diameter is placed in the space. The smaller tubes are used to evacuate a pneumothorax while the larger tubes are used to evacuate fluid, blood, or pus. A heavy, nonabsorbable suture of silk or nylon is used to tightly close the incision around the chest tube insertion site and to tie the chest tube in place. The tube is immediately connected to the underwater drainage system (figure 21–1). The disposable Pleur-evac® system is most commonly used in the United States. A chest radiograph is taken following the chest tube insertion to confirm the appropriate positioning and reexpansion of the lung.

The Pleur-evac® contains three chambers. The first chamber to which the chest tube is connected contains the drainage collection chamber. This chamber has graduated markings to allow measurement of the amount of fluid that has

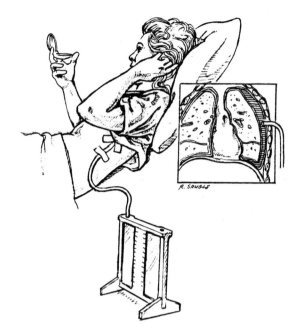

Figure 21–1. Chest tube draining left pleural cavity.

drained from the pleura. The second chamber is the water seal chamber in which 1 to 2 cm of water provides a seal between the intrapleural space and the outside air. The third chamber is the suction control chamber in which a larger volume of water determines the amount of suction delivered when it is necessary to provide continuous suction to promote continuous drainage of thick fluid or blood from the chest or to promote drainage of a continuing air leak. The water seal chamber serves as an interpleural manometer, that is, the fluctuations of the fluid level in this chamber reflect the compliance of the lung and gauge the interpleural pressure. Normal inspiratory tidaling of water in the inspiratory chamber varies form 2 to 6 cm.

The negative pressure in the interpleural space produced by deep inspiration or coughing will cause the fluid level in the water seal chamber to rise markedly. During the cough itself on expiration the fluid level will drop markedly. When there is increased respiratory difficulty such as with upper airway respiratory disease or atelectasis, the degree of tidaling in the water seal chamber is accentuated. The patient on positive pressure respiration will have fluid level fluctuations that are reversed because the lungs are filled with positive pressure from the machine instead of negative pressure from the diaphragm.

When chest tubes are used to drain the mediastinum (e.g., following open heart surgery) tidaling will be absent or diminished because negative pressure in the mediastinum is not as great as the pressure in the interpleural space during inspiration.

When the time comes for removal, the suture holding the chest tube in place will be cut and the tube will be easily extracted.

POSTPROCEDURE INFORMATION

The patient will have some incisional pain after the anesthetic wears off. There will also be some chest pain in many cases because of the presence of the chest tube itself. If the pain is excessive, this may indicate improper placement of the chest tube or advancement of an excessive amount of the chest tube into the pleural space.

COMPLICATIONS

Sudden removal of an excessive amount of fluid from the pleural space may cause syncope caused by a vasovagal response or may be followed by pulmonary edema on the same side as the chest tube. Symptoms of these complications include cough, bradycardia, other arrhythmias, and hypotension.

Most complications of chest tube insertion are related to the underlying condition for which the chest tube has been inserted. Patients with spontaneous pneumothorax may develop a recurrence in the future that may eventually require thoracotomy. Empyema may occur following chest tube insertion, but is most often related to a underlying pleural infection.

Other, less common complications of chest tube insertion may include diaphragmatic perforation, empyema formation, lung laceration, inadvertent insertion of the chest tube into the abdomen with or without laceration of the liver, massive intercostal bleeding, and unilateral pulmonary edema due to extreme negative pressure to the interpleural space or rapid reexpansion of a lung that has been collapsed for a prolonged period of time.

PATIENT QUESTIONS

Why is a tube being inserted into my lung?

The tube is not being inserted into the lung but into the space around the lung. Its function is to remove air or fluid that does not belong in this space in order to allow the lung to expand normally with respiration. When the air and fluid accumulation has stopped, the chest tube can be removed. This can take from several days to several weeks. Generally, if the chest tube is required for more than 2 weeks, a new site is selected and a new tube is placed before removing the old tube. The appropriate time for removal of the chest tube is determined by the decrease in drainage in the Pleur-evac® chamber or the amount of air leak noted in the suction control chamber.

Why is the collection chamber so noisy?

Bubbling that occurs in the suction control chamber is expected and is related to the suction device attached to promote passage of fluid and air from the pleural cavity.

Will the chest tube allow my lung to expand and remain that way?

The utility of the chest tube is to remove fluid and air present at the time of insertion. The underlying pathology will determine whether the lungs will remain totally inflated after the chest tube is removed.

Can I move around with the chest tube in place?

The chest tube is anchored to the chest wall by a suture. The tube must remain connected to the water-sealed collecting apparatus. The patient can get out of bed and sit in a chair. Care must be taken to keep all the connections intact. If the collecting apparatus falls on its side, it should be returned to an upright position and the water seal should be checked. The patient may intermittently be asked to cough or breath vigorously in order to force out any accumulated pleural air. The patient can eat normally but will probably have to use a bed pan or a commode.

My chest tube has not caused me any problems until now when I have developed new chest pain. What might be happening?

The problem may be related to the chest tube or the underlying pathology. The pain may be caused by incisional discomfort, anxiety, myocardial infarction, pulmonary embolism, or other causes of chest pain that might be unrelated to the chest tube. The physician should listen for breath sounds to confirm that the chest tube has allowed complete expansion of the lung.

Will the hole into my lung heal properly?

Usually, the incision through the skin and the pleura will heal properly. The lung itself is not being cut or injured in any way. However, pneumothorax can recur, especially in smokers who continue smoking. Recurrent pneumothorax may require surgery.

CONSENT

Informed consent is required for insertion of a chest tube except in emergency circumstances.

SELECTED BIBLIOGRAPHY

Dalbec DL, Krome RL: Thoracostomy. *Emer Med Clin North Amer* 1986;Aug:4(3):441.

Erikson R: Solving chest tube problems. *Nursing* 1981;June:62.

Kersten L: Chest tube drainage system—indications and principles of operation. *Heart and Lung* 1974;Jan–Feb:3(1):97.

Richards V: Procedures in family practice: tube thoracostomy. *J Fam Pract* 1983;6(3):629.

Van Way CW: Persisting pneumothorax as a complication of chest suction. *Chest* 1980;77:815.

22

Mediastinoscopy

RICHARD SADOVSKY

Mediastinoscopy permits the examiner, through an exploring scope, to directly visualize mediastinal structures and to biopsy paratracheal and carinal lymph nodes. Cervical mediastinoscopy allows exploration of the superior mediastinum and biopsy of lymph nodes in the anterior aspect of the subcarinal space, around the proximal main stem bronchi and lower trachea, and in the paratracheal region. Lymph node examination and biopsy can detect lymphoma (including Hodgkin's disease), sarcoidosis, and aid the staging of lung cancer. Contents of the mediastinum that can be visualized with anterior mediastinoscopy include surface views of the heart and its vessels, the trachea, esophagus, thymus, and lymph nodes.

Exploration of the right side of the mediastinum is relatively easy and is commonly used to stage lung cancer. Exploring the left side is less satisfactory and more hazardous because of the closeness of the aorta.

INDICATIONS

Mediastinoscopy is done to detect bronchogenic carcinoma, lymphoma, other mid-mediastinal tumors and extrathoracic malignancies, and sarcoidosis, and to determine staging of lung cancer. Its role in diagnosing such mediastinal masses as thymoma or germ-cell tumors is arguable because diagnosis may involve breaking the capsule of a potentially curable malignant lesion. It should be remembered that, in most patients, the limit of the mediastinoscope extends to the initial portions of the right and left mainstem bronchi and the hilar areas, but the anterior mediastinum is generally beyond reach.

Other less frequent indications for mediastinoscopy include testing the pressure measurements from the heart or great vessels, and the placing of pacing wires on the left atrium. Selected patients with mesothelioma, esophageal carcinoma, and other tracheal lesions may benefit from the procedure. Diagnosis of the lesion causing superior vena cava syndrome is critical to relieve the pressure on the vessels.

The routine use of mediastinoscopy for indications other than the staging of bronchogenic carcinoma is controversial. Even with this condition, it is unclear as to whether a determination of positive mediastinal lymph nodes are a criteria for nonresectability.

The results of mediastinoscopy for diagnosis of unknown mediastinal masses, whether benign or malignant, remains quite good. This procedure has a sensitivity of 93% and a diagnostic accuracy (specificity) of up to 100%. Mediastinoscopy can often provide tissue for the diagnosis of superior mediastinal masses, whether they are lymphadenopathy or a mediastinal tumor. Yield of this procedure has been high in benign lymph node disease such has infection or sarcoidosis. Unknown mediastinal masses indicate the need for this procedure if the mass is clearly not vascular, if the mass is accessible to the mediastinoscope, and when biopsy, rather than excision, is most appropriate.

Malignant lymph nodes usually indicate inoperable, but not necessarily untreatable, lung or esophageal cancer, or lymphomas. Staging of lung cancer helps to determine therapeutic regimens. Multiple nodular involvement may contraindicate surgery. Preoperative mediastinoscopy may obviate the need for staging procedures by lymph node biopsy during thoracotomy.

Posterior mediastinoscopy can be performed through a small incision with resection of the posterior aspect of a rib. This will identify direct tumor invasion of the posterior mediastinum. This procedure is rarely performed because of the accuracy of computerized axial tomography (CT) scanning and the availability of fine needle biopsy techniques.

ALTERNATIVES

Less invasive techniques used to evaluate mediastinal masses and lymph nodes include mediastinal tomography, gallium scanning, computed tomographic (CT) scan, MRI or transbronchial needle aspiration. The benefits and shortcomings of each of these procedures have been discussed in numerous reports. Many argue that, if a preoperative CT scan shows no enlargement of mediastinal lymph nodes, thoracotomy should be advised without invasive staging. The overall sensitivity of standard chest radiographic analysis has been reported to be around 75%, demonstrating greater accuracy when the radiograph is normal (90% agreement between a normal radiograph and negative mediastinoscopy) than when it is abnormal (43% agreement between an abnormal radiograph and positive mediastinoscopy). Many study groups have recommended avoidance of mediastinoscopy in patients with a peripheral lesion and a radiologically normal mediastinum. The number of equivocal radiographs, however, causes problems in the studies that have used this technique.

Tomography has a reported sensitivity of 52% to 67%, a specificity of 79% to 90%, and a diagnostic accuracy of approximately 80%. This technique requires great expertise in order to obtain reproducible results. This procedure has been helpful in staging of patients with small peripheral lesions who are free from systemic metastasis by clinical and biochemical investigations (liver function tests and calcium). Tomography is useful in evaluating the hilum, but it generally fails to distinguish between a benign or malignant mediastinal adenopathy.

Pulmonary angiography has been used for staging of tumors and appears to have a role in assessing pulmonary artery, pericardial, and atrial involvement. However, these factors are infrequently the deciding factors in terms of resectability, and a significant proportion of patients with abnormal angiograms have resectable tumors.

Gallium scintigraphy has been extensively used for detection and staging of bronchogenic carcinoma. The type and quality of scanning machinery is very important with sensitivity varying greatly between the large-field Anger camera (high) and the rectilinear scanners (low). Observer experience is also an important factor. Scanning cannot differentiate hilar from mediastinal masses, and in addition, gallium is taken up by primary and secondary lung tumors as well as by inflammatory lesions.

CT scanning has a greater sensitivity and specificity than does gallium scanning. The use of scans alone to evaluate mediastinal lymph nodes appears inadequate. The gallium scan cannot always differentiate between inflammation and malignancy, and the CT scan does not distinguish hyperplastic, anthracotic, or granulomatous nodes from malignant nodes. Neither method is effective in detecting intranodal metastases to lymph nodes 2 cm or less in diameter.

With the advent of enhanced CT and MRI, the mediastinum is frequently being evaluated by these modalities. Numerous reports recently have shown increasingly, that if there is no evidence of mediastinal abnormality demonstrated by CT scanning or MRI, the yield of mediastinoscopy will be very low. On the other hand, if the CT scan or MRI is positive for significant lymphadenopathy, this would be an indication for mediastinoscopy and would help to direct the biopsy. The question as to whether this will be a more cost-effective way of staging the patients than doing routine mediastinoscopies remains to be answered.

The role of flexible transbronchial needle aspiration needs further clarification. Early reports show a sensitivity of 76% and a specificity of 100% with this procedure.

In the near future we will see the advent of scanning radioactive, tumor specific monoclonal antibodies, which may make invasive staging of the mediastinum no longer necessary.

POSSIBILITY OF FAILURE

In inexperienced hands, mediastinoscopy can be unsuccessful at visualizing the appropriate structures and morbidity can be unacceptably high.

CONTRAINDICATIONS

Relative contraindications to mediastinoscopy include aortic arch aneurysms, previous mediastinoscopy (although some reports demonstrate that repeated procedures can be done without complication), superior vena cava obstruction, previous median sternotomy, or a coagulopathy.

PREPROCEDURE PREPARATION

Routine laboratory tests including a coagulation profile are performed. The patient's history should be checked for hypersensitivity to anesthetics. The patient is asked to fast from midnight before the procedure, and a sedative is often administered the night before the test.

PATIENT EDUCATION

The procedure should be described to the patient, the administration of general anesthesia should be given, and the patient informed that the procedure will take about 1 hour. Advance warning about temporary chest pain, tenderness at the incision site, or a sore throat will help the patient understand these possible after effects.

PROCEDURE

An endotracheal tube is placed to ensure adequate respiration since almost all mediastinoscopic examinations are performed under general anesthesia. The surgeon then makes a small transverse suprasternal incision. Finger dissection is used to form a channel and to palpate the lymph nodes. A mediastinoscope is inserted into the mediastinum and tissue samples are collected for analysis (figure 22–1.). All biopsies should be preceded by needle aspiration of the structure to make certain that it is not vascular. Some physicians report the use of needle aspiration biopsies instead of punch biopsies and report a higher yield because of the increased range of the needle and decreased complications, including procedures done on patients with superior vena cava syndrome. Frozen section may be performed if indicated and a thoracotomy and pneumonectomy may follow immediately.

A chest radiograph should be done following the procedure to be certain that no pneumothorax has occurred.

The entire procedure requires 15 to 20 minutes and can be done in conjunction with bronchoscopy.

POSTPROCEDURE INFORMATION

This procedure is always done on an inpatient basis with general anesthesia. The patient's postprocedure care will be provided by the hospital.

COMPLICATIONS

Mediastinoscopy can generally be performed safely and with minimal mortality when the technique is performed by experienced personnel who can tend immediately to any complication.

Complications can include fever (mediastinitis), crepitus (subcutaneous emphysema), dyspnea, cyanosis, diminished breath sounds on the affected side (pneumothorax), recurrent nerve injury, and tachycardia and hypotension (hemorrhage). Life-threatening complications, including severe hemorrhage or tracheobronchial and esophageal injury are rare.

PATIENT QUESTIONS

Will mediastinoscopy determine whether my lung tumor is resectable?

The determination of resectability of lung tumors is based on many factors, including the report of the mediastinoscopy. Other evidence of metastasis, including results of radiographs and scans, are taken into consideration. The size

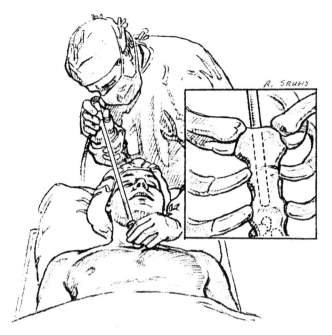

Figure 22–1. Mediastinoscopic examination.

of mediastinal metastatic lesions are important as is the histology. In many centers, mediastinoscopy is a useful tool in determining resectability while in others, less invasive tests are given greater consideration. Mediastinoscopy has a high predictive value with no false positives and a very low false-negative rate.

Will the procedure hurt?

Mediastinoscopy is usually done under general anesthesia. The patient feels no pain during that period, but may awaken while still intubated. This requires some prior patient preparation. In addition, the patient may have chest soreness and/or a sore throat when the procedure is completed because of needed manipulation.

CONSENT

Mediastinoscopy is an invasive procedure and informed consent is required. The patient should understand the reason for doing the test and the potential complications.

SELECTED BIBLIOGRAPHY

Ginsberg RJ: Evaluation of the mediastinum by invasive techniques. *Surg Clin North Am* 1987;Oct:67:5:1025.

Rhoads AC, Thomas JH, Hermreck AS, George EP: Comparative studies of computerized tomography and mediastinoscopy for the staging of bronchogenic carcinoma. *Amer J Surg* 1986;Dec:152:588.

Trastek VF, Piehler JM, Pairolero PC: Mediastinoscopy. *Brit Med J* 1986;42:3:240.

23

Pulmonary Function Testing

MICHAEL J.H. AKERMAN AND RICHARD SADOVSKY

Pulmonary function tests (PFTs) are used to quantitate respiratory status. Undiagnosed patients with respiratory complaints can be objectively evaluated. The severity of known pulmonary disease can be measured and followed for both prognosis and the response to medication or other therapy. PFTs are also useful for disability evaluation as well as for identification of patients at risk for postoperative pulmonary complications.

Pulmonary function tests are grouped into several categories based upon the fact that different methodologies are necessary to evaluate different aspects of pulmonary physiology and function. PFTs can measure (1) a combination of dynamic lung volumes and airflows (spirometry); (2) static lung volumes and capacities; (3) diffusion across the pulmonary membrane; (4) effectiveness of matching of ventilation to perfusion and gas transfer; and (5) airway resistance.

Spirometry is the most commonly ordered pulmonary function test. It includes measurement of forced inspiratory and expiratory air movement, dynamic lung volumes, and graphical plotting of the air flow versus lung volumes (flow volume loops). The results are classified into normal, obstructive, and restrictive patterns. The maximum volume of air that is exhaled in the first second is called the forced expiratory volume in one second (FEV_1). It is then expressed as a percentage of the forced vital capacity (the total amount of air that can be exhaled after a maximal inspiration). Another measurement made by spirometry is the maximum voluntary ventilation. This is the maximum amount of air that can be breathed by the person over a period of 12 to 15 seconds. The results are then extrapolated and reported as a 1 minute value.

Tests of **lung volumes and capacities** are among the oldest measures of pulmonary function. Lung volumes are divided into two broad categories based on the measuring technique involved. These are (1) dynamic lung volumes, including the tidal volume (usual volume of air moved with normal relaxed breathing) and vital capacity. These are measured by spirometry. (2) Static lung volumes including the residual volume (the amount of residual air left in the lungs after a total exhalation), functional residual capacity (the residual volume plus the inspiratory reserve volume), and the total lung capacity (vital capacity plus the residual volume). Static lung volumes are measured by the more complicated technique of gas dilution or by body plethysmography.

Normal values for these tests are predicted based upon age, height, sex, and race. The normal range was formally defined as ranging from 80% to 120% of predicted. However, newer normal values have been developed that use a more valid statistical approach to define the specific normal range for the test (based upon the concept of the 95% confidence interval).

Tests for diffusion capacity are usually measured by the single-breath carbon monoxide test. This measures the lung's ability to conduct a gas from the alveoli to the capillaries. Abnormal results may reflect damage to the pulmonary interstitium, such as infiltration by inflammatory cells, fluid, or fibrosis. Abnormal results may also reflect damage on the vascular side of the pulmonary membrane due to vasculitis or embolism, or vascular destruction such as in emphysema.

Tests for gas exchange reflect the overall uniformity of the match between pulmonary ventilation and blood circulation. The easiest measurement is the taking of an arterial blood sample on room air breathing. The sample is analyzed for oxygen and carbon dioxide pressures and for pH, and the results are compared to established normal values. Once an abnormality is detected, a blood-gas study done on oxygen breathing can inform the physician whether the abnormality is correctable and caused by mild ventilation-perfusion mismatching, (or if not correctable with low-flow oxygen, that the abnormality is very severe and caused by a blood shunt).

Pulmonary exercise testing can further evaluate the effectiveness of pulmonary ventilation-perfusion matching, especially when the PFT results do not match the severity of the patient's complaints. When conducted in its most comprehensive form this test will usually be able to identify the patient's problem as belonging to the lungs, pulmonary vasculature, heart, peripheral circulation, or musculoskeletal organ systems, or as being due not to any pathology but rather to obesity or anxiety. The equipment and expertise necessary for this test is becoming widely available.

Airway resistance is measured by body plethysmography. It is a useful procedure for diagnosing occupational asthma or cough-equivalent asthma by bronchial challenge techniques. Resistance measurements are a more sensitive indicator of this problem than are spirometric measurements. However, the equipment for this testing is much more expensive and more technically demanding and, therefore, not as widely available as spirometry. It is mostly used as a research tool.

INDICATIONS

The use of pulmonary function testing for screening healthy patients is controversial. Many question the value of screening because of the uncertainty of its ability to intervene and correct early airflow problems that might be discovered. However, portable, accurate spirometers have recently become widely available to physicians in general practice in a price and sizes comparable to that of ECG equipment.

PFTs should generally be done as part of the diagnostic work up for shortness of breath, since they are clearly indicative of the presence of disease. In addition, in high-risk populations, PFT are indicated as screening tests to determine whether there is significant pulmonary damage.

In early interstitial involvement of the lungs, PFTs may provide early evidence of disease and thus the only indication for the need for further evaluation. Examples of this include decreased diffusion capacity in sarcoidosis, or in an intravenous drug addict who is injecting crystals and/or fibers mixed with the drug into his vein, or in a worker exposed to asbestos.

In patients with obstructive disease, expiratory flow rates are decreased. Therefore their lung volumes are exhaled in a longer period of time. Mild airway obstruction may prolong only the peak expiratory flow rate. As the obstruction worsens, all flow rates fall lower then predicted. In nonsmokers, forced expiratory volume declines gradually with age. Smokers seem to fall into susceptible and nonsusceptible groups with the former showing a more rapid decline in forced expiratory volumes and therefore becoming disabled with obstructive lung disease while the latter follow a pattern of decline similar to that of nonsmokers. In persons who stop smoking, the rate of decay in forced expiratory volume may revert to nonsusceptible levels and less disability may result.

In patients with restrictive lung disease there is a marked decrease in lung volumes, including the forced vital capacity, total lung capacity, and residual volume. This can be mimicked by conditions causing abdominal distention such as ascites, hepatomegaly, obesity, and pregnancy.

Patients with obstructive lung disease may occasionally have a reduced forced vital capacity, also, because of a physiologic phenomenon known as air trapping. Therefore, spirometry alone may not always differentiate the obstructive lung diseases from the restrictive lung diseases. Pulmonologists then rely on tests of lung capacity (residual volume and total lung capacity) to differentiate whether the patient has obstruction, restriction, or both. (Grading of restrictive impairment is based on total lung capacity.)

Flow volume loops are determined by the elastic recoil of the lungs and by the flow-resistive pathways of the small airways. Therefore, obstruction and restriction show different patterns on the flow volume loop. The graphical pattern of the flow volume loops can further distinguish between different types of airway obstruction that cannot be distinguished by other spirometric criteria. For instance, fixed obstruction (as in tracheal stenosis or goiter), variable extrathoracic obstruction (as in vocal cord paralysis or polyps), tracheal masses or foreign bodies, and variable intrathoracic obstruction as caused by tumors can be distinguished from each other and from bronchial obstruction due to asthma or chronic obstructive pulmonary disease (COPD). This differential may come up occasionally with regard to the recently intubated asthma patient who now complains of dyspnea. The flow volume loop may distinguish laryngeal obstruction due to scar tissue from the lower airway obstruction of asthma. Patients with goiters can be evaluated by a flow volume loop in the supine position to determine if the thyroid gland causes compression to the trachea and obstruction to airflow in the supine position.

Tests for diseases of the small peripheral airways are helpful in the determination of early chronic obstructive lung disease. Most commonly, this information is derived from the maximal midexpiratory flow rate (MMEF or FEF25-75), which is measured by spirometry. There is debate among pulmonologists with regard to the utility and sensitivity of other tests that may be used to detect small airways obstruction. These other tests are commonly used as epidemiologic or behavioral modification tools and are not discussed further here.

Typically, patients with chronic obstructive pulmonary disease have slower flow rates and lower peak flow rates than other persons. In contrast, restrictive lung disease decreases lung volumes, but flow rates remain normal. Therefore, portable, inexpensive, hand held peak flow meters can be used by asthma patients at home to assess fluctuations in disease. This can help guide patients in management of their own problems because a decrease in peak flow may warn them early of a new worsening of their obstructive lung disease. It therefore gives patients a chance to adjust their medications and avoid a catastrophic, full-blown, asthma attack.

Testing with meter-dosed bronchodilator sprays allows the clinician to recognize patients who will definitely improve with bronchodilator therapy. However, lack of a bronchodilator response on the day of testing does not rule out a clinical response to bronchodilators. Therefore, bronchodilators should still be tried if the patient has obstructive lung disease.

There are predictable changes in lung volumes and breathing patterns after surgery. Therefore, diagnostic pulmonary function testing is indicated preoperatively for surgical patients in several situations. Thoracotomy and upper abdominal operations are associated with the largest decreases in lung volume and therefore have the most risk of postoperative pulmonary complications. Lower abdominal surgery is associated with smaller changes in pulmonary function; peripheral surgeries are not associated with any significant changes in lung function. The lung function changes may be caused by marked alterations in diaphragmatic excursions that are only partially explained by the presence of pain from the surgery. Therefore, screening pulmonary function tests (spirometry and the MVV) are indicated for smokers, or patients with suspected pulmonary disease who are scheduled for thoracotomy or abdominal surgery. Additional risk factors for these complications include obesity, advanced age, smoking, sepsis, and shock.

A second indication for preoperative pulmonary function testing is for the evaluation of patients who are to undergo lung resection. The purpose of the testing is to assess operability by assuring that adequate pulmonary function reserve exists to allow satisfactory respiratory function after the lung resection. Spirometric results, when combined with the results of a nuclear medicine perfusion lung scan, frequently allow the pulmonologist to answer this question. In borderline cases, pulmonary exercise testing can help predict postoperative function and guide the physician in deciding whether to go ahead with the thoracotomy.

Pulmonary function tests are helpful in assessing pulmonary disability or quantitation of disease. For example, in patients with chronic bronchitis, it is apparent that a greater-than-expected decrease in pulmonary function (even as simple a test as forced expiratory volume) offers the best guide to prognosis. However, at times, abnormalities on resting pulmonary function testing may not fully explain and diagnose the patient's complaints anymore than resting ECGs can diagnose exercise-induced angina. Therefore, pulmonary exercise measurements may be indicated in these cases to further evaluate the cause and extent of the disability.

Surveillance of pulmonary function (vital capacity as measured by spirometry) can help the practitioner to predict the advent of respiratory insufficiency in patients with chronic chest bellows impairment such as amyotrophic lateral sclerosis, or kyphoscoliosis. In hospitalized patients with acute muscular weakness such as the Guillain-Barré syndrome, serial measurements of peak inspiratory and peak expiratory pressures may be more sensitive than serial vital capacity measurements in predicting imminent respiratory failure.

It is important to emphasize that pulmonary function tests do not establish a diagnosis any more than does a chest radiograph. Sometimes a pattern is revealed that might be highly characteristic of a common disease and is therefore likely to be diagnostic, while other times the findings might be compatible with a long list of etiologically unrelated diseases with vastly different prognoses. The physician must therefore correlate the results of the PFTs with the patient's total clinical picture in order to arrive at the appropriate diagnosis.

ALTERNATIVES

For many reasons, chest radiographs correlate poorly with most pulmonary function tests. However, lung-volume measurements do show some correlation with lung volumes calculated by planimetry from standard posterior-anterior chest roentgenogram.

A CT scan of the lung represents axial sections and is generally considered to be more sensitive in detecting early interstitial thickening, small nodules, and bullae than plain radiography. Therefore some studies have suggested that, in some diseases, chest CT scans may correlate with diffusion measurements.

An alternative to blood sampling for the measurement of arterial oxygen pressure is the noninvasive measurement of arterial oxygen content by ear oximetry. This is a device that is attached by a clip onto the ear or fingertip and measures the oxygen saturation of hemoglobin. However, it is not as sensitive nor as accurate as the actual blood gas measurement. Therefore, its use is usually reserved for patient monitoring during long hospital procedures, or out-of-hospital screening by therapists.

There are several simple tests that can be done in the physician's office to provide a qualitative idea of the patient's current level of pulmonary function. Perhaps more important though, these can be used to serially follow and compare the patient's function from one visit to another. Some of these tests are also useful for pediatric patients or those who cannot cooperate in PFT testing. However, the obvious disadvantage of these tests are their occasional lack of precision and their inability to detect early or small changes in function.

The forced expiratory time (FET) can be determined by placing a stethoscope over the patient's trachea. The patient is instructed to inhale maximally and then exhale as fast and as long as possible. In asthma or other obstructive lung diseases, the FET will be prolonged (usually to greater than 5 seconds).

Other office tests have the patient blow out a match held at a measured distance from the mouth, take a maximal inhalation and count as high as possible on the single breath, walk upstairs counting the number of steps that can be climbed before experiencing shortness of breath, or walk as far as possible in a 12 minutes then measure the distance. The first test estimates degree of obstructive lung disease, the second estimates vital capacity (or restrictive lung involvement), and the last 2 tests reflect cardiopulmonary integrated function.

POSSIBILITY OF FAILURE

Quality control is essential to pulmonary function testing and requires frequent checks and calibrations of all instruments. The test results are also very dependent on patient effort. The technologist performing the examination must be well trained and able to obtain good patient effort and cooperation. The physician must realize that the values obtained from pulmonary function testing present problems in interpretation that are far greater than those presented by the results of many other commonly used laboratory tests. Reliability depends strongly on the consistency of testing techniques.

CONTRAINDICATIONS

There are no absolute contraindications to pulmonary function testing. Patients with acute coronary insufficiency, angina, or recent myocardial infarction should not be tested until they are stable and several weeks postinfarction. However, if it is absolutely necessary to test them, the test must be done carefully, observing them closely for respiratory distress, changes in pulse rate and blood pressure, coughing or bronchospasm. PFTs should not be done any sooner than 24 hours postcardiac catheterization or bronchoscopy.

Conditions that may interfere with the accuracy of the examination include lack of patient cooperation, recent surgery, hypoxia, pregnancy or gastric distention displacing lung volume, analgesic or sedative medications, and recent use of bronchodilators.

PREPROCEDURE PREPARATION

Pulmonary function tests can be affected by irritants and bronchodilators. Doctors must emphasize to their patients the importance of not smoking because smoking may aggravate obstruction or elevate blood carbon monoxide and affect diffusion, of not drinking coffee because caffeine is a bronchodilator, and of not inhaling respiratory irritants in the 6 hours preceding pulmonary function testing. The patient who is currently taking bronchodilating medications should be informed whether the medications need to be discontinued and for how long before the test. The test should be performed several hours after meals to avoid impaired results caused by abdominal distention. Restrictive clothing should be avoided and the patient should avoid fatiguing activity for 4 hours immediately before the test. In addition, any medications that may depress respiration should be avoided if possible, (such as sedatives or tranquilizers) because they will affect the patient's ability to follow instructions.

Psychological preparation is important to allay the patient's fears and to ensure good patient cooperation with the testing. If body plethysmography is to be used, then assure the patient that there is no danger of suffocation and that someone will be present at all times. If possible, it is often helpful for the patient to see the laboratory beforehand and to learn something about the equipment. The patient should also be informed in advance if there will be arterial blood gas sampling.

PATIENT EDUCATION

Patients should be told that many factors affect the predicted "normal values." Among these are race and sex—blacks and women having lower vital capacities. Most reputable laboratories do adjust their normal values for these factors. However, good normal value data does not exist for all races. Variability among patients may result from random, unexplained causes. Pulmonary function seems to be at its worst in the morning, and forced expiratory volume usually improves as the day progresses. However, overall daytime variability is less than 10%. Therefore, it is not necessary to be rigorous and insist that a patient's comparative tests be done at the same time of day.

The physician must encourage the patient must attempt to be compliant and request the patient to follow instructions as closely as possible for the best results.

PROCEDURE

Pulmonary function testing, which may require several hours for comprehensive studies, requires the patient to wear a nose clip and to breathe through a mouth piece (figure 23–1). In spirometry, the most common test, the mouthpiece is attached by tubing or wires to a device that measures the volume of air exhaled and the rate of exhalation. In body plethysmography, the patient sits in an air-tight "body size box" with a transparent wall that enables measurement of functional residual capacity and airway resistance. For both these tests, the patient will be asked to inhale and exhale with different amounts of force, speed, and frequency. Inspiratory and expiratory excursions are recorded on calibrated paper or in a computer. A respiratory therapist or other trained person will be there to coach and assist the patient. In order to obtain accurate and reproducible results, the technician will inevitably ask the patient to repeat the maneuvers several times.

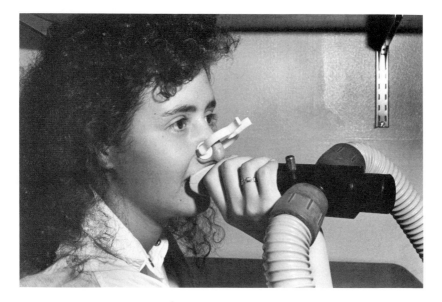

Figure 23–1. Preparing for pulmonary function testing.

The patient is permitted to rest if necessary. In some cases, repeat visits might be needed to complete the study. Reproducibility is essential and the therapist will be reporting the extent of the patient's cooperation and effort.

For some problems or diseases, sampling of venous and arterial blood may be needed.

Pulmonary exercise testing is usually done on a bicycle or treadmill. The basic setup is similar to that described in chapter 10 on cardiac exercise testing. However, in addition to ECG monitoring, the patient will also be breathing through a mask or mouthpiece during the entire exercise period. Many laboratories will also draw blood samples during exercise through a small arterial catheter inserted into a radial or brachial artery.

POSTPROCEDURE INFORMATION

The patient may be short of breath following a comprehensive battery of pulmonary function tests if some pulmonary pathology is present. If an arterial blood gas has been obtained, the site of puncture should be observed for continued bleeding or hematoma formation.

COMPLICATIONS

Morbidity and mortality are generally limited to anxiety, fatigue, and shortness of breath. These are all temporary and should resolve soon after the test is concluded. If an arterial puncture is performed to obtain a blood gas, precautions must be taken to avoid bleeding, hematoma formation, or arterial occlusion.

PATIENT QUESTIONS

Should I have a pulmonary function test to help encourage me to stop smoking?

This question should be answered on a case-by-case basis, depending on the patient's motivations and medical history. Studies have shown that, when persons in a screening program are found to have abnormal results on spirometry and are notified of this situation, they stop smoking at a rate approximate to that achieved at smoking cessation clinics. Surgeons who see middle-aged patients with abnormal results on preoperative screening spirometry may be able to combine this information with the drama of the preoperative period to convince the patient to stop smoking.

Will I have fewer postoperative pulmonary complications if I stop smoking before surgery?

Yes. In patients with obstructive lung disease, cessation of smoking a week or two preoperatively, combined with optimizing bronchodilator medications and pulmonary toilet, does decrease the incidence of postoperative pulmonary complications. It is, however, beneficial to try to convince the preoperative patient to stop smoking even for a short period since smoking worsens a patient's oxygen-carrying capacity by increasing carboxyhemoglobin.

Can pulmonary function testing be performed on my infant or young child?

Testing can be carried out in newborns and small infants without sedation. Generally, the tests are performed during quiet breathing using a tightly fitting mask and a respiratory jacket, but these are cumbersome to perform. Usually only arterial blood gas tests are performed. In many cases, children as young as 4 years of age may be able to cooperate with the same procedures as adults. It is a misconception that pulmonary function testing in children under 10 years of age is of limited value because of their shortened attention span. Results in children with proper training are as reproducible as results in adult tests.

Can pulmonary function tests be used to confirm my diagnosis of asthma and to see if my medication is really helping?

Yes. Asthma can usually be diagnosed by spirometry. Exercise-induced asthma can usually be diagnosed by several minutes of exercise on a bicycle or treadmill followed by spirometry. Results of treatment can also be monitored by pulmonary function testing. Decisions as to whether to increase an already prescribed medication or to change to an alternate drug can be facilitated by objective quantitative data. Monitoring a simple test such as peak flow rate can assist in adjusting medication. Prebronchodilator and postbronchodilator tests can be done in one session to make therapy decisions easier. Occasionally, spirometry may not confirm a clinically suspected case of asthma. In that case, specialized bronchoconstrictor challenge testing may be necessary. This is an arduous test and requires the use of a body plethysmograph.

Why should I have a pulmonary exercise test if I have already had a cardiac stress test?

Cardiac stress testing looks only at certain aspects of cardiac function. If the patient's symptoms have not been explained, exercise function of the lungs and pulmonary circulation should be evaluated. Exercise PFTs can also help to determine whether exercise ability is normal, and whether the symptoms are caused by anxiety, obesity, or other normal physiologic causes such as aging.

CONSENT

Consent is not required for pulmonary function tests if only noninvasive procedures are performed. It is, however, a good idea to document the physician's explanation of the test to the patient.

SELECTED BIBLIOGRAPHY

Chan YM, Lam S, Enarson D: Pulmonary function measurement in the industrial setting. *Chest* 1985;Aug:88:2:270.

Ganesthananthan M, Fink RJ: Pulmonary function testing in the pediatric outpatient. *Pediatr Ann* 1986;Apr:15:4:323, 328.

Levinson RM, Ramsdell JW: Pulmonary function testing: An under-used office tool. *J Resp Dis* 1988;May:23.

Neuberg GW, Friedman SH, Weiss MB, Herman MV: Cardiopulmonary exercise testing. *Arch Int Med* 1988;Oct:148:2221.

Williams DO, Cugell DW: Pulmonary function testing: indications and interpretation. *Hosp Med* 1988;May:23.

V
Gastrointestinal System Procedures

24

Endoscopic Retrograde Cholangiopancreatography

RICHARD SADOVSKY

Endoscopic retrograde cholangiopancreatography (ERCP) involves the use of a duodenoscope to visualize the upper gastrointestinal tract, identify the ampulla of Vater, and enter the orifice of the ampulla. Contrast material is then injected, allowing the evaluation of the pancreatic and bile ducts by means of fluoroscopy and radiography.

Endoscopic biliary tract surgery without laparotomy, or endoscopic sphincterotomy of Vater's ampulla, allows the removal of stones in the biliary tract through spontaneous passage or basket extraction.

INDICATIONS

ERCP has been shown to be of value in all diseases that involve the pancreatic duct system as well as in the evaluation of extrahepatic obstructive causes of jaundice. The causes of obstruction that are easily demonstrated include stone, tumor, benign stricture, and inflammation. The procedure is particularly valuable in jaundiced patients where, if the bilirubin is too high, oral cholecystography and intravenous cholangiography are usually unsuccessful. ERCP is helpful for patients with upper abdominal complaints with no demonstrable stomach, duodenum, liver, or gall bladder disease in the hope of avoiding unnecessary, diagnostic laparoscopy. One of the major indications for ERCP is the necessity to look for residual or recurrent common bile duct stones following cholecystectomy. Diagnosis and evaluation of pancreatic disorders are enhanced by viewing the ductal anatomy, obtaining secretory material, and by the identification of pseudocysts or other mass lesions such as carcinoma of the duodenal papilla, the pancreas, and the biliary ducts. The obtaining of biopsies, brushings, and aspirations allow almost 100% accuracy in the hands of the experienced operator.

Endoscopic sphincterotomy can be performed under fluoroscopy and following ERCP when small stones are noted in the biliary tract.

The duodenal papilla can be easily located as the site of emptying of the pancreatic and hepatobiliary ducts in the ampulla of Vater. The presence of a pancreatic pseudocyst, or the distortion or dilatation of pancreatic ducts caused by pancreatitis, calculi, pancreatic tumors, carcinoma of the duodenal papilla, and papillary stenosis may be revealed by ERCP. Viewing the hepatobiliary tree permits evaluation of these canals for lesions, calculi, and irregular deviations suggesting biliary cirrhosis, primary sclerosing cholangitis, or carcinoma of the bile ducts.

ALTERNATIVES

Although the differentiation of surgical and nonsurgical jaundice can usually be made by computerized tomography (CT) scan or ultrasonography, ERCP plays a unique role by obtaining finer resolution of the site and type of obstruction of the biliary tree because it is the only nonsurgical method capable of defining the pancreatic ductal system, and it allows the operator to obtain tissue and fluid samples. ERCP has been reported to be as sensitive (if not more so) as ultrasonography in the diagnosis of biliary dilation or stones if unsuccessful examinations are excluded. CT scanning has approximately the same sensitivity, if unsuccessful ERCP examinations are excluded. Arteriography is significantly less sensitive than ERCP in diagnosing resectable pancreatic cancers, but, unlike ERCP, angiography is a useful tool to assess operability.

New techniques using nonionic surfactant added to the contrast material during ERCP has demonstrated increased sensitivity in cases of more peripherally located pancreatic tumors.

It is possible that percutaneous transhepatic cholangiography may be a simpler alternative to ERCP but it may be contraindicated if coagulation disorders are present; it has the added risk of hemorrhage, biliary leakage, and peritonitis.

POTENTIAL FOR FAILURE

ERCP is the most specific and sensitive test available for pancreatic and hepato-biliary disease. The ability to obtain tissue and fluid samples under direct visualization in conjunction with detailed radiographs of the involved ducts makes the procedure optimal. There is no test more specific, although unsuccessful ERCP can occur because of difficulties with endoscopy or duct cannulation. When this occurs, less specific tests must be used.

CONTRAINDICATIONS

ERCP cannot be performed in patients with obstructions of the esophagus or the pylorus. Recent bouts of pancreatitis contraindicate ERCP because of the possibility of recurrence. Under certain circumstances, however, such as pancreatitis caused by choledocholithiasis or an undiagnosed pseudocyst, ERCP can be performed safely. The known presence of a pancreatic pseudocyst is a relative contraindication, although the study may have some clinical utility and has been shown to be safe when carefully performed. Acute cholangitis precludes the safe performance of ERCP unless the procedure is done immediately preoperatively or is performed for drainage via sphincterotomy. Other types of infectious disease as well as severe or acute cardiorespiratory disease also contraindicate this procedure.

Generally, the procedure is not indicated for patients who are not considered surgical candidates at the time of the procedure.

Allergy to contrast material may also cause serious problems although even patients who are allergic to iodine have safely undergone ERCP using water-soluble contrast materials because the volume entering the bloodstream is unlikely to be enough to cause allergic reactions.

Contraindications to endoscopic sphincterotomy include a coagulation disorder, long strictures of the distal bile duct, abnormalities of the proximal bile ducts, a large stone (bigger than 2.5 cm), and acute pancreatitis.

PREPROCEDURE PREPARATION

Patients should have an empty stomach in order to prevent vomiting and aspiration. Dentures must be removed, and, if the examinee is a child, the teeth should be examined for any loose teeth that might become dislodged during the procedure.

The patient's history should be examined for hypersensitivity to iodine, seafood, or contrast material used for any other diagnostic procedure.

PATIENT EDUCATION

Patients should understand the procedure as thoroughly as possible. A description of the endoscope is helpful with emphasis on its narrowness. Patients should understand that they must be kept awake so that they can move when requested by the examiner in order to optimize viewing of various aspects of the gastrointestinal tract mucosa.

Patients should also be forewarned of the mildly uncomfortable feeling of "fullness" from the instillation of air or gas. Mild abdominal cramps may also result, most frequently when air is introduced into the duodenum.

The side effects of the anticholinergics that will be used to decrease peristalsis should be explained including dry mouth and blurred vision. Patients may also note transient flushing on injection of the contrast medium.

PROCEDURE

ERCP is generally performed in the radiology suite by a gastroenterologist and it generally requires 30 minutes to 2 hours. It is generally an inpatient procedure with the patient being observed for 24 hours following completion, although more centers are doing ERCP on an outpatient basis.. Precautions including monitoring of vital signs and continuous ECG monitoring is needed in some patients. Sedation with a benzodiazepine and meperidine is usually given. Atropine is often given to decrease salivary and gastric secretions and to prevent vagal bradycardia during the insertion of the scope. A local anesthetic is used to relax the throat and appropriate doses of intravenous sedation help the patient to relax.

The patient is asked to swallow the scope and the physician inspects the mucosa as the scope passes through the esophagus and the stomach. This is generally done with the patient in a left-lateral position. Gas or air is introduced into the lumen to obtain good views of the surface.

Once the duodenum is entered (figure 24–1), the patient is assisted to the prone position. At this stage, compazine and/or glucagon may be used to hinder peristalsis movement and the cannula, filled with contrast material, is passed through one of the channels of the endoscope. Approximately 2 to 5 ml of contrast material is injected under fluoroscopic guidance, initially, to visualize the pancreas. The hepatobiliary tree is then viewed by injection of 10 to 15 ml of contrast material into the common bile duct. When the needed radiographs have been taken, the cannula is removed. Before the endoscope is removed, tissue or fluid samples can be obtained for examination.

Endoscopic sphincterotomy involves diathermy cutting of the sphincter, allowing passage of the stones. Stones smaller than 10 mm usually pass within 1 to 2 weeks. A thin wire with a basket-like end covered by a plastic sheath can be inserted through the endoscope if spontaneous passage of the stones does not

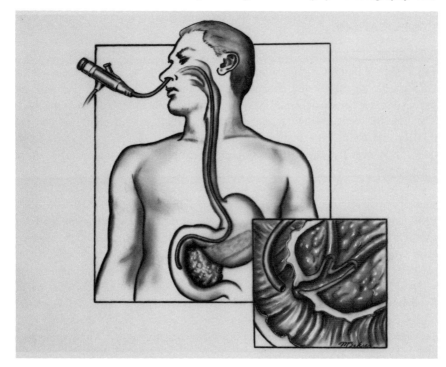

Figure 24–1. Endoscopic cannulation preparing to enter the pancreatic duct.

occur. Basket retrieval is difficult in cases in which there is inadequate room to open the basket or when there are large numbers of stones. Surgery is generally indicated for these patients.

Antibiotics may be indicated if stones or a stricture have been found.

POSTPROCEDURE INFORMATION

The patient is told to rest in bed for several hours following the examination and will require assistance in getting home if the procedure has been done on an outpatient basis. Food and fluids are withheld until the gag reflex recovers and the anesthetic effects disappear. A sore throat may remain for 24 to 48 hours after the procedure. Lozenges or appropriate gargles can be used to relieve the discomfort. Antibiotics may be indicated if a stone or a stricture has been found.

The patient should be observed for symptoms of shock or hemorrhage, including hematemesis, melena, tachycardia, pain, cough, abdominal distention, fever, and hypotension.

COMPLICATIONS

Surveys of complications of endoscopic procedures have demonstrated that ERCP has the highest complication rate (1.0% to 8.0%) of any diagnostic procedure. Only the therapeutic procedures of colonoscopy with polypectomy and pneumatic esophageal dilatation have rates comparable to those seen with ERCP. The mortality rate following the diagnostic ERCP examination lies between 0.001% and 0.8%. The majority of the fatalities are due to to bacterial infections. It is clear that the complication rate is proportional to the expertise of the endoscopist.

A rare mechanical complication is perforation or tear of the mucosa. Patients should watch for evidence of bleeding, especially if a biopsy has been done. Pain may also indicate perforation, and its localization may give a hint as to the site of the perforation. Neck and throat pain require evaluation of the cervical area, epigastric pain hints at trauma to the esophagus in the thoracic region, and shoulder pain or dyspnea may indicate perforation of the distal esophagus.

Other complications can include arrhythmias and syncope from endoscopy. Symptoms of ascending cholangitis following infection or obstruction of the biliary tree can occur and should be monitored for fever, chills, abdominal pain, and jaundice (if it is not already present). Gram negative sepsis with hypotension may subsequently develop. Pancreatitis may occur following contrast injection, of the pancreatic duct with severe epigastric pain, nausea and vomiting, fever, shock, elevated serum amylase levels, and transient hyperbilirubinemia. The complication of pancreatitis has been found to be diminished with the avoidance of repeated pancreatic duct injections. After injection pancreatitis and cholangitic sepsis, drug reaction (as in routine endoscopy) is the most common complication.

Other signs of complications can include respiratory depression, diaphoresis, bradycardia, and laryngospasm.

Another complication is infection of a pancreatic pseudocyst.

PATIENT QUESTIONS

Will I be able to breathe during the test?

Patients should be assured that they will be able to breathe during the entire test. The mouthguard used for protection of the patient and the endoscope will not obstruct the airway. Swallowing may be difficult, and the patient should allow the saliva to simply drain from the side of the mouth.

Can my pancreas be evaluated by a noninvasive test?

In symptomatic patients presenting for evaluation, ERCP has proved sensitivity and specificity in making the diagnosis of pancreatic cancer. Successful ERCPs are as accurate or more so than ultrasonography or CT scanning, but the latter two tests are much less expensive, easier to perform, and are associated with a lower morbidity. Most physicians do an ultrasound first, then an ERCP or a CT scan for clarification of an indeterminate ultrasound examination. The most cost effective screening test for early diagnosis of pancreatic cancer remains to be discovered.

Should my gallstones be removed endoscopically or by surgery?

Endoscopic retrograde sphincterotomy is a new therapeutic modality for stones less than 2.5 cm in diameter. Recurrent stenosis does not seem to be a major problem, and the complication rate compares favorably with that of surgical treatment of choledocholithiasis. Clearly, if surgical contraindications exist, endoscopic sphincterotomy is a viable option. More studies are needed, however, to determine ways to make the procedure safer, and to determine which patients will benefit most from nonsurgical intervention. Chemical dissolution of bile duct stones as an adjunct to endoscopic sphincterotomy is being investigated. At present, much depends on the skill of the endoscoper.

CONSENT

Informed consent is required with this invasive procedure.

SELECTED BIBLIOGRAPHY

Carr-Locke DL, Cotton PB: Biliary tract and pancreas. *Br Med Bull* 1986;Jul:42(3):257.

Classen M, Phillip J: Endoscopic retrograde cholangiopancreatography (ERCP) and endoscopic therapy in pancreatic disease. *Clin Gastroenterol* 1984;Sep:13(3):819.

Neoptolemos JP, London N, Slater ND, Carr-Locke DL: A prospective study of ERCP and endoscopic sphincterotomy in the diagnosis and treatment of gallstone acute pancreatitis. A rational and safe approach to management. *Arch Surg* 1986;Jun:121(6):697.

Paternel E: A high tech approach to a GI problem. Endoscopic retrograde cholangiopancreatography (ERCP) for gallstones. *RN* 1985;June:48(6):44.

25

Gastrointestinal Endoscopy

RICHARD SADOVSKY

Diagnostic endoscopy in the esophagus, stomach, and duodenum is the most commonly performed endoscopic examination of the gastrointestinal tract. The early 1960s saw the development of a flexible scope based on fiberoptic technology and, today, a 120 cm flexible scope is the standard unit for evaluation of the upper gastrointestinal tract.

Rigid proctosigmoidoscopy was first introduced in 1895 for investigation of rectal symptoms of bleeding, change in bowel habits, mucus discharge, and painful defecation. Rigid instruments changed little until the development of the flexible fiberoptic scopes in the late 1960s. Proctosigmoidoscopy has become the outpatient diagnostic tool of choice in the evaluation of rectal or colonic symptoms while colonoscopy permits evaluation of the entire bowel up to the cecum.

INDICATIONS

Upper gastrointestinal (GI) endoscopy has a very high rate of accuracy in diagnosing peptic ulcers, cancer, and causes of upper gastrointestinal hemorrhage. Indications include persistent symptoms not diagnosed on upper GI series, evaluation of the postoperative stomach, or a radiologic abnormality needing further clarification. Many practitioners are using endoscopy as the initial means of evaluating a dyspeptic patient who is unresponsive to treatment. Upper GI hemorrhage evaluation, and re-evaluation of patients who have been treated for peptic ulcers can be done endoscopically. Endoscopic findings may include esophagitis, esophageal cancer, esophageal varices, gastric ulcers, neoplasms, other gastric lesions such as mucosal changes and gastritis, duodenal ulcers, arteriovenous malformations, and duodenal tumors. A variety of therapeutic maneuvers including electrocoagulation, sclerotherapy, esophageal dilation, foreign body removal, laser therapy, and polypectomy have become available.

Proctosigmoidoscopy, using a short fiberoptic flexible scope 30 to 65 cm in length, views the rectum, sigmoid colon, and often the lower portion of the descending colon. This procedure is important because it can visualize the lower 10 cm of the rectum not seen on barium enema and allows mucosal examination of the bowel. The procedure can be easily learned by the operator. Flexible fibersigmoidoscopes are clearly superior to the rigid scopes in detecting both benign and malignant lesions. A rigid scope can view an average distance of approximately 20 cm of the lower bowel, while the flexible scope can view much more. Indications include evaluation of lower colon symptoms such as rectal bleeding, diarrhea, constipation, or abdominal pain, and the procedure can be used as a screening procedure to detect colorectal polyps and cancer in patients over 40 or 50 years of age depending on the guidelines the practitioner chooses to follow. Patients with familial polyposis or other risk factors should be scoped regularly at a younger age. Some authorities advise flexible sigmoidoscopy prior to barium enema studies in all circumstances. Flexible sigmoidoscopes have virtually replaced the rigid scopes because of the inability of the latter to truly evaluate the sigmoid colon.

Colonoscopy using 140 to 180 cm scopes allow total examination of the bowel to the cecum. The reasons for performing colonoscopy are somewhat different from those for proctosigmoidoscopy because the procedure is more expensive and involves greater discomfort to the patient. Indications include (1) the evaluation of an abnormality revealed on a barium enema, (2) unexplained rectal bleeding, diarrhea, or other rectal discharge, (3) evaluation of inflammatory bowel disease, (4) pre-operative and postoperative assessment, (5) the evaluation of patients with polyps detected on proctosigmoidoscopy to look for other lesions above 50 cm, and (6) in order to perform a therapeutic procedure such as polypectomy or destruction of vascular malformations. Colonoscopy is generally not helpful in patients with unexplained abdominal pain.

Future indications for endoscopy may be the need to mount ultrasound equipment on the endoscope tip to allow dramatic views of organs around the stomach. The placement of prosthesis through malignant strictures obviating the need for surgery may also became more routine in the future as larger channel scopes are perfected. The use of percutaneous endoscopic gastrostomy is also being explored.

ALTERNATIVES

The recent development of increased accuracy and detail of examination by endoscopy has stimulated radiologists to improve barium studies so that high quality, double-contrast barium studies have increased diagnostic yields tremendously. A well-prepared double-contrast barium enema may be less expensive to perform than colonoscopy, but problems in interpretation may occur. Barium may better track through fistulas and strictures that may be invisible to the endoscopist, but errors in the radiographic reading of the sigmoid and the cecum are frequent. Proctosigmoidoscopy does, however, allow a better view of the distal colon, which is a weak point of the barium radiographic examinations. Colonoscopy has a higher detection rate for mucosal abnormalities, colitis conditions, and polyps than does the barium enema, but approximately 5% of colonoscopic evaluations are difficult, severely painful, or impossible even in expert hands. These patients may require a repeat examination or further study using some other diagnostic modality. In addition, colonoscopy is unpredictable from patient to patient and, in the hands of inexpert examiners, can have an unacceptable complication rate.

POSSIBILITY OF FAILURE

Colonoscopy is difficult in the patient who has had prior pelvic surgery or who has diverticular disease because of the relative fixation of the sigmoid colon.

CONTRAINDICATIONS

The only contraindication to upper endoscopy is the presence of an esophageal stricture that will not allow passage of the endoscope. Potential hazards may be encountered with cervical kyphosis, anterior osteophytic proliferation on the cervical spine, Zencker's diverticulum, and thoracic or abdominal aneurysms, but proper precautions can allow a safe examination. The patient who is agitated or in shock, who has had caustic injury to the esophagus, or who has an aortic arch aneurysm requires care on the part of the endoscopist.

Sigmoidoscopy is relatively contraindicated in patients with acute inflammatory bowel disease, toxic megacolon, or acute intraabdominal conditions.

Contraindications to colonoscopy include evidence of peritonitis, impending perforation, or acute diverticulitis, and it is not recommended during the unstable period for several weeks following a myocardial infarction. The possibility of bacteremia is an indication for using antibiotics if there is heart valve disease or replacement.

PREPROCEDURE PREPARATION

The preparation for upper GI endoscopy requires a fast for at least 6 hours. Simethicone may be administered to eliminate bubbling in the stomach.

Preparation for proctosigmoidoscopy is minimal, requiring the use of one or two disposable phosphate enemas, or a similar preparation, immediately prior to the procedure. The precise preparatory regimen may depend on the age of the patient, the bowel transit time, and the specific indication for the procedure. The sigmoidoscopes with larger suction channels allow greater removal of any solid material remaining in the bowel than do the colonoscopes.

Preparation for colonoscopy involves liquefaction of bowel contents together with colonic lavage. This is usually accomplished by 2 to 3 days of a low-residue diet followed by a liquid diet for 24 hours prior to the procedure. On the day before the procedure, the patient takes some type of laxative preparation to clean the bowel and release the contents. On the day of the examination, a colonic enema is usually administered leaving the colon well cleansed and allowing for a relatively pain-free procedure. The recently introduced of effective total gut irrigation solution allows safer cleansing of the gut and the avoiding of laxatives. These electrolyte preparations, however, must be drunk at a rate of at least 1 liter each hour for several hours until a clear rectal effluent is obtained. Some patients may have difficulty drinking this large quantity of liquid. Following the bowel cleansing with these electrolyte solutions, the patient is placed on a liquid diet until colonoscopy is performed.

Laboratory evaluations including electrolytes, blood count, and bleeding and coagulation profiles should be done prior to colonoscopy. A rectal inspection and digital examination should be done before to every sigmoidoscopy and colonoscopy to determine the possible presence of a rectal mass because the initial 6 cm insertion of the scope is done blindly. In addition, the examination helps to relax the sphincter.

PATIENT EDUCATION

The patient should have a good understanding of the procedure. A well-motivated patient can be tremendously helpful to the examiner and will facilitate the procedure. The patient who understands the possibility of a feeling of fullness or bloating will be able to better tolerate the discomfort.

Colonoscopy is generally performed under sedation with one of the benzodiazipines and with the addition of an analgesic although the use of these medications varies among centers. Patients with prosthetic heart valves, ascites, or severe immunodepression should probably be given appropriate prophylactic antibiotic coverage.

PROCEDURE

Esophagogastroduodenoscopy for diagnostic purposes can be done as an outpatient procedure. The pharynx may be anesthetized with a spray or gargle. The patient then lies in the left lateral decubitus position and a plastic mouthpiece is placed between the teeth. Under direct vision, the practitioner then introduces the endoscope as rapidly as possible into the duodenum. As the endoscope is withdrawn, the descending duodenum and the duodenal bulb are studied. Moving the scope further outward allows examination of the stomach esophagus, pharynx, epiglottis, and the vocal cords.

Proctosigmoidoscopy is performed with minimal, if any, sedation, and takes approximately 10 minutes to perform (figure 25–1). The patient lies on the left side. The patient's comfort is important and the precise position may vary depending on the patient's preference. The instrument is well lubricated and the tip is advanced, under direct visualization, following the bowel lumen by angulating the scope tip. After maximum insertion, which should not cause great discomfort, the instrument is slowly withdrawn with the operator scanning the circumference of the bowel.

Colonoscopy generally requires about 20 to 45 minutes and can be done as an outpatient procedure. The basic technique of colonoscopy involves insertion of the tip of the scope into the rectum, advancing the colonoscope into the rectum, managing bends by using the up-and-down control and rotating the instrument with slight use of the right-to-left control. The use of insufflation and suction with air and the appropriate positioning of the patient allows the colon to stretch on the colonoscope, usually avoiding large loops. Views of the colon mucosa are obtained both during insertion and withdrawal.

Therapeutic procedures such as polypectomy or destruction of vascular malformations can be done through the scope by fulguration or by snare with or without a diathermy current.

POSTPROCEDURE INFORMATION

Upper GI endoscopy and proctosigmoidoscopy are relatively benign procedures, and the patient should be able to leave the examiner's office shortly after the examination concludes. If some invasive therapeutic or diagnostic procedure has been done through the scope, the patient may be uncomfortable and will require assistance returning home. Following colonoscopy, the patient is allowed to rest for 1 or 2 hours to permit the medications to wear off and to be monitored for complications. Hospitalization might be recommended if an unanticipated complication occurs.

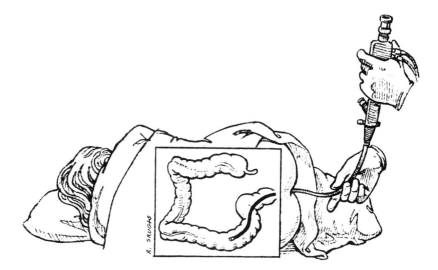

Figure 25–1. Flexible sigmoidoscopy.

The patient can return to work the next day following an uneventful diagnostic endoscopy. Therapeutic endoscopes may require longer observation and recuperative periods. Evidence of prolonged bleeding as determined by the presence of blood in the stool, fever, malaise, pain, abdominal distention, or changes in eating habits should be reported to the physician.

COMPLICATIONS

Upper GI endoscopy has the potential major complications of (1) perforation, (2) bleeding, (3) cardiopulmonary accidents, (4) adverse reactions to the premedications, and (5) infections. Perforation occurs rarely and generally is due to instrument trauma to an inflamed area. Bleeding may follow polypectomy but rarely requires transfusion. Cardiac arrhythmias may occur in patients with cardiac disease and these patients should be monitored appropriately. The most common complication, i.e., respiratory depression, is generally seen in the elderly or the cirrhotic patient and results from the premedication.

Flexible sigmoidoscopy has one major potential complication, that of colonic perforation. The incidence of this is rare, probably less than 1 in 5,000 cases. Bacteremia is another possible complication, but appears to occur much less with the use of the flexible scopes because of the smaller diameter of the instrument.

Preparation for colonoscopy can cause fluid and electrolyte imbalance with dehydration and hypovolemia cause by the ingestion of hypertonic solutions.

Recently developed inert osmotic electrolyte solutions may decrease this complication. The use of intravenous valium may cause respiratory depression or apnea. Thrombophlebitis or pulmonary embolism are also rare complications of diazepam usage. Hypotension, nausea, and vomiting may occur concurrently with narcotic analgesic.

Colonoscopy is a major procedure and can result in perforation or serious hemorrhage. Perforations resulting in death following colonoscopic post-polypectomy surveillance have occurred. Less serious, but more frequent complications such as a vasovagal reflex and a postcolonoscopy distension syndrome can occur. These are particularly distressing to the patient and may be associated with excessive air insufflation during the examination.

The majority of the complications of colonoscopy occur as a result of polypectomy or biopsy during the endoscopy. Hemorrhage may be primary or may be delayed for up to 1 to 14 days, and perforation is more likely to occur and may even be initially silent.

PATIENT QUESTIONS

Is endoscopy safe for my child?

Pediatric practice has approached adult practice in the use of gastrointestinal endoscopic procedures. Recent studies have even confirmed the safety and efficacy of upper gastrointestinal endoscopy on infants less than 25 months of age using minimal or no anesthesia. Smaller caliber instruments have been developed that can negotiate the gastrointestinal tract of children with great ease. General anesthesia may be needed when endoscoping a child because of increased dangers of stretching and possible perforation of the intestine or bowel, but many more centers are using intravenous sedation or no sedation at all when appropriate.

Is endoscopy painful?

Upper GI endoscopy and proctosigmoidoscopy are uncomfortable, but are often accomplished with a minimum of anesthesia. While colonoscopy involves some discomfort, the sensations are fairly well tolerated by most patients, and experience has shown that most patients will consent to the procedure a second time or more if necessary. Additional medication can be provided during the procedure if the patient cannot manage the cramping and uncomfortable sensation.

Why do I need to have repeat examinations?

When endoscopy is used judiciously as a screening tool, it can help to locate tumors and other pathology of the bowel early enough for potentially successful treatment. Endoscopy is also used posttreatment in a number of situations to preclude recurrence of disease. Some examples of this are postgastrectomy for cancer, postcolectomy for colon tumors, postpolypectomy in high-risk patients, and posttreatment of duodenal and gastric ulcers. Direct visualization of a viscus is the most effective way to recognize the development of pathology.

CONSENT

Consent is generally required for upper endoscopy and for colonoscopy. Consent for polypectomy should be obtained along with that for colonoscopy in case an unexpected polyp is encountered. Proctosigmoidoscopy is a relatively benign procedure and, at this time, consent is obtained at the discretion of the examiner. It is certainly a good idea to obtain informed consent before performing all invasive examinations and procedures.

SELECTED BIBLIOGRAPHY

Gibb SP, Laney JS, Tarshis AM: Use of fiberoptic endoscopy in diagnosis and therapy of upper gastroenterological disorders. *Med Clin North Am* 1986;Nov:70:6:1307.

McSherry CK, Cwern M, Ferstenberg H, Ghazi A, Sekons DH, Shinya H, Wolff WW: Interventional endoscopy. *Curr Prob Surg* 1985;Jul:22:7:1.

Neugat AI, Forde KA: Screening colonoscopy: has the time come? *Am J Gastroenterol* 1988;Mar:83:3:295.

Norfleet RG: Endoscopy: lower GI tract. *Hosp Med* 1986;Mar:30. 20:6:26.

Schuman BM: Endoscopy: upper GI tract. *Hosp Med* 1986;Feb:22:2:111–114, 116–117.

Turner JM: Flexible sigmoidoscopy. *Fam Pract Recert* 1988;July:10:7:20.

26

Gastrointestinal Motility Studies

RICHARD SADOVSKY

Gastrointestinal motility studies can be done grossly using radiographic contrast imaging or, more precisely, by manometric studies. The upper gastrointestinal series with small bowel follow through can offer some information about motility problems such as achalasia and cardiospasm. Manometry, utilizing measurements of intraluminal pressure events by means of pressure sensitive transducers, offers more precise data about esophageal spasm and competency of the cardiac sphincter.

INDICATIONS

Symptoms related to gastrointestinal motility are extremely common in medical practice. Most knowledge of gastrointestinal motility has been obtained in animal experiments.

Oropharyngeal dysphagia is a problem with the movement of solids or liquids from the oropharynx into the upper esophagus. Symptoms include hesitancy in initiation of swallows, food or liquid sticking in the throat, nasal or oral regurgitation, and coughing after swallowing. This can be caused by neuromuscular diseases, local factors, and by dysfunction of the upper esophageal sphincter. Swallowing disorders are evaluated by cinematographic visualization and manometry. Manometry provides helpful information about pharyngeal motility, resting pressure, relaxation of the sphincter, and coordination between contraction and relaxation phases.

Esophageal motility disorders may present as chest pain, dysphagia, or a choking sensation and can sometimes be qualitatively seen on conventional barium studies. Manometry is very useful in evaluating esophageal motility disturbances. Motor activity of the esophagus can be determined and precise information is obtained concerning the function of the esophageal body and of the upper and lower sphincter. Esophageal motility disorders may be secondary to several systemic diseases including scleroderma, and diabetes mellitus. Manometric studies may be helpful in these patients and may even document systemic disease long before esophageal involvement is clinically evident.

Gastroesophageal reflux presents with symptoms of dysphagia, frequent nocturnal regurgitation of undigested food, and nocturnal wheezing, coughing, and choking due to aspiration of regurgitated material from the dilated, obstructed esophagus. This condition is not an indication for motility studies since these examinations have a low level of sensitivity and specificity and manometry demonstrates poor sphincter pressure in only a small number of these patients.

Stomach motility disorders can be evaluated using manometry. Pressures can be measured and intubation allows for measurement of gastric emptying of known quantities of marked liquid.

Duodenogastric reflux is not well evaluated by contrast radiography or manometry. Endoscopic gastritis, mucosal biopsy evidence of gastritis, and intubation measurements of gastric emptying and duodenogastric reflux provide the diagnosis.

Small intestine motility problems can be observed by barium flow under cinefluorography, but observation time is limited. Manometric studies can be done from multiple sites of the small intestine, but prolonged recording of intestinal motility by intubation is uncomfortable for the patient.

The gross pattern of **colonic movements** can be studied by radiocinematography after barium ingestion. Colonic transit can be measured after ingestion of radiopaque markers. Manometry has recently been used in the rectum and the sigmoid of patients with irritable bowel syndrome with some conflicting results at present. The use of motility studies in irritable bowel syndromes still requires further study as the precise nature of the motility disorder in this syndrome has not yet been firmly established.

An esophageal source of **chest pain** should be sought after cardiac evaluation has been completed and following an upper GI series and gall bladder series. If the source of chest pain has not been determined, patients can be studied with 24 hour ambulatory esophageal motility and a pH system. Abnormalities in pH are associated slightly more often with noncardiac chest pain than motility abnormalities. However, the majority of episodes of chest pain do not correlate with either abnormality and may be the result of decreased esophageal pain threshhold for distention.

Manometric studies appear to be useful in the evaluation of fecal incontinence and, utilizing visual cues from the direct-writing display recorder, patients with fecal incontinence can be taught sphincter strengthening exercises to increase the tone of the external sphincter.

ALTERNATIVES

Electromyography has been used to study the sequence of buccal and pharyngeal contractions and may be helpful if the motility disorder is neuromuscular in origin.

Esophageal motility problems can be studied in many ways including measurements of clearance of instilled acid, 24-hour pH ambulatory monitoring (still in the testing and standardization stages), and esophageal scintigraphy (utilizing a bolus of water labelled with technetium 99m sulfur colloid or radiolabelled test meals). This latter technique allows quantitative assessment of therapy and has been used to test the efficacy of administration of nifedipine and isosorbide dinitrate and pneumatic dilatation on esophageal emptying. At present, esophageal scintigraphy is the most sensitive test for evaluating esophageal emptying and appears to be useful in regularly evaluating medical management of motility problems such as achalasia. Its use in routine practice, however, is limited by the need for expensive equipment and radioisotopes.

Stomach motility disorders evaluated by gastric emptying measurements via intubation and aspiration are qualitative at best and can be enhanced by use of radionuclide scintigraphy. Recently, real-time ultrasonic imaging of the stomach has been described enabling the study of gastric contractions in response to a test meal.

Small bowel transit can be measured in a noninvasive way by the appearance of hydrogen in expired air after ingestion of a nonabsorbable carbohydrate, usually lactulose. This technique measures mouth-to-cecum transit time, and so the rate of gastric emptying greatly influences the results.

POTENTIAL FOR FAILURE

Conventional barium studies are of low sensitivity in detecting esophageal motility disorders and the results are difficult to quantify.

Motility disorders, such as esophageal spasm, are usually difficult to detect by radiologic study since spasms may be transient and erratic. Manometry is a better tool for detecting such disorders, especially when various provocative agents are used during manometry such as edrophonium and bethanacol. However, achalasia (cardiospasm) is strongly suggested on conventional radiographic study when the esophagus has a beaking appearance (caused by the smoothly tapered narrowing at the distal end of the esophagus), and gastric reflux appears as a backflow of barium from the stomach into the esophagus. Manometric evaluation in these patients is not confirmatory and does not correlate with symptoms In patients with achalasia, manometric studies may be more diagnostic.

Barium studies and manometry have low sensitivity and specificity in the evaluation of heartburn and reflux esophagitis. The symptom complex is usually established from the patient's history, and can be confirmed by endoscopy and biopsy of the distal esophagus. Confirmation of the presence of acid-mediated chest pain can be obtained by an acid perfusion (Bernstein) test. This involves administering infusions of 0.1 N hydrochloric acid alternating with saline into a nasoesophageal tube while the patient is in an upright sitting position. If the patient notes chest pain regularly during acid perfusion and no pain during saline perfusion, the test is positive. The acid perfusion test does not identify esophagitis but it does show the sensitivity of the esophagus to acid. Reproduction of the patient's symptoms suggests esophageal origin. Endoscopy is important in the diagnosis of secondary complications such as stenosis or esophagitis. The use of manometry in patients with heartburn should be reserved for patients in whom a surgical antireflux procedure is planned.

Gastroesophageal scintigraphy is a sensitive noninvasive test for detecting gastroesophageal reflux and it also allows the reflux to be quantified. The 24-hour esophageal H monitoring identifies the presence of abnormal gastroesophageal reflux and can distinguish whether the patient's symptoms are being caused by reflux. This can be done as an outpatient and, with the future improvement of radiotelemetric recording systems, patient compliance and physician's diagnostic skills will improve.

CONTRAINDICATIONS

The upper GI series and small bowel series is contraindicated in patients with obstruction or perforation of the digestive tract. In these patients, barium may worsen the obstruction or leak into the abdominal cavity.

Manometry done through a catheter placed in the gastrointestinal tract through the nose or the mouth has no contraindications.

The acid perfusion test is contraindicated in patients with esophageal varices, congestive heart failure, acute myocardial infarction, or other cardiac disorders.

PREPROCEDURE PREPARATION

Patient preparation for contrast motility studies is the same as that for the upper GI contrast study. A low-residue diet is recommended for 2 to 3 days prior to the test, and the patient is advised to fast and not smoke after midnight before the test. Most oral medications should be withheld after midnight, and anticholinergic and narcotics withheld for 24 hours before.

These instructions are the same prior to manometry.

PATIENT EDUCATION

Motility evaluations done by contrast material may take up to 6 hours to complete, and the patient should be advised to bring along some reading material to the test site. The test may involve rotation of the x-ray table putting the patient into various positions. The patient is securely placed on the table and may, in addition, be asked to move into supine, prone, and side positions. The barium mixture will taste chalky but must be completely ingested. A cathartic and/or a saline or tapwater enema may be advised the evening before the test.

Manometry procedures require the use of a catheter to enter the gastrointestinal tract. The patient should be advised of the possible discomfort of the procedure and the tendency to gag or retch. Reassurance should be given that the operator will be gentle and not cause pain.

PROCEDURE

Gastrointestinal motility studies done using radiography involve monitoring the passage of barium through the upper intestine (figure 26–1). The patient is asked to ingest the barium at appropriate intervals that will allow careful study of all the upper gastrointestinal structures. As the barium passes through the digestive tract, fluoroscopy reveals the outlines of peristalsis and the mucosal contours. The evaluation of the upper gastrointestinal tract generally takes several hours and concludes when the barium reaches the ileocecal valve and the region around it and enters the cecum.

Approximately 6 hours following contrast ingestion, the head of the barium column is usually in the hepatic flexure; the tail in the terminal ileum. The barium causes complete opacification of the large bowel 24 hours after ingestion. Spot films are taken 24, 48, and 72 hours after barium ingestion to evaluate motility and movement of the contrast column. When spot films suggest intestinal abnormalities, more specific studies such as colonoscopy and additional contrast procedures may be helpful.

Manometry involves passage of the catheter either through the nose or mouth using topical anesthesia when needed (figure 26–2). Passage of the catheter into the esophagus is best performed in the sitting position. The catheter is then

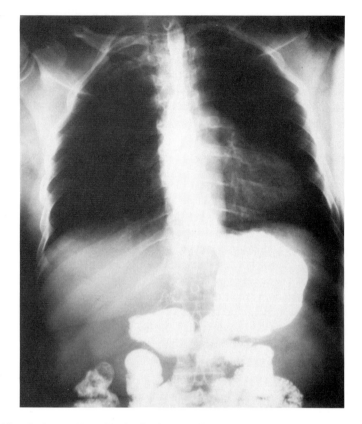

Figure 26–1. Barium swallow with visualization of a dilated esophagus.

passed further to the desired location. A mouthpiece is often used to prevent the patient from biting the tubing. This also helps to keep the tube steady and minimizes movement during the study. The pH may be recorded at this time. Pressure measurements are taken intermittently usually as the tube is being slowly withdrawn.

Pressure transducers for manometry may be present in the catheter itself, or a water perfusion system may be used with externally located transducers. Pressure waves are recorded on a multichannel pen writer.

POSTPROCEDURE INFORMATION

Following radiographic gastrointestinal study, the patient should be allowed to rest because the procedure exhausts most patients. If the test is being done on an

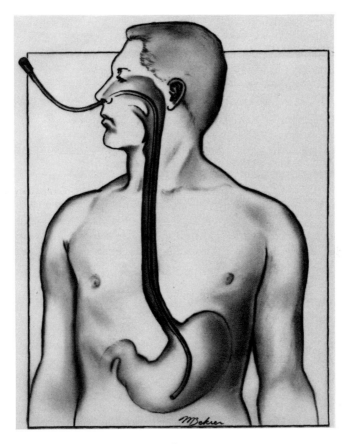

Figure 26–2. Nasogastric tube entering the stomach.

outpatient, it is advisable, although not absolutely necessary, for someone to accompany the patient and to assist in the return home.

Stool may be lightly colored for 24 to 72 hours. If fecal impaction occurs due to barium ingestion for more than 2 to 3 days, the physician should be notified.

Following intubation for manometry, the patient may complain of a sore throat. Soothing lozenges can be recommended.

COMPLICATIONS

Barium studies may cause discomfort and constipation in some patients. Administration of contrast for radiography is considered a benign procedure when done properly.

Manometric evaluation done through a narrow catheter has minimal morbidity and mortality. Care must be taken to determine that the catheter enters the esophagus and not the trachea. Rarely, episodes of arrhythmia have been reported during intubation. Vomiting may cause aspiration of fluid into the lungs as may improper removal of the catheter from the esophagus.

PATIENT QUESTIONS

Will I gag or have difficulty breathing when the tube is put in my throat?

Patients generally have great fear of gagging, of not being able to breathe with the tube in place, or of being unable to swallow the tubing at all. It is helpful to inform the patient that a certain amount of gagging is commonly experienced by all patients. If care is taken to allay the patient's fears prior to the study, the patient's cooperation will be greatly enhanced.

If the procedure results are abnormal, does that mean the cause of my symptoms has been found?

It should be noted that many abnormal motility patterns may not produce symptoms or be otherwise clinically significant. There is also no totally reliable way to determine the relationship of discovered abnormalities to the patient's symptoms. Findings can be regarded only as a clue to the possible gastrointestinal etiology of symptoms. Certainly, the occurrence of symptoms during the documentation of abnormal motility may strengthen the diagnosis, but certainty is not possible.

Why are multiple tests needed to evaluate gastrointestinal motility?

Patients presenting with dysphagia generally have a barium contrast study as the first procedure of choice. Hints of structural lesions are then studied and biopsied by endoscopy. If the radiograph is normal, manometry is the next procedure of choice. If manometry does not give the answer, radionuclide transit studies might be performed.

If chest pain is the presenting symptom, coronary artery disease should be ruled out. Then barium contrast radiographs are done and, possibly, an oral cholecystogram. If no structural lesions are identified, certain clinical circumstances may indicate endoscopy and then manometric studies.

The tests are done in this general order to minimize patient risk, to complete the tests that give the broadest information first, and to obtain hints that may localize the pathology allowing greater manometric accuracy.

CONSENT

Consent is not currently required for contrast radiography of the gastrointestinal tract.

Manometric studies or other evaluations that require the use of a tube placed into the gastrointestinal tract are considered invasive studies. Patients should understand the procedure, the accompanying sensations, the probability of obtaining information useful for diagnosis and treatment, and the potential complications. Signed consent is needed.

SELECTED BIBLIOGRAPHY

Anuras S, Loening-Baucke V: Gastrointestinal motility in the elderly. *J Amer Geriatr Soc* 1984;May:32(5):386.

Cohen LB: Clinical application of gastrointestinal motility studies. *Mt. Sinai J Med (NY)* 1984;Sep:51(5):620.

Dabaghi RE, Scott LD: Evaluation of esophageal diseases. *Am Fam Physician* 1986;Jan:33(1):119.

Gelfand MD, Botoman VA: Esophageal motility disorders: a clinical overview. *Am J Gastroenterol* 1987;Mar:82(3):181.

McCallum RW: Diagnosing motility disorders of the upper gastrointestinal tract. *South Med J* 1984;Aug:77(8):947.

27

Gastrointestinal Radiographic Dye Studies

DAVID H. GORDON

Barium swallow or esophagography is the cineradiographic examination of the pharynx and the esophagus following ingestion of barium mixtures. This test is usually performed as part of an upper gastrointestinal series. **The upper gastrointestinal series and small bowel follow through** examines the esophagus, stomach, and the small bowel. Peristalsis and mucosal outlines are traced with spot films recording significant findings. **Barium enema** is the radiographic examination of the large bowel after rectal instillation of barium (single contrast technique) or barium and air (double-contrast technique). **Hypotonic duodenography** is the fluoroscopic examination of the duodenum after instillation of barium and air through an intestinal catheter and injection of glucagon to distend the duodenum.

Oral cholecystography works on the principle that orally administered Telopaque®, which is an iodinated contrast material, is absorbed through the bowel, excreted by the hepatocytes in the liver into the biliary tree and stored in the gall bladder where it is concentrated. Following adequate opacification of the gall bladder, radiographs are taken to view the gall bladder.

INDICATIONS

Indications for **upper and lower gastrointestinal tract contrast studies** can include symptoms derived from any part of the entire tract. Esophageal symptoms such as dysphagia, reflux, inability to swallow, hematemesis, repeated pulmonary infections possibly caused by reflux or abnormal peristalsis of the food bolus, and heartburn warrant an esophagram to outline the lining of that structure. Gastric and duodenal symptoms of pain, persistent vomiting, hematemesis, feelings of early satiety, gastric outlet obstruction, reflux and/or heartburn or the presence of a mass on physical examination may be evaluated by upper GI series. Small bowel symptoms such as absorption problems, fatty or bulky, floating stools, blood or mucus in the stool, recurrent small bowel obstruction, weight loss, and repeated bleeding with no definable lesion warrant performing a small bowel series. Hypotonic duodenography is indicated in patients with clear evidence of duodenal or pancreatic pathology such as severe upper abdominal pain.

Large bowel studies or barium enemas are indicated to evaluate symptoms arising from the region of the ileocecal valve to the anus. Indications include gastrointestinal bleeding that appears to originate in the lower bowel, lower abdominal pain, iron deficiency anemia of unknown etiology, change in bowel habits, change in size or consistency of stool, excessive flatulence, or postcolostomy evaluations. Symptoms of obstruction also require evaluation of the colon.

Oral cholecystography is indicated for suspicion of gallstones. Symptoms may include right upper quadrant pain, jaundice, dyspepsia, or other ill-defined right upper quadrant symptoms. The presence of gall stone ileus or the presence of cholecystitis also requires evaluation of the gall bladder although this technique is not of value in acute cholecystitis.

Contrast study of the esophagus (esophagram) includes an assessment of the esophageal mucosa and the presence of any anatomic abnormality. Ulcerations and mucosal destruction from any cause can be clearly seen. Impingement on the esophagus by extrinsic lesions such as vascular anomalies or masses can be ascertained as can narrowing at any point. Pulsion and traction diverticuli can be well defined by esophogram. Hiatal hernia and reflux can be distinguished. Enlargement of the left atrium may be found on esophagram although echocardiography and magnetic resonance imaging (MRI) are less invasive methods of defining the left atrium.

Upper gastrointestinal series with small bowel follow through (figure 27–1) can reveal inflammatory diseases including ulcers, gastritis, diverticula, malabsorption syndromes, motility disorders, hiatus hernia, and Crohn's disease. In addition, masses can be evaluated with some ability to determine malignancy by the effect of the mass on peristalsis. Malignant masses usually interrupt peristalsis while benign masses do not. Small bowel evaluations look closely at the

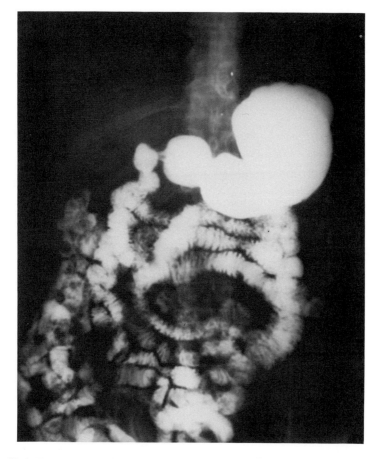

Figure 27–1. Upper gastrointestinal series demonstrating the stomach and the small intestine.

mucosal patterns. A specific diagnosis is unlikely and biopsy through an endoscope is required when mucosal abnormalities are found. Anatomic abnormalities such as internal hernias and partial obstruction or kinks in the bowel can be seen. Occasionally, hints about pancreatitis or pancreatic masses are noted by alterations in the loops or in the duodenal mucosa. These findings mandate further study of the pancreas. Hypotonic duodenography can demonstrate small duodenal lesions and tumors of the head of the pancreas that press on the duodenal wall. Positive findings require further tests such as amylase determinations, endoscopic retograde cholangiopancreatography (ERCP), pancreatic ultrasound, or pancreatic computerized tomography (CAT) scanning. Barium enemas allow visualization of the large bowel mucosa and walls (figure 27–2). Inflammatory diseases can be detected as well as polyps, mass lesions, congenital malforma-

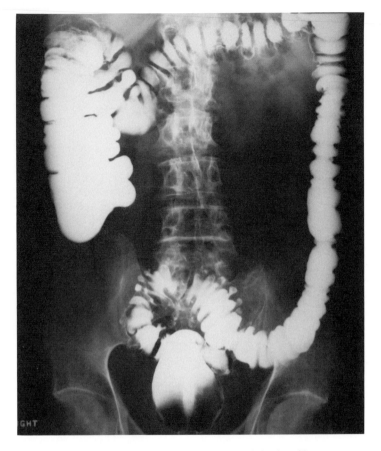

Figure 27–2. Barium enema demonstrating the large intestine and the sigmoid.

tions of the colon, and structural changes in the bowel such as intussusception and volvulus.

Air-contrast studies of the upper and lower gastrointestinal tract are considered to be the best procedure for evaluation of the mucosal surface although for wall exophytic lesions the CT scan is of greater benefit. Hypotonic duodenography may be employed when specific symptoms point to the duodenum.

Oral cholecystography demonstrates the morphology of the gall bladder including septations and other filling defects in the gall bladder such as polyps. Gall bladder carcinoma is occasionally revealed usually as an incidental finding in the presence of gall stones. Nonvisualization of the gall bladder may mean the presence of acute cholecystitis, with or without gall stones. An additional explanation may be the obstruction of the cystic duct preventing the contrast material from entering the gall bladder.

ALTERNATIVES

Information about the esophagus can be learned in many other ways. The introduction of endoscopic techniques has permitted direct visualization of the gastrointestinal mucosa allowing diagnosis in the esophagus of varices and other intraluminal abnormalities. A biopsy can be done at the same time allowing tissue diagnosis of the abnormality when indicated. Angiography and CT scanning can also reveal varices and mass lesions. Esophagoscopy also permits direct visualization of the mucosa, but it is less effective in defining fistulae that are better outlined by contrast studies.

Upper gastrointestinal studies are being replaced in many centers by endoscopy. Initial CT scans of the stomach and generally not of value especially when the mucosa is of special interest. Wall lesions, however, may be better evaluated by the CT scan. CT scans of the small bowel are possible and can reveal evidence of internal hernias, sites of bowel obstruction, inflammatory changes, and diverticuli.

The barium enema is a relatively definitive test, but a specific diagnosis may not be possible from the morphologic appearance of the mucosa. Various colitic conditions will appear similar on the radiographs. Colonoscopy allows direct visualization of the colon and biopsy. Where this procedure is readily available, it has largely replaced barium enemas.

The presence of gallstones and other gall bladder pathology is being more commonly determined by ultrasound. In many centers, ultrasound has become the preferred initial procedure. CT scans will reveal gall stones but, because of ionizing radiation, CT scans are not done to look specifically at the contents of the gall bladder.

POSSIBILITY OF FAILURE

A properly performed esophogram will coat the mucosa well and delineate both intrinsic and extrinsic masses impinging on the esophagus. Endoscopy does give the opportunity for a biopsy. Vascular rings are defined more clearly by angiography or by MRI. Motility studies will often require manometry to achieve a definitive diagnosis.

An upper gastrointestinal series is a highly sensitive technique. The presence of a mass lesion requires endoscopy and biopsy. Wall lesions can often be evaluated more precisely with CT scanning. Evaluation of the small bowel is a difficult task. Changes in the mucosal pattern is the main objective of the small bowel series. Clarification of an abnormality is usually by biopsy unless the picture is typical of Crohn's disease. Sprue and celiac syndromes are less specific.

Large bowel disorders are being diagnosed primarily by colonoscopy at present with the exception of arteriovenous malformations that often require angiography. Current thinking is that a CT scan is more accurate at defining diverticulitis especially when complications such as abscess formation or fistulas have developed.

Oral cholecystography is a highly accurate test with a 97% sensitivity. It is comparable to ultrasound in its efficacy. For the diagnosis of gall stones, it is rare that any additional test will be needed. There are equivocal results in which suboptimal visualization occurs and ultrasound or a CT scan will be required. Impaired hepatic function with jaundice (a serum bilirubin level greater then 3 mg/dl) result in decreased excretion of the contrast material into the bile. This prevents adequate visualization of the biliary tract. These patients must be studied using ultrasound or transhepatic cholangiography.

CONTRAINDICATIONS

An esophogram can be performed under any circumstances as long as the procedure is done carefully. The patient who has difficulty swallowing may regurgitate some of the contrast material with the potential for aspiration into the lungs. If there is the possibility of a fistula between the esophagus and the trachea, barium should be used instead of Gastrografin® because the latter is highly irritating to the tracheobronchial tree.

There are no specific contraindications to performing an upper gastrointestinal series. Obstructions or perforation of the bowel is a marginal contraindication and, under these circumstances, the procedure must be done with caution. In the rare cases in which glucagon is to be administered for hypotonic duodenography, contraindications to the administration of glucagon include pheochromocytoma, severe cardiac disorders, and diabetes.

Relative contraindications to barium enema include a large rectal mass wherein placement of the enema tube may perforate the rectum. In addition, barium enema is contraindicated in patients with serious tachycardia, fulminant ulcerative colitis associated with systemic toxicity, and toxic megacolon. Suspicion of bowel perforation is not an absolute contraindication for barium enema, but Gastrografin® instead of barium should be used with careful fluoroscopic instillation of the contrast material. Barium and feces released into the abdominal cavity can cause barium peritonitis with serious results. Barium enema should be performed with caution in patients with obstruction, acute inflammatory conditions such as ulcerative colitis and diverticulitis, acute vascular insufficiency of the bowel, and severe bloody diarrhea.

Hypersensitivity to iodine or Telopaque® is a contraindication to oral chole-cystography. Patients with severe renal or hepatic disease should not have oral cholecystography. Severe diarrhea or malabsorption may interfere with the ab-sorption of the oral contrast.

PREPROCEDURE PREPARATION

Preparation for an ingested dye study is minimal. The patient is asked to eat a liquid breakfast to avoid solid material being in the gastrointestinal tract. Per-formance of an upper gastrointestinal series, a small bowel study, or a barium enema requires the patient to have nothing by mouth after the previous midnight as the presence of retained gastric contents may cloud the diagnostic picture by making it difficult to clearly view the stomach wall. Many radiologists recom-mend a low fiber diet for 3 days before the procedure if this is possible. Prepara-tion for a barium enema also includes the use of cleansing enemas before the procedure and a laxative is given the night before the test. The better the cleans-ing of the bowel, the more likely that the test will be accurate and reliable. Stool in the colon must be completely removed as it may simulate polypoid defects.

Digital examination of the rectum must always precede a barium enema to define large rectal masses that may result in perforation when the enema tube is inserted.

Most gastrointestinal medications should be withheld including antacids for 1 to 2 days prior to the evaluation. Anticholinergics and narcotics should be with-held for 24 hours prior to the procedure, since these drugs can affect small intestinal motility.

PATIENT EDUCATION

The patient should understand the specific procedure for which he/she is being referred. In the case of hypotonic duodenography, the patient should be aware that a nasogastric tube will be inserted and that glucagon will be given by intramuscular injection. If barium or gastrografin is going to be swallowed, the patient should be warned not to drink too fast as this may cause vomiting.

Preparation for a barium enema involves understanding that the procedure may be uncomfortable and even painful at times. Excessive flatulence may occur during or immediately following the procedure. The patient must keep the anal sphincter tightly closed around the enema tube to prevent leakage of the barium material.

PROCEDURE

Dye-contrast studies are begun by obtaining scout films in multiple views. Esophograms may be done using cine esophagography with the patient swallowing the barium while a cine x-ray is obtained. This demonstrates the physiology of swallowing and the sphincter mechanisms of the upper esophagus. The lower esophagus is studied using a thick barium paste (esophotrast®), which has a chalky flavor. The swallowing of a "barium marshmallow" may be needed to discern small strictures. Films are then taken by both overhead and spot technique in various projections with the patient being asked to turn into various positions while holding the breath. The procedure requires about 30 minutes.

An upper gastrointestinal series involves the performance of a scout film and then the administration of the contrast material by mouth. Views are obtained with the patient erect, and then supine on a tilt table. Multiple projections are taken with particular attention to any region depending on the presenting symptoms. Spot external compression may be performed to make areas of the stomach or the duodenum more visible. Hypotonic duodenography involves the use of a nasogastric tube for the instillation of air and glucagon administration by injection in order to paralyze and distend the bowel allowing maximal visualization of mucosal detail because of the double contrast of both air and barium.

Small bowel examination requires the ingestion of several cups of contrast material while radiographs are taken at 15 minute intervals to follow the course of the contrast material through the small intestine to the ileocecal valve. This procedure can take up to 6 hours so the patient should be encouraged to bring some reading material to the examination.

A barium enema involves the instillation of several cups of barium through an enema tube into the lower bowel and requires 30 to 45 minutes. Air may be also forced into the bowel to allow for double contrast. The procedure is performed under fluoroscopic control and, if a perforation is seen, the procedure is immediately halted. When a tight, constricting lesion is noted, it is unwise to force barium above the constriction because, if it is retained with water absorption from the bowel, a barium concretion can form. Both dilute barium and air can be introduced to promote good contrast. The patient is turned in multiple directions to coat the mucosa and to facilitate passage of the barium and air mixture around the colon in an even manner.

Oral cholecystography involves the taking of 6 pills containing the contrast material 24 hours before the procedure, a light fat dinner that evening, a laxative at night, and nothing by mouth from the midnight before the procedure. The pills can be taken at five minute intervals with one or two mouthfuls of water. Thereafter, water should be withheld. The procedure involves overhead and spot filming of the gall bladder with pressure spots obtained to demonstrate detail of any filling defects.

POSTPROCEDURE INFORMATION

The performance of an esophogram is fairly simple and will not affect the patient in any way. Bedrest is wise since the procedure will probably tire the patient. Following any gastrointestinal contrast procedure the stool may be white for one or two days. The patient may be constipated and laxatives should be given to avoid a barium concretion in the colon. The physician should be notified if there are still symptoms of retained barium 3 days after the procedure.

Patients who have received glucagon or an anticholinergic in preparation for hypotonic duodenography should be observed for normal urination and clearing of vision. These patients probably need to be accompanied by another person who can help them get home.

Assistance may be required with the preparation for the oral cholecystography procedure in terms of taking the contrast pills and eating a low-fat dinner the day before the test.

COMPLICATIONS

Esophograms can be performed under any circumstance if done with care. The entry of Gastrografin® into the trachea can cause severe tracheitis and inflammation. Barium extravasation into the mediastinum can cause formation of barium granulomas. Extravasation often mandates immediate surgery, both for the underlying fistula as well as for the problems of the intrathoracic barium.

Acute reactions to the contrast material used in oral cholecystogram have been reported. These can be prevented by careful screening of the patients for prior reactions or allergies.

PATIENT QUESTIONS

Why might I be asked to have a contrast study as well as some other study of the same area?

The ability of several diagnostic modalities to view the same organ or tissue allows an increased sensitivity of the testing regimen to various abnormalities. Therefore, the likelihood of detection of a specific abnormality may be increased by the performance of more than one diagnostic test. An example of this is with esophageal varices that are missed in about 20% of the cases when an esophagram, an endoscopic exam, or an angiogram is performed alone. The performance of two of these procedures, when the first did not define the abnormality and the clinical picture indicated further evaluation, increases the diagnostic yield.

Is the procedure uncomfortable?

The patient will feel uncomfortable sensations during the studies at various times such as when drinking the contrast material, at the insertion of an enema tube, the insertion of a nasogastric tube when indicated, the instillation of air, and, when asked to change positions. The patient should be encouraged to withstand the discomfort as patient cooperation is essential for a successful study.

Is there any special order in which I should have these gastrointestinal tests performed?

When there is a high likelihood that more than one gastrointestinal contrast procedure will be needed, the tests involving the lower part of the bowel should be performed first. This is done because of the likelihood of previously administered contrast material confusing the results if the procedures are done in the reverse order and some of the contrast material has been retained in the bowel prior to the actual bowel examination. Oral cholecystography should precede upper gastrointestinal series in order to avoid retention of barium obscuring detail of the gall bladder.

CONSENT

Consent is not required for dye-contrast studies that involve instillation of the contrast material through the mouth or the anus.

Consent is not required for oral cholecystogram.

SELECTED BIBLIOGRAPHY

Jaffe MH, Goldstein HA, Zeman RK, Choyke PL: Noninvasive imaging of the gastrointestinal tract. *Med Clin North Am* 1984;Nov:68:6:1515.

Maglinte DD, Lappas JC, Kelvin FM, Rex D, Chernish SM: Small bowel radiography: how, when,and why? *Radiology* 1987;May:163:2:297.

Margulis AR, Thoeni RF: The present status of the radiologic examination of the colon. *Radiology* 1988;Apr:167:1:1.

Trenkner SW, Laufer I: Doublecontrast examination. Part I: Oesophagus, stomach, and duodenum. *Clin Gastroenterol* 1984;Jan:13:1:41.

VI
Neurologic Procedures

28

Electroencephalography

RICHARD SADOVSKY

The electroencephalogram (EEG) is used to evaluate the functional status of the central nervous system. Abnormalities too minimal to produce anatomical changes can be localized with some precision. Spontaneous inherent activity of the brain, primarily that of the cerebral cortex, can be examined.

An EEG is a register of electrical activity generated in the cerebral cortex. An electroencephalograph is the machine used to make the recordings and consists of 6 to 20 amplifiers, each with its own pen, recording electrical activity from electrodes attached to the scalp.

INDICATIONS

An EEG can be helpful in a variety of situations. In patients with seizure disorders, the EEG may be the only test demonstrating any pathology. The test is often used to screen for patients whose symptoms suggest the possibility of brain disease and to decide which patients require further evaluation. The EEG is also often used to confirm brain death.

Patterns in a normal EEG are determined by many factors including age, level of consciousness, and individual characteristics. There is a normal rhythm, called alpha rhythm, that is the major property of the normal, relaxed adult. This rhythm appears at about 1 year of age and increases during childhood. This rhythm is absent during sleep and is lost if a patient becomes comatose. This alpha activity is generally constant throughout adult life.

Diseases or abnormalities of the brain produce a variety of changes in the EEG. Since the EEG is a measure of brain function, it should be clear that different diseases can cause similar EEG abnormalities. Only a characterization of the abnormality can be made. Usually other tests are required to determine the precise cause or etiology. The three major forms of abnormalities include (1) epileptiform abnormalities generally thought to be associated with seizures, (2) focal, or localized, slowing usually associated with a localized disease process, and (3) diffuse or bilateral abnormalities that can result from many different primary or secondary diseases of the brain. These types of abnormalities may occur together and demonstrate a combination of aberrant wave forms.

EEG is uniquely useful in the diagnosis of seizure disorders and the determination of initial treatment. Depending on the type of seizures, there is a 50% to 80% probability that an abnormality will be detectable on the EEG between seizures. The type of epileptiform abnormality can help to distinguish localized from generalized etiologies.

Focal slowing suggests the presence of a localized process such as a tumor, abscess, trauma, or vascular disease. Superficial lesions are easier to recognize than deeper ones. The change in the EEG over time may allow monitoring of progress or improvement of the lesion.

Diffuse or bilateral abnormality is probably the most frequent pattern seen and can be caused by any significant change in cerebral function. Metabolic diseases (such as hepatic or renal insufficiency), drugs, a variety of primary brain diseases such as degenerative diseases and panencephalitis all can produce a diffusely abnormal EEG. This pattern is also characteristic of Jakob-Creutzfeldt disease and Alzheimer's disease. The EEG does not make the diagnosis, but can help in estimating the severity of disease. Usually, any condition that causes a decreased mental state in the patient will alter the EEG pattern in proportion to the degree of wakefulness lost. In brain death, no activity is recorded at high amplification.

Treatment of seizure disorders can be monitored by EEG. In petit mal, or absence-type seizures, anticonvulsant medication can eliminate or reduce the epileptiform activity. In other seizure disorder types, the abnormalities often persist. Return to normal of the EEG with treatment may be a sign of remission of underlying diffuse disorders.

EEG testing may also be helpful in deciding whether to withdraw the patient from anticonvulsants by looking for persistent epileptiform activity. Continuous or ambulatory monitoring may help to distinguish real from factitious seizures.

ALTERNATIVES

When used for the diagnosis of intracranial space-occupying lesions, careful EEG studies can provide fairly good localization information in cases of cerebral hemisphere tumors, giving results comparable to cerebral angiography, but lacking the precision available with computerized tomography. EEG may provide the first hint that altered states of consciousness may be caused by a space-occupying lesion but, in contrast to EEG, arteriography, CT scans, and magnetic resonance imaging all have the advantage of indicating structural effects and edema produced directly by a tumor or mass. The CT scan has restricted the use of EEG for the detection and localization of brain lesions, but it has allowed the EEG to focus appropriately on physiologic rather than anatomic issues. Clinically important electroencephalographic abnormalities may occur in the presence of a normal CT scan, and clinicians must be aware of the possible significance of such dissociations.

The development of positron emission tomography may provide another way of looking at brain physiology. At present, EEG is the only examination performing this job.

POSSIBILITY OF FAILURE

Electrical discharges are dependent on neural activity, but they do not necessarily indicate the integrity of the cerebral structure. Little diagnostic specificity exists. There is also a certain amount of subjectivity depending on who is interpreting the EEG. Sensitivity is also limited with some normal subjects having an abnormal EEG. These problems can be reduced by having someone familiar with the clinical problem for which the patient has been referred interpret the EEG.

In psychiatric illnesses, the practical value of the EEG is not very great, although it maybe helpful in providing the diagnosis in cases of delirium or unrecognized seizure disorder.

Electrical activity from the brain can be obscured by the activity occurring with facial or other head movements. This makes recording very difficult in uncooperative patients. Sedation can be used, but the value of the EEG may be limited in these situations.

CONTRAINDICATIONS

There are no contraindications to electroencephalography.

PREPROCEDURE PREPARATION

Patients should be instructed to wash their hair before the test and not to use hair sprays or oils on the day of the examination. This helps to permit good electrical contact between the electrode and the scalp. The patient can and should eat prior to the examination since prolonged fasting resulting in low blood sugar can cause abnormalities in the recording. Caffeine-containing beverages should be avoided. Medications can be taken as usual although sedative drugs should be avoided because they may alter the examination and limit its usefulness. If the examination is scheduled to include a sleep EEG, the amount of rest time the night before the examination should be reduced.

PATIENT EDUCATION

The patient should be reassured that the test is neither painful nor harmful. Mental tensions should be diminished since brain wave patterns can be affected.

Patients should understand that this test does not read their mind and does not make any determination about their intelligence.

PROCEDURE

Electrodes, usually consisting of disks 4 to 5 mm in diameter are attached to the clean scalp with either collodion or special conductive paste (figure 28–1). Needle electrodes are rarely used in conscious patients. Generally, from 16 to 22 electrodes are placed in locations determined by the natural anatomic landmarks of the skull. This technique allows reproducibility and accurate localization of abnormal activity.

An EEG generally requires 1¹/₂ to 2 hours to do, with a recording activity done over a 20 to 30 minute time span. Sometimes it is desirable to do this while the patient is both awake and asleep. Sedation may be needed to induce sleep, and is frequently given with minimal after effects. Performing a sleep EEG significantly increases the amount of time needed to perform the examination.

The patient may be tested in various stress situations to elicit abnormal patterns not seen on the resting recording. For example, the patient may be asked to breathe deeply for several minutes or be subject to bright lights blinking rhythmically. Recordings are made with the patient's eyes open and closed. Recordings can also be made for a 24 hour period while the patient is doing normal daily activities.

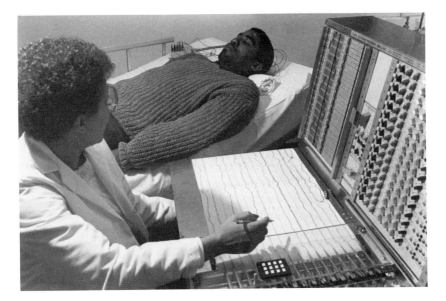

Figure 28–1. Electroencephalography

EEGs done to confirm brain death are generally done at the patient's bedside. Monitoring equipment and movement around the patient needs to be minimized to reduce artifacts on the recording. Pavulon®, a neuromuscular blocking agent, may be required to eliminate uncontrollable muscle activity.

POSTPROCEDURE INFORMATION

Adult patients who are coming for sleep EEG testing should be accompanied by someone in case sedation is required. Driving should not be attempted within 8 to 12 hours of sedation. Children should have dry diapers with them, some favorite juice or formula, and perhaps a favorite toy in order to feel more secure.

COMPLICATIONS

The patient should be observed for seizure activity especially if the procedure involves the use of a stressful stimulus. Assistance should be available in the event that a seizure occurs during the EEG.

PATIENT QUESTIONS

Will I receive a shock from the electrodes?

The patient should be assured in advance that the electrodes will not give a shock. If needle electrodes are used, some sticking sensations will be felt when they are introduced. Flat electrodes, however, are more commonly used.

Must I lie completely still during the examination?

All movements of the patient that might cause an artifact on the recording should be noted by the examiner. The recording may be stopped periodically to allow the patient to find a more comfortable position. This may be important, since fatigue and restlessness can cause changes in the brain wave pattern.

Does a normal EEG mean that I have no disease?

A normal EEG can never be accepted as precluding any disease. A degree of certainty is possible when looking for conditions such as cerebral abscess but the finding of a normal EEG only diminishes the probability of a lesion or disease process being present, but it does not exclude it.

CONSENT

Generally, consent is not needed for electroencephalography, but many laboratories are now obtaining informed consent.

SELECTED BIBLIOGRAPHY

Brenner RP: The electroencephalogram in altered states of consciousness. *Neurol Clin* 1985;Aug:3:3:615.

Fisch BJ, Pedley TA: Evaluation of focal cerebral lesions. *Neurol Clin* 1985;Aug:3:3:649.

Fisher J: What you need to know about neurological testing. *RN* 1987;Jan:50:1:47.

Niedermeyer E: Cerebrovascular disorders and EEG In Niedermyere E, Lopes da Silva, F. eds: *Electroencephalography: Basic Principles, Clinical Applications, and Related Fields.* Baltimore: Urban and Schwarzenberg, 1982.

Westmoreland BF: The electroencephalogram in patients with epilepsy. *Neurol Clin* 1985;Aug:3:3:599.

29

Electromyography

ROGER W. KULA AND RICHARD SADOVSKY

Electromyographic (EMG) studies complement the neurological exam by assessing standardized electrophysiologic parameters of nerve conduction, neuromuscular transmission, and muscle excitation. Nerve conduction is assessed by surface electrical stimulation of peripheral nerves at various points and by an analysis of the characteristics of evoked responses in muscle or in a sensory nerve at another point along the nerve. The distance between the points of stimulation divided by the difference in the interval time from stimulus to muscle response is typically determined and expressed as a conduction velocity (m/sec.). This basic measure of nerve function is compared with standardized values. Reduced conduction velocities generally reflect disturbance in the myelination of peripheral nerve axons.

Assessing the sustained reproducibility of the evoked muscle response with repetitive nerve stimulation reflects the intactness of neuromuscular transmission. As a complement to the analysis of the compound muscle action potential recorded with surface electrodes, needle recordings from within the muscle at rest and with minimal and maximal voluntary effort provide a more detailed analysis of size, distribution, irritability, and recruitment of motor units. This information provides for a broad distinction of pathological processes into those disrupting the innervation of muscle (denervative) and those causing primary muscle cell damage (myopathic).

Relaxed, healthy muscle generally shows no spontaneous activity except in the region of its endplates, but activity can be provoked by insertion of a needle electrode or by muscular activity. Varying kinds of spontaneous activity may be found in diseased muscle, and the insertion and voluntary activity of such muscles may differ in several ways from that found in normal muscle.

INDICATIONS

Electromyography offers a visual and auditory recording of changes in electrical potential in muscle. This is helpful in delineating a number of muscle and nerve problems that cause symptoms of pain, weakness, gait alterations, deformity of a part, or disability in the performance of a given task.

The motor unit is the basic element of motor activity. This motor unit is comprised of the anterior horn cell, its axon and branching terminals, the neuromuscular junctions, and the 10 to 2000 muscle fibers innervated by that axon. The recruitment or regulation of motor unit firing at the spinal cord level controls muscle function. Muscle activation is produced by release of acetylcholine into the neuromuscular junction as a result of nerve activation. The interaction of acetylcholine with postsynaptic receptors on muscle results in muscle cell firing. The muscle fiber responds by initiating biochemical reactions (excitation-contraction coupling) causing the muscle to shorten either in a twitch or in a more sustained manner producing work.

Surface electrical stimuli close to a nerve can cause the nerve to be actively stimulated. The delay (or latency) in muscle activation following the electrical nerve stimulation results from the physiological conduction of the nerve impulse along the intervening nerve segment. Analysis of the change in latency upon stimulation at various distances along a nerve allows for the calculation of a **conduction velocity** expressed in meters per second for various segments along the nerve. The measurement reflects the function of the most rapidly conducting nerve fibers, characterized by a large fiber diameter and thick myelinization. Similar studies can be carried out in sensory nerves, although with more difficult recording of evoked nerve, rather than muscle, potentials.

Nerve conduction studies are standardized for particular stimulus and recording techniques, various sensory and motor nerve regions, limb temperatures, and age. Nerve conduction can be measured with relatively good accuracy although its sensitivity is frequently overrated. In some cases, damage to as many as 50% of fibers may occur without significantly altering nerve conduction measurements. What is more, in some disorders such as motor neuron diseases, amyloidosis, or porphyria where axonal damage is primary, abnormalities in nerve conduction occur very late in the disease process. Abnormalities in nerve conduction should not be considered as a measure of functional activity. Patients with chronic hereditary neuropathies or these recovering from Guillain-Barré syndrome may demonstrate very slow conductions with normal functional strength while an individual with motor neuron disease may have a normal conduction study but be quite weak. Conduction studies may be helpful in localizing damage to a peripheral nerve as in various compression syndromes (carpal tunnel, tarsal tunnel, ulnar nerve palsy, and plexus lesions). Isolated root compression, as in lumbar or cervical disk disease, may be obscured by the confluence of root levels expressed in peripheral nerve trunks.

Under normal physiological conditions, neuromuscular transmission has a high degree of reserve capacity and plays no role in limiting functional muscle strength or endurance. In diseases such as myasthenia gravis or botulism, however, compromised neuromuscular transmission can be life threatening. **Repetitive stimulation studies** assessing repetitive muscle contraction can demonstrate disorders of neuromuscular transmission occurring when individual neuromuscular synapses fail. This results in a significant reduction or decrement in the surface recorded contraction over time.

Electromyographic or needle recordings from muscle represent a sensitive way of assessing the individual physiologic activity of motor units. An analysis is made of three basic aspects of motor unit function: (1) the response to needle insertion and movement, (2) activity recorded with the muscle completely at rest, and (3) activity recorded with minimal and maximal sustained voluntary muscle contraction. Normal muscle produces no spontaneous muscle activity when at rest. If spontaneous activity is present, it is usually abnormal and results from injured or denervated muscle fibers and poorly regulated or reinnervated motor units. Abundant fibrillations are abnormal and may be indicative of neuropathic or denervating disorders (peripheral neuropathy, radiculopathy, and motor neuron disease), as well as certain myopathic disorders such as muscular dystrophy, polymyositis, some metabolic disorders, and botulism.

Large potentials on minimal muscle movement are derived from large reinnervated motor units in chronic denervating diseases. Small polyphasic potentials may result from fragmentation or diminution of motor unit potentials by inflammatory, toxic, or metabolic injury to muscle fibers.

Recruitment of motor unit potentials during forceful contraction are observed for orderly development and amplitude. Early recruitment and reduced overall patterns are characteristic of primary muscle diseases in which a greater number of fragmented or depleted motor units must be brought into action to produce a given muscular force.

The final EMG report should contain nerve conduction velocity determinations in both sensory and motor nerves. Accessible nerves in the upper extremity include the median, ulnar, radial nerves and the entire brachial plexus. Accessible nerves in the lower extremity include the femoral, posterior tibial, common peroneal, and the sural. The amplitude, duration, and configuration of motor unit potentials are described. The appearance of excessive polyphasic potentials or presence of giant units is indicated and the interference pattern is described. The concluding analysis provides an interpretation based on pathophysiological aspects as related to clinical problems. It may be possible to determine whether the cause of weakness is myopathic or neuropathic, and in the latter case, whether it may be due to a root, peripheral nerve, or motor neuronal lesion. EMG and nerve conduction studies alone cannot be used to provide a definitive clinical diagnosis because they relate to physiological function only and are neither sufficiently specific nor sensitive to underlying etiological processes.

Additional indications currently being explored for EMG include the diagnosis of chronic back pain and biofeedback for both pain and stroke victims.

ALTERNATIVES

There are no alternatives to EMG for determining the physiological properties of nerve conduction and motor unit activation. These studies significantly extend the observations of muscle strength, reflexes, and sensation in the routine neurological examination. In addition, the precision necessary to make accurate localizations and diagnostic decisions is dependent on the EMG.

Studies have been done to compare the diagnostic yield of the electromyographic examination compared with that of a biopsy in the contralateral muscle in patients with myopathy diagnosed by clinical features, serum levels of enzymes, and nerve biopsy. In over 85% of patients with myopathy, the EMG confirmed the clinical classification. In 79%, the biopsy was diagnostic and, in 77% of the patients, both electromyographic and histologic findings confirmed the classification. The highest incidence of discrepancy between EMG and biopsy was found in patients with disorders in neuromuscular transmission. In most patients with myasthenia gravis, the EMG may appear normal.

The EMG proved superior to biopsy in cases with marked electrophysiologic abnormalities indicating "loss of fibers" but without structural change in the biopsy. This is sometimes the case in patients with thyrotoxic myopathy. In addition, in systemic lupus erythematosus, a large number of patients with EMG abnormality have no clinical signs or symptoms of muscular involvement and, in some of these patients, the biopsy shows only slight or borderline changes.

While muscle biopsy is limited to the sampling of a relatively discrete area of a single muscle, EMG provides the security of assessing a wide variety, as well as multiple areas, of muscles. Conversely, there are conditions in which involvement of the muscles might be suspected, but in which the electromyogram offers no assistance. These include some instances of disuse atrophy, severely wasted muscles in anorexia nervosa, and in endocrine exophthalmic ophthalmoplegia.

POSSIBILITY OF FAILURE

If cooperation is limited because of pain, poor comprehension, or emotional overlay, the interference pattern during maximal effort may be reduced because only a small number of units is activated. Lack of patient cooperation not only compromises the quality of the recordings but it also limits the extent of testing that may be needed to fully explore a particular clinical problem. Muscle biopsy may be the diagnostic test of choice if a lack of cooperation obscures proper testing.

It is important to recognize the need for a highly qualified electromyographer. Both the administration of the examination and its interpretation require appropriate skill, training, and experience.

CONTRAINDICATIONS

The most common contraindication is the patient's inability or unwillingness to cooperate. The uncooperative patient will cause inaccuracies that will make the procedure minimally useful.

Since the needles are placed through the skin, superficial and contagious skin infections should delay the performance of electromyographic and conduction studies. If the study is urgent, it should be done in these circumstances under extreme aseptic conditions. Lymphedema may preclude needle insertion in the affected area.

Attention should be paid to the possibility of an electrical hazard in patients who have cardiac pacemakers. Certainly blood dyscrasias characterized by easy bleeding such as hemophilia may preclude the examination, but the study can be performed with care to observe the post-examination needle sites and with the application compression bandages when necessary. Patients on Coumadin may be managed in a similar manner.

PREPROCEDURE INSTRUCTIONS

The patient may be requested to restrict the use of cigarettes, coffee, tea, or cola for 2 to 3 hours before the test. The patient's usual medications can be continued, since the examination is not affected by any medication other than heavy sedation that may cause stupor. The skin should be clean without any creams or emollients.

PATIENT EDUCATION

The patient should be reassured that a small-gauge needle is used, but should understand that electrical currents may be uncomfortable or painful. A patient who understands the importance of the procedure will be more cooperative and better physiologic data will result.

PROCEDURE

An electromyographic examination is performed by a trained physician or technician. The patient is placed in a supine position on the examining table where the examination is performed both on the affected extremity and on the contralateral part for comparison (figure 29–1). The limbs to be examined should be warm unless low temperature is desired to bring out a specific abnormality such as myotonia. The skin is cleaned with isopropyl alcohol and sterile or disposable needles are used. Occasionally, slight abrasion of the epidermis is required to reduce the extremely high resistance of the skin in surface electrode recordings. The surface electrodes are used both to stimulate electrical current and to record the current moving through the nerve fiber (the conduction velocity). The patient may be moved to the prone position if necessary for completing the examination.

The number of insertions of the needle electrode in an EMG may vary from a minimum of 3 to 10 in the upper extremity or to 15 or 20 in the lower extremity on the affected side. Examination of the unaffected side may require half as many insertions of the needle. The cervical, dorsal, lumbar, and lumbosacral paraspinous muscles may require 3 to 6 insertions on the affected, and fewer on the unaffected, side. Measurements of muscle activity are taken at rest, with minimal muscle activity, and with forceful voluntary contractions. The duration of the typical electromyographic examination varies from a half hour to 2 hours.

Electromyography is more difficult in children because they do not tolerate the pain well and they do not have a clear understanding of the procedure. Needles can cause anxiety and cooperation may be poor. It is probably best if the parent is not present, the nurse or technician provides reassurance and support, and the child is restrained, if necessary. Passive movements of the extremities by the examiner may be needed to obtain the proper recordings. Nerve conduction studies should be done prior to electromyography because the latter procedure often causes more distress.

POSTPROCEDURE INFORMATION

The patient should be able to get off the examination table by himself and leave the examination area without any assistance. Evidence of subcutaneous or intra-

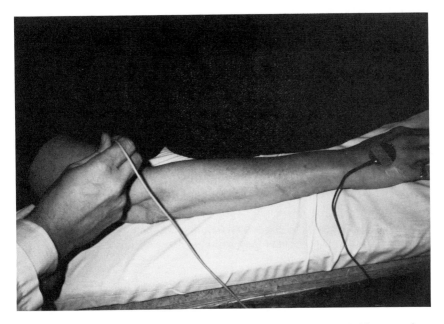

Figure 29–1. Inserting a needle electrode for electromyographic study of the right biceps muscle.

dermal bleeding (most likely to occur in the first 24 hours) should be noted and reported to the physician. The patient should be instructed to apply warm compresses to tender areas and to use analgesics as needed.

COMPLICATIONS

Muscle or skin paresthesias can occur indicating temporary alteration of nerve function. Long-term parasthesias suggesting extensive disruption of nerve fibers is uncommon but have occurred, in the few reported cases, following lengthy and detailed recording sessions of over 2 hours. The absence of permanent after effects following EMG suggests that any disturbance of nerve tissue is minimal and reversible.

Pneumothorax is a rare but potential complication of EMG of the thoracic cage musculature in the paraspinal or scapular regions. This can be avoided by careful needle placement.

PATIENT QUESTIONS

Will the procedure hurt?

A small-gauge needle is used and the feeling will be like pinpricks. This can be very uncomfortable in distal, small muscles when the patient is required to exert force with the muscle. Many electromyographers choose to use unipolar as opposed to bipolar needles because they are smaller and less painful. Patients should be reassured that the discomfort is not harmful. They may also feel shocks from the surface applied electrical stimulation. It should be emphasized that the shocks may seem severe but are not damaging.

The factors that contribute to the sensory input of pain are not clear. Studies suggest that needles in the back, neck, and hand are more painful than in other areas. There appears to be no correlation between such factors as anxiety or the number of areas studied and the perceived amount of pain. For some patients the experience is so unpleasant that they will not submit to further testing.

Is electromyography safe?

Although the apparatus used for electromyography has become increasingly sophisticated, the principles underlying the procedure have not changed. Important safety considerations have become standard. Care is taken to avoid component failure and to be certain than even if there is failure, no current that can constitute a hazard to the patient will pass through the recording electrodes. Stringent criteria are applied to the manufacture of the equipment and all apparatus is checked for electrical safety prior to installation. With respect to the electrodes in use, most labs are now using disposable needles because of the perceived risk of disease transmission.   Nevertheless, sterilization procedures in practice are safe and effective.

Will this test provide a diagnosis?

This examination will help clarify the location and pathophysiology of disease. The actual diagnosis will be made by the clinician using the EMG report, clinical observation, other serum serology and enzyme tests, and possibly a muscle and/or nerve biopsy.

CONSENT

A consent form is requested in some laboratories because of the invasive nature of the examination.

SELECTED BIBLIOGRAPHY

Aminoff MJ: *Electromyography in Clinical Practice.* Boston:Addison-Wesley;1978.

Buchthal F: Electromyography in the evaluation of muscle diseases. *Neurol Clin* 1985;Aug:3(3):573p–598. (Review).

Jablecki CK: Electromyography in children and infants. J Child Neurol 1986;Oct:1(4):297–318. (Review).

Lenman JA, Ritchie AE: Clinical electromyography, third edition, Pitman; 1984.

30

Brain Stem Evoked Potentials

RICHARD SADOVSKY

Evoked potential (EP) is the transitory electrical response of the nervous system to a stimulus. EPs are constantly being produced as a result of internal and external stimuli. In diagnostic studies, EPs are evoked by repetitive discrete external stimuli. Their latency, or time delay, following the stimulus reflects their transmission along the central nervous system (CNS) pathways. Three major modalities have been examined by this technique. These include visual (VEP), auditory (BAEP), and tactile, or somatosensory (SEP) evoked potentials.

INDICATIONS

EPs are useful in examining the function of sensory pathways in patients difficult to examine otherwise, such as infants and comatose patients. The provision of an objective measure of sensory function may allow localization of the site of abnormality within the nervous system producing sensory symptoms. Evoked potentials appear to be most sensitive to diseases that affect the white matter tracts. It should be noted that EPs evaluate only the neural pathways that convey information in the brain. Symptoms may be present with a normal EP study.

Visual evoked potentials (VEP) are generated using alternating checkerboard patterns and will be abnormal in disorders affecting the anterior portion of the visual pathway, such as the optic nerve and chiasm. Demyelinating lesions such as optic neuritis can be distinguished from compressive or destructive nerve lesions by changes in the amplitude, configuration, and latency periods of the VEP configuration. This technique appears to be the most sensitive and shows the highest incidence of abnormal results including abnormalities indicating subclinical lesions.

Brainstem auditory evoked potentials (AEP) are generated using click-like auditory stimuli. Most attention is being placed on the early elements of the AEP, which have been shown in humans to originate from brainstem structures. Lesions at any point along the auditory pathway from the ear to the inferior colliculus may produce abnormalities of the AEP. Demyelinative, compressive, and destructive lesions involving the brainstem all tend to prolong the latency differences, and, if severe, may cause the later waves of the AEP to be lost.

Somatosensory evoked potentials (SEP) are generated using percutaneous pulse electrical stimulation of a mixed peripheral nerve. Recording is usually done from scalp electrodes with a lesion at any point along the conduction pathway likely to cause an abnormality. The lesion can be better localized by recording from multiple sites along the pathway. This allows identification of the segment of the pathway in which the lesion occurs. This technique can help distinguish early demyelinating disease, but specificity is lacking in this procedure.

Clinical applications include (1) quantitation of sensory dysfunction and the ability to follow changes over time, (2) localization of CNS lesions, (3) diagnosis of multiple sclerosis, (4) hysteria, (5) coma, (6) trauma, and (7) perceptual and cognitive disorders. Complaints of visual or hearing impairment can be localized to the sensory organs or to the central nervous system. Identification of a point at which conduction fails or deteriorates may permit localization of the lesion. Multifocal abnormalities occurring in areas of clinical dysfunction as well as normal areas may be indicative of multiple sclerosis. This is more frequently seen in the VEP.

EP analysis is most useful in confirming clinical impressions. Normal findings may imply psychogenic etiology under certain circumstances. In the comatose patient, the integrity of these central nervous system pathways can be evaluated, offering information not otherwise obtainable. Traumatic injuries and the severity of injuries to nervous systems can be evaluated and localized by EP. Additional uses of EP include intraoperative monitoring during neurosurgical procedures to avoid damage to vital structures, and the use of analysis of intermediate and late-wave components in relation to psychological processes such as perception, cognition, reasoning, and motivation. This latter area, that of so-called event-related potentials, is being explored and does not yet have clear application in clinical medicine.

ALTERNATIVES

A good neurological exam measures neural function, but involves subjective patient responses and physician interpretations. EPs provide objective and repro-ducible measurements. The two approaches are best thought of as complimentary.

The EEG provides a great deal of information about the functional status of the cerebral cortex, but does not allow evaluation of specific sensory systems. EPs performed by means of sophisticated electronic averaging techniques allow analysis of specific sensory input systems. Neither test allows specific diagnosis of the disease process.

Depending on the indications, other procedures that can be helpful include analysis of cerebrospinal fluid, myelography, or even surgical exploration. The EP technique is noninvasive, relatively inexpensive and safe while providing extremely sensitive measurement of the functional integrity of distributed CNS pathways. In many cases, changes can be appreciated before clear structural changes (as measured by CT scanning or biochemical alterations) can be documented.

The diagnostic value of EP examinations can be expressed by the number of neuroradiological examinations or exploratory operations that might be avoided in the patients tested.

POSSIBILITY OF FAILURE

It is important not to use EPs as the independent variable in neurologic evalua-tions. The procedure is highly dependent on a number of physiologic and techni-cal factors. Each lab needs to operationally define the EP variability for itself, using its own methods.

Reasons for negative results in patients with a history and/or signs indicating lesions in the regions forming the target of the examination might be (1) lesions that do not involve the pathways examined, (2) the lack of complete sensitivity of technique, or (3) the evaluating criteria do not sufficiently discriminate be-tween normality and abnormality.

AEPs may suggest the reversibility of coma even when the EEG is flat, as is the case in drug overdose. Conversely, they can imply the irreversibility of an unresponsive state when the EEG is still relatively normal, by suggesting diffuse structural brainstem injury.

CONTRAINDICATIONS

There are no contraindications to the measurement of evoked potentials.

PREPROCEDURE PREPARATION

There is no specific preprocedure preparation. The patient should be told that the procedure is neither painful nor harmful. Sedative medications should be avoided prior to the examination.

PATIENT EDUCATION

The patient should understand, when possible, the nature of the examination and its specific indications.

PROCEDURE

EPs are usually recorded with the same type of electrodes as used for electroencephalography (EEG). Metal discs are applied to the scalp with electrolyte paste. Electrode locations are set by the sensory system anatomy. For visual EPs, electrodes are placed over the occipital region of the head (figure 30–1), for SEP recordings, electrodes may be placed over the spine and the proximal segments of peripheral nerves.

The various stimuli used are described above. There is some variation among various laboratories, but the basic procedures are the same.

POSTPROCEDURE INFORMATION

There are no specific instructions for this examination. The family should understand that further evaluation may be necessary if there is not clear clinical correlation between symptoms and the EP recording results.

COMPLICATIONS

There are no after effects or complications following EP recording.

PATIENT QUESTIONS

Will the stimuli used be uncomfortable?

Generally, stimuli causing no or only minor discomfort are chosen. For brain stem evoked potentials, an audiometer is used to give approximately 75 dbl clicks through an earphone. Visual evoked potentials are brought on by viewing

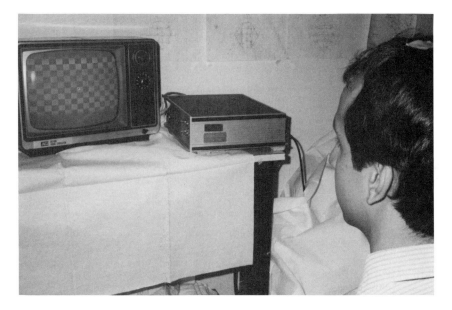

Figure 30–1. Patient prepared for visual evoked potential testing.

a checkerboard of white and black squares that reverses at a predetermined speed. Somatosensory evoked potentials are delivered by a surface electrode applied to the skin and giving small, barely perceptible, electrical stimulations.

How accurate is evoked potential testing?

When successful and reliable recordings can be obtained, the results are highly accurate. Recording and filtering techniques, however, are variable, and standards for each laboratory must be rigorously established in order to meaningfully assess the comparative significance of results.

AEP abnormality is considered specific for brain stem lesions. VEP abnormality is considered specific for lesions in or influencing the optic pathways. SEP abnormality is considered specific for cervical cord, brain stem, and hemispherical lesions.

CONSENT

Consent is not required for this evaluation, but it is obtained at many centers.

SELECTED BIBLIOGRAPHY

Cassvan A: Electrodiagnosis: central evoked potentials. *Arch Phys Med Rehabil Suppl* 1987;May:68(5-S):S13, S28.

Dorfman LJ: Sensory evoked potentials: clinical application in medicine. *Annu Rev Med* 1983;34:473.

Hughes JR, Fino JJ: A review of generators of the brainstem auditory evoked potential. *J Clin Neurophysiol* 1985;Oct:2:4:355.

Newlon PG: Utility of multimodality evoked potentials in cerebral injury. *Neurol Clin* 1985;Aug:3:3:675.

31

Lumbar Puncture

ROGER W. KULA AND RICHARD SADOVSKY

Sampling of cerebrospinal fluid is useful in the diagnosis of a variety of neurologic problems. Cerebrospinal fluid (CSF) serves both a protective and a transport function in the subarachnoid space. Fluid is usually obtained by lumbar puncture as a simple diagnostic procedure, or during other invasive diagnostic tests such as myelography and pneumoencephalography.

INDICATIONS

Lumbar puncture has been shown to be helpful in diagnosing four major classes of disease: meningeal infection, subarachnoid hemorrhage, central nervous system (CNS) malignancy, and demyelinating disease. The use of spinal taps during or at the end of treatment for meningitis is usually reserved for those patients with the rarer chronic meningeal infections such as cryptococcus or tuberculosis or if there is clinical suspicion of treatment failure.

Lumbar puncture and cerebrospinal fluid analysis allow measurement of pressure as well as the collection of fluid samples for analysis. Specimens are sent to the laboratory for analysis of protein, glucose, and cell count with differential, as well as for cytology, culture, and serologic testing for neurosyphilis or crypto-coccus as the clinical circumstances dictate. Special culture techniques for fungi, anaerobic organisms, or mycobacteria may need to be requested.

In the immediate investigation of possible infection, Gram staining and India ink preparations for cryptococcus may be critical. Opening pressure with the patient in a lateral decubitus position should be less than 20 cm of water, and the fluid should be clear and perfectly colorless. Low CSF pressure in a dehydrated patient may confound observation of CSF flow making an initial upright posi-tioning advantageous. Early bloody return with clearing usually signals a slightly traumatic tap. On centrifugation the supernatant will be clear. In situations of subarachnoid bleeding such clearing is not observed, and when centrifuged the supernatant will be yellow, or xanthochromic, because of the presence of oxyhe-moglobin and, later, bilirubin. Such xanthochromia requires approximately 6 to 12 hours to develop and is indicative of subarachnoid bleeding. Turbidity of the spinal fluid is caused by the presence of white cells usually in concentrations of greater than 200 per mm^3. The CSF should contain no more than 5 mononuclear cells per mm^3 and no polymorphonuclear cells should be present.

Elevations of white cells and the relative numbers of lymphocytes and neutro-phils may allow for the diagnosis of bacterial meningitis, viral infections, and tuberculous or mycotic meningitis. Protein values in the spinal fluid may be increased by inflammation, primary or metastatic CNS malignancy, intraspinal block, or damage to the brain or spinal cord. Increased gamma globulin concen-trations with normal total protein levels can be helpful in the diagnosis of multi-ple sclerosis, but can also be seen in syphilis, Guillain–Barre syndrome, other inflammatory conditions of the central nervous system, and some peripheral neuropathies. Glucose values are a function of serum levels and should be 60% to 80% that of the serum. A low CSF glucose, generally less than 45 mg%, is seen in bacterial meningitis.

Gram stain results should be confirmed by appropriate cultures. Stains dem-onstrating bacteria or yeast require rapid action with appropriate antibiotics. Cultures should be held for 3 to 4 days before a negative report is issued while cultures for tuberculosis may need to be held for several weeks.

Therapeutic indications for lumbar puncture include the administration of intrathecal antineoplastics, spinal anesthesia, and occasionally for administration of antifungal agents. Lumbar puncture itself also plays a therapeutic role in the treatment of pseudotumor cerebri, in which serial lumbar punctures and removal of aliquots of CSF help reduce elevated pressures.

ALTERNATIVES

Indications for lumbar puncture have changed with the advent of the computer-ized tomography CT scan and magnetic resonance imaging MRI. Scanning has become the preferred method for examining patients with apparent ischemia or hemorrhage causing a stroke. Subarachnoid bleeding can frequently be observed with CT scan obviating the need for, and risk of, lumbar puncture. Lumbar puncture can add nothing to the evaluation of intraparenchymal cerebral bleeding and is usually contraindicated in such circumstances. In the face of a normal CT scan, however, lumbar puncture is often the only method of diagnosing subarachnoid hemorrhage. Cerebrospinal fluid spectrophotometry may, in the future, prove to be more highly sensitive in detecting cerebral hemorrhage.

Cytologic examination of CSF is helpful in the diagnosis of primary and more common secondary CNS malignancies. This is especially true in patients with leukemia and lymphoma, and in those malignancies that have a predilection for CNS metastases or malignant meningitis such as breast and lung cancer. Cytologic studies in suspected cases of metastatic disease or malignant meningitis should be obtained on at least 5 to 10 cc of fluid. Unless this is done, there is a high rate of false negatives in initial taps in these situations.

POSSIBILITY OF FAILURE

The specificity and sensitivity of cerebrospinal fluid analysis for central nervous system infections and subarachnoid hemorrhage are fairly good. With the advent of more precise scanning techniques, the use of lumbar puncture has been relegated to a secondary role in diagnosing lesions impinging on nearby structures. In attempts to diagnosis malignancies, localized infections such as brain abscesses, and subdural bleeds, lumbar puncture is probably not the appropriate test to initiate the evaluation.

CONTRAINDICATIONS

The rapid evolution of a lateralizing hemispheric process is the clearest contraindication for lumbar puncture. The presence or absence of papilledema is not a good predictor of risk in an evolving acute neurologic process, although it is more reliable in chronic disorders. All contraindications are relative especially when the risk of meningitis is high. Infections at the puncture site contraindicate lumbar puncture as does the presence of increased intracranial pressure associated with focal neurological findings. Suspected intracranial mass lesions including brain abscess and subdural hematoma may contraindicate lumbar puncture. The significant risk (approaching 40%) of herniation with all intracranial mass lesions makes lumbar puncture rarely justified if the presence of a mass is known.

Evidence of a bleeding disorder is a relative contraindication. Platelet counts of greater than 40,000 and prothrombin times less than 50% above control are generally considered safe.

PREPROCEDURE PREPARATION

The patient does not need to restrict food or fluid intake. The bladder and bowel should be emptied out before the procedure. A complete neurologic examination should be performed with careful observation of the fundi.

Coumadin, if used, should be omitted and prothrombin time normalized before lumbar puncture. Heparin should be discontinued 4 to 6 hours before and not resumed until at least 1 hour after the procedure.

PATIENT EDUCATION

The procedure should be described to the patient. The patient's cooperation will make the test much easier and reduces the likelihood of post-tap headaches. Patient activity during the puncture can alter CSF pressure and the patient should be urged not to cry, cough, or strain. During the procedure, the patient should be encouraged to report periods of pain or discomfort after the initial insertion of the needle through the dura mater as these may indicate lateral needle placement and irritation or puncture of a nerve root. The patient should be advised to lie still and breathe normally.

PROCEDURE

The patient is positioned on his side at the edge of the bed with his knees drawn up to his chest and his chin on his chest. In this flexion position, the curve of the spine allows easy access to the lumbar subarachnoid space (figure 31–1). Having an assistant present to help the patient maintain this position will be extremely helpful but may raise the patient's anxiety level. Lumbar punctures can be done in a sitting position with the head bent forward resting over a bedside stand (figure 31–2).

The skin is prepared with an appropriate antiseptic solution and the anesthetic is injected at the skin site. The spinal needle with the stylet in place is inserted between the spinous process of the vertebrae below L3 since the spinal cord terminates at L1 to L2. Using lower interspaces may make the tap more difficult because of narrowing of the subarachnoid space. If the needle has entered the subarachnoid space, a slight pop is experienced and fluid will drip from it when the stylus is removed. A manometer is used to measure the initial CSF pressure and a stopcock is attached to the needle to allow control of CSF flow. After adequate sampling has been done, a closing pressure is obtained and the needle is removed.

Spinal fluid sampling can also be done through cisternal puncture by inserting a needle below the occipital bone or laterally in the high cervical region under fluoroscopy. This is hazardous because of proximity to the brain stem but may

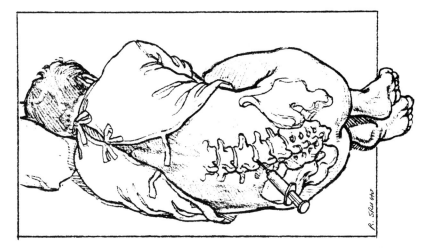

Figure 31–1. Spinal tap in the lateral position.

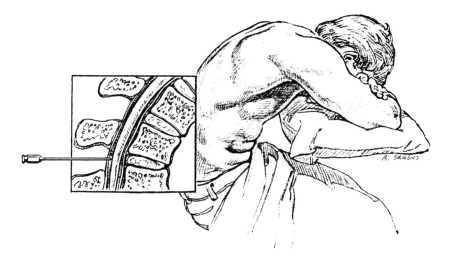

Figure 31–2. Spinal tap in the upright position.

be indicated if there is infection at the lumbar puncture site or if myelographic documentation of the upper extent of a spinal cord compressive lesion is necessary.

Ventricular puncture is a neurosurgical procedure used primarily for the management of CSF-obscuring lesions and for placement of reservoirs for intrathecal drug administration.

POSTPROCEDURE INFORMATION

Following the procedure, the patient should be kept lying flat and preferably prone for at least 3 hours. The patient should be encouraged to drink fluids and is advised to remain in bed for 6 to 12 hours. The puncture site should be checked for evidence of induration or infection. The need for monitoring of vital signs and postprocedure surveillance are dictated by the circumstances of the diagnostic evaluation.

Diagnostic lumbar puncture in a thoroughly investigated patient completing workup for syphilis, demyelinating disease, or peripheral neuropathy can be appropriately carried out on an outpatient basis. In such cases, someone should accompany the patient to provide transportation and supervision.

COMPLICATIONS

Complications of lumbar puncture include anesthetic reactions, bleeding into the spinal canal or epidural space, and rare cranial nerve palsy. Possible, but rare, danger signs include fever, neck rigidity, and irritability, decreased levels of consciousness, altered vital signs, or respiratory failure.

Postpuncture headaches can occur caused by leakage of the cerebrospinal fluid into the epidural space. This occurs in 10% of patients and is seen most frequently after multiple lumbar puncture attempts and it correlates with the diameter of the needle used. The onset of the headache is usually within 24 to 48 hours and is striking for its positional nature. The headache is immediately relieved by lying flat. The majority of headaches resolve in 1 week. Fewer than 1% of headaches last as long as a month.

Transtentorial or tonsillar herniation may occur, usually caused by inadequate preprocedure evaluation. Herniation may not occur until 24 to 48 hours after the lumbar puncture. This complication requires immediate intervention with steroids, mannitol, and neurosurgical consultation.

Other complications can include septic meningitis and epidural empyema due to faulty aseptic technique, backache caused by injuries to the spinal ligaments, vascular trauma caused by perforation of local vessels, and the development of a intraspinal epidermoid cyst caused by the introduction of epithelial cells into the spinal canal by the use of a needle without the stylet. This latter complication can be avoided by always introducing the needle with the stylet in place.

PATIENT QUESTIONS

Will I have a headache or other discomfort after the lumbar puncture?

About 10% of patients who have lumbar punctures develop headaches. The incidence of this complication can be decreased by carefully following the doctor's instructions, by cooperating with the procedure and the postprocedure instructions of bedrest and increased fluid intake. Generally the headaches are minor and transient, and can be relieved with analgesics. Headaches rarely last for longer than one week. Other complications include nausea, vomiting, local irritation, or temporary leg pain caused by nerve root irritation.

Can I become paralyzed by the lumbar puncture?

In the early years of spinal anesthesia, the incidence of arachnoiditis was high and some women receiving this anesthesia prior to childbirth became paralyzed. This situation has made everyone anxious about this complication following lumbar puncture. A simple, diagnostic spinal tap should not cause paralysis.

Should I agree to a repeat lumbar puncture following treatment for meningitis?

Following antibiotic treatment for acute bacterial meningitis, a lumbar puncture is generally not needed. This is especially true when the clinical course of disease has been as expected and there has been as good response to therapy. Patients who have completed treatment for chronic meningitis such as tuberculosis or cryptococcus should probably have a repeat lumbar puncture as should patients who have not responded to antibiotic treatment. The determination of the need for a repeat procedure at the end of therapy requires correlation with clinical judgment.

CONSENT

The patient or responsible member of the family must sign a consent form prior to lumbar puncture.

SELECTED BIBLIOGRAPHY

Brooker RJ: Technique to avoid spinal tap headache. *J Amer Med Assoc* 1958;168:261.

Gorelick PB, Biller J: Lumbar puncture. *Postgrad Med* 1986:79.

Marton KI, Gean AD: The spinal tap: a new look at an old test. *Ann Int Med* 1986;104:6:840.

Marton KI, Vender M: The lumbar puncture: patterns of use in clinical practice. *Med Decis Making* 1981:1:331.

Petito F, Plum F: The lumbar puncture (Editorial) *N Engl J Med* 1974;290:225.

VII
Eyes, Ears, Nose and Throat

32

Fluorescein Angiography of the Eye

RICHARD SADOVSKY

Fluorescein is a unique dye that fluoresces, emitting a yellow-green color. It is eliminated by the liver largely within 1 hour and entirely within 24 hours. The use of intravenous peripheral injections of this dye has given ophthalmologists the ability to see fine details of the retinal and choroid vasculature. Angiography can play an important role in the diagnosis and monitoring of the progression of certain macular diseases.

INDICATIONS FOR PROCEDURE

The use of angiography in the evaluation of patients with visual problems has been narrowed by the use of computerized tomography (CT) scans and magnetic resonance imaging (MRI) evaluations. Angiography remains valuable in cases in which visualization of vascular structures is needed and is unobtainable by any other procedures. Visual disturbances may result from ischemia of any portion of the visual pathway. Referrals for fluorescein study often are for patients with descriptive, nonspecific diagnoses such as macular edema or macular hemorrhage. Fluorescein angiography is helpful also in evaluating the ophthalmologic consequences of certain systemic diseases such as diabetes.

During a normal study, the entire retinal vasculature is sharply defined. Choroidal and disc vasculature are also visualized. Normal arm to retina circulation time is approximately 10 to 13 seconds. The flow of the dye and the vascular filling and blushes produced allow recognition of diseases, characterized as a breakdown of the normal anatomic and physiologic relationships of these vascular patterns. Vascular abnormalities such as arteriovenous shunts, neovascularization, and microaneurysms can be detected in the early filling stage, while vascular leakage can be observed later.

These disturbances can be classified according to changes seen in the disc, retina, retinal pigment epithelium, and choroid. In the disc evaluation, papilledema will cause fluorescence of the disc with indistinct margins. Hemangiomas are visualized as well as congenital vascular problems and other optic disc problems.

The presence of fluid within the retinal tissue caused by trauma or inflammation will cause fluorescence of that tissue. Neovascular formations will be detectable because of abnormal permeability that causes leaking of fluorescein.

Choroidal pathology such as arterial occlusive disease and tumors can be clarified by this technique. Choroidal neovascularization can be localized and diagnosed with great accuracy allowing laser treatment to be reasonably effective.

In addition, the value of selected treatments can be determined. Assessment of fundus disease is essential prior to treatment with photocoagulation. Angiography may show the potential value of laser treatment by demonstrating competence or the loss of surrounding capillaries.

ALTERNATIVES

Intraorbital masses generally do not require angiographic evaluation. The CT scan will even reveal such vascular tumors as hemangiomas. Intravenous digital subtraction angiography, most helpful in outlining the extracranial carotid system, has been shown to reveal venous stasis retinopathy secondary to carotid disease and acute arterial retinal emboli. Retinal hemorrhages, infarcts, and retinal vein obstruction can also be detected. The use of fluorescein, however, remains more sensitive in the diagnosis of intra-optic vascular abnormalities.

Refinements in ophthalmoscopy using restricted spectral light do allow improved visualization of atrophy of the nerve fibers and abnormality of the blood vessels. Measurements of the fundus and fundal photography are allowing greater evaluation of the depth of the fundus and evaluation of the disc margins. These techniques are becoming more refined. Fluorescein angiography remains the most effective way to visualize fundal abnormalities, new vasculature, vascular obstructions, leaking capillaries, and pigment epithelial disorders.

POSSIBILITY OF FAILURE

Care must be taken to evaluate the results of fluorescein angiography. This requires expertise and knowledge about the anatomic and physiologic relationships of the vasculature and structures of the eye.

The use of fluorescein angiography to determine episodes of retinal vascular occlusion is helpful only when the evaluation is done within a few hours of the presumed occlusion. Done any time later, the examination may not demonstrate any abnormality once circulation has been restored.

CONTRAINDICATIONS

Fluorescein angiography should be avoided in patients who have experiences a life-threatening type of anaphylactoid reaction because even the administration of prednisone and diphenhydramine do not seem to prevent a recurring reaction. Pregnancy is not a contraindication to fluorescein angiography although certain operators avoid doing the procedure when possible.

Patients with a history of a seizure disorder should be observed carefully during the use of a flashing blue light during photography. Caution should be exercised in these patients.

PREPROCEDURE PREPARATION

A careful history should be obtained to determine any prior history of severe anaphylactoid reaction to any foods or drugs in the past. In addition, a complete medical history and examination should be performed.

PATIENT EDUCATION

The patient should understand the nature and reason for the procedure. Discussion of common, transient after effects, such as yellowing of the skin at the injection site and discoloration of the urine, will help to decrease later anxiety. The flashing lights that may occur with photography should be noted.

PROCEDURE

Fluorescein angiography can be performed as an office procedure. Following pupillary dilation with a topical cycloplegic, the patient is positioned comfortably in a sitting position with one arm extended to receive an intravenous injection. A slit lamp or an ophthalmoscope is used to observe the study. While direct observation occurs, approximately 5 cc of fluorescein is injected peripherally over a 2 to 3 second period. The area should be directly observed for the first 30 seconds, at 3 to 5 minutes, and at 20 to 60 minutes from the time of injection.

Most operators take photographs of the angiograms obtained for further study and comparison (figure 32–1).

POSTPROCEDURE INFORMATION

It is not essential that the patient be accompanied to the examination, but it would certainly be comforting. The possibility of side effects such as allergic reactions or slightly blurred vision should be recognized.

COMPLICATIONS

The most common complication is extravasation of dye locally around the injection site. This is an innocuous problem and may result in parasthesias of the thumb. Thrombophlebitis, perivenous necrosis, sloughing of the skin, and pain have also been infrequently reported following injection.

The complication rate is higher in patients undergoing multiply dye injections than in those who had a single injection. Toxicity to fluorescein dye is rare, with reactions ranging from mild itching, erythema, or nausea and vomiting due to an anaphylactic reaction. These reactions are generally transient. Respiratory allergic reactions such as wheezing and laryngeal edema have occurred. Fever may be present for 24 hours following the procedure.

The incidence of unexpected, significant reactions are thought to be less than 1%. Shock, pulmonary edema, myocardial infarction, and death have been known to occur. The incidence of complications has been reported to be higher in males than in females but it is uncertain that this is correct. Some studies have indicated that younger patients are more likely to develop severe nausea and vomiting.

PATIENT QUESTIONS

Will this procedure affect my vision?

Fluorescein is a unique dye that is cleared from the circulation entirely with 24 hours. There have been no reported episodes of loss or decrease of visual acuity following fluorescein angiography that were not attributable to other underlying ophthalmologic problems. The patient should be able to leave the office following the procedure with the same visual acuity as before the procedure. The only difficulty may be a sensitivity to light caused by pupillary dilation.

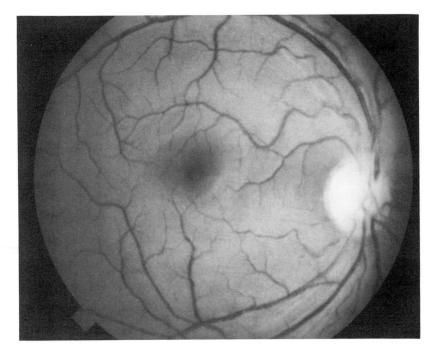

Figure 32–1. Fluorescein angiogram of retinal vessels.

What symptoms might I get that are indicative of an allergic reaction?

Cases of numbness of the thumb, pruritus of the soles and hands, and "hay-fever"-like reactions have been noted. Redness of the skin accompanied by a feeling of warmth may also be a transient problem. Skin testing does not seem to be of value in determining who will have an allergic reaction to the injection of fluorescein.

CONSENT

Informed consent should be obtained prior to performing fluorescein angiography.

SELECTED BIBLIOGRAPHY

Hedges TR, Jr., Giliberti OL, Magargal LE: Intravenous digital subtraction angiography and its role in ocular vascular disease. *Arch Ophthalmol* 1985;May:103:5:666.

Pacurariu RI: Low incidence of side effects following intravenous fluorescein angiography. *Ann Ophthalmol* 1982;Jan:14:1:32.

Singerman LF: Fluorescein angiography. Practical role in the office management of macular disease. *Ophthalmology* 1986;Sept:93:9:1209.

Zimmerman RD, Russell EJ: Angiography in the evaluation of visual disturbances. *Int Ophthalmol Clin* 1986;Fal:26:3:187.

33

Intraocular Foreign Body Removal

RICHARD SADOVSKY

Foreign fragments in the eye can be a serious problem and should be suspected when any traumatic eye condition occurs. Careful examination to evaluate the extent of perforating injury must be done using local anesthetics and lid retractors. Early care by untrained personnel should be limited to rinsing the eye and then firmly patching the affected eyes and transporting the patient to a location where definitive care can be offered.

INDICATIONS

The entry of a foreign body into the eye can be a painful and upsetting experience for the patient. The patient will note irritation almost instantly in most cases, possibly along with photophobia and a scratching sensation especially severe on blinking. Pain is much more severe with corneal foreign bodies than with conjunctival ones. Painful superficial ocular foreign bodies are either on the cornea or on the tarsal surface of the upper lid that covers the cornea.

CONTRAINDICATIONS

There are no contraindications to removal of a foreign body from the eye.

PREPROCEDURE PREPARATION

Tetanus toxoid should be administered as soon as possible. Lacerations from the entry of the foreign body can be seen with fluorescein staining. Often systemic antibiotics are begun early and are continued into the postoperative course. Accurate localization of the foreign body is essential before removal or surgical procedure is attempted. Careful x-ray studies can be done to determine the general location. Occasionally dental film is used to pick up foreign bodies in the anterior portion of the eye, especially when they are small or nonmetallic. Ultrasound may also be used for localization of the particles.

An electronic localizer is also a valuable tool to locate the foreign body. This tool uses transformers to detect current disturbances caused by foreign particles and the strength of the disturbances can be used to locate the foreign particle until it is directly under the point of the localizer.

Assessment of associated damage is obtained at the same time as localization. Ultrasound can help determine the presence of hemorrhage, detachment, organization, and even encapsulation.

Foreign bodies that are wood cause more problems in localization because ultrasound sees wood and the surrounding inflammation as having the same density. CAT scanning may be of some assistance in these situations.

PATIENT EDUCATION

The patient should be advised to avoid rubbing the eye. The patient can be advised to try to remove foreign bodies that are easily visible by dabbing with a clean handkerchief or by irrigating the eye with a salt water solution. The physician should be contacted if these efforts do not work or if the nature of the eye injury appears more severe.

PROCEDURE

Intraocular foreign bodies should be removed as rapidly as possible, generally within 48 to 72 hours.

Patients will more rapidly calm down with relief of the acute pain using topical anesthesia. Fluorescein dye introduced topically will assist in the identification of mucus or tears surrounding a foreign body. Superficially embedded corneal foreign bodies are removed by irrigation using a squeeze bottle of sterile solution, or picked out with a cotton spindle (avoided by some clinicians who claim that the cotton causes irritation of the surrounding tissue) or a needle without anesthetic (figure 33–1) or with minimal superficial anesthesia. The procedure should be done with careful attention to aseptic technique. In cases of intraocular foreign bodies, a single antibiotics instillation in the office may be sufficient, but most clinicians give topical antibiotics for several days. Danger signs include a deeply lodged foreign body, a penetrating wound, or blood in the anterior chamber. The presence of a rust ring is also an indication for the need for extreme care in adequately removing the rust without scarring the cornea.

Deeply embedded corneal foreign bodies and foreign bodies that partially invade the anterior chamber are removed by making a corneal incision under anesthesia. This allows careful removal of the foreign body with as little trauma as possible. Corneal sutures may be required. A magnet can be used to assist in the removal of appropriate foreign bodies. As corneal resistance to infection is low, prophylactic use of topical anesthetics is advised until the epithelium is healed.

In the anterior chamber foreign bodies should optimally be removed through the original corneal wound if possible. If this cannot be done, a small incision is made. Either a magnetic tool is used for removal or a small forceps is inserted when needed.

In the iris, an iridotomy or iridectomy removing the a section of the iris and the particle may be necessary.

In the lens, inert material can be allowed to remain until cataracts develop. If the lens is seriously damaged, or if infection or glaucoma results, the foreign body should be removed. Iron and copper particles should be removed immediately to avoid loss of the eye from chemical damage.

Posterior chamber foreign bodies may be removed carefully through the anterior chamber or they may require an iridectomy.

Complicated foreign body extraction may require a vitrectomy, especially in the case of posteriorly located foreign bodies associated with retinal detachment.

POSTPROCEDURE INFORMATION

The patient should understand that the topical anesthetic effect may dissipate within 15 to 30 minutes, and some irritation and itching may be noted. A single eye dressing is occasionally used, but may not be needed if the foreign body is superficial and easily removed. The patient should remain relatively inactive depending on the amount of eye damage. Steroids, local or systemic, as well as local antibiotics, are often administered if there is considerable corneal abrasion. The length of hospital stay, if any, will vary depending on the extent of the damage. Anesthetics should not be used postoperatively because of their inhibitory effect on reparative activity of corneal epithelium. Corticosteroids are not indicated in the management of minor corneal abrasions.

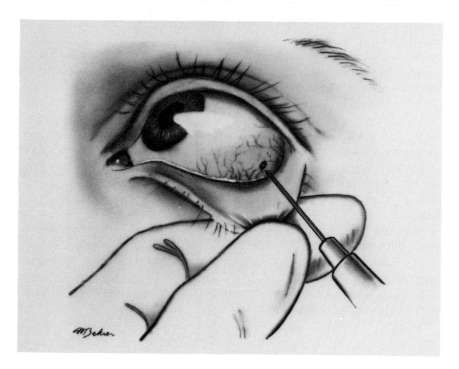

Figure 33–1. Conjunctival foreign body removal using a needle.

Patients with severe pain after an eye injury may require systemic analgesia or even sedation, in addition to the routinely prescribed moist compresses.

Repeat evaluation with fluorescein may be needed to evaluate the progress of healing.

COMPLICATIONS

Prognosis is generally good with small, easily identifiable, superficial foreign bodies. Prognosis is more serious if the foreign body is deep within the eye and serious infection has already begun.

PATIENT QUESTIONS

Is it possible that some of the foreign body will be left behind after surgery?

Even with the most careful surgical procedure, small pieces of foreign body, especially those that are difficult to detect by localizers and ultrasound, may remain in the eye. These may cause an inflammatory reaction leading to further problem or may remain quiescent. Certain materials such as wood may be brought to the surface over time and the patient may be surprised at the size of the remnant remaining. For this reason, foreign body removal procedures require careful follow up.

Will I have to wear a patch?

Generally, a patch is used after removal of a foreign body to prevent scuffing of the anesthetized eye and for at least 24 hours after. Healing proceeds at the same pace whether the eye is patched or not. Since patching encourages infection, it has no place in the management of bacterial conjunctivitis or keratitis.

Will my vision be impaired?

Most superficial foreign bodies do not cause any lasting problems. It is important that the foreign body be managed appropriately and an evaluation be done to determine the nature of the offending material. Copper and iron particles require special management. The prognosis for a nonmagnetic foreign body, being larger in general than the others, is considerably worse with approximately 50% of patients obtaining a final visual acuity of 20/200. The relationship of visual outcome to size of the intraocular foreign body has been expressed as 85% with relatively good vision with a foreign body smaller than 2 mm^2, as opposed to only 15% good vision for those foreign bodies greater than 10 mm^2. Postoperative visual acuity studies are complicated by a number of factors including variations in the reporting method, variations in case groupings, and the existence of clinical variables.

CONSENT

Consent should be obtained for the ambulatory or operative removal of a foreign body in the eye.

SELECTED BIBLIOGRAPHY

Coleman DJ, Lucas BC, Rondeau MJ, Chang S: Management of intraocular foreign bodies. *Ophthalmology* 1987;Dec:94:12:1547.

Colvin JL, Reich JA: The missed intraocular foreign body. *Aust Fam Physician* 1986;Dec 15:12:1599.

Holt GR, Holt JE: Management of orbital trauma and foreign bodies. *Otolaryngol Clin North Am* 1988;Feb 21:1:35.

Newell SW: Management of corneal foreign bodies. *Amer Fam Physican* 1985;Feb:31:2:149.

34

Laryngoscopy

RICHARD SADOVSKY

Laryngoscopy involves the visualization of the larynx through the oral cavity. Indirect laryngoscopy allows visualization of the larynx using a warmed mirror positioned at the back of the throat. Direct laryngoscopy uses a fiberoptic scope or laryngoscope passed through the mouth and the pharynx permitting direct visualization of laryngeal structures and the obtaining of biopsy specimens.

INDICATIONS

Laryngoscopy should be performed on patients with symptoms of laryngeal or pharyngeal disease. A history of smoking accentuates the need for inspection. These symptoms can include cough, persistent hoarseness (for more than 2 weeks), hemoptysis, dysphagia, or stridor. Unilateral otitis media in an adult over 40 years of age may indicate the possibility of a tumor of the nasopharynx.

Laryngoscopy includes visualization of laryngeal structures and the collection of secretions or tissue for further study. Direct laryngoscopy allows inspection of the entire endolarynx including the true or false vocal cords, anterior commissure, laryngeal ventrice, epiglottic tubercle, and subepiglottic region. A normal larynx shows no inflammation, lesions, strictures, or foreign bodies. Foreign bodies, when present, can often be removed through this procedure. Laryngeal, hypopharyngeal, or nasopharyngeal carcinoma may be diagnosed by laryngoscopy and biopsy.

Indications for direct laryngoscopy include children who cannot cooperate with an indirect examination, patients with a strong gag reflex, the need to obtain a biopsy specimen, and the therapeutic treatment of certain laryngeal lesions. Laryngological surgery can be performed through the direct laryngoscope.

The fiberoptic laryngoscope is currently being utilized to enhance visualization of laryngeal structures. New uses of these scopes include videolaryngoscopy, which allows evauation of the physiologic function of the larynx. These scopes are commonly being used in pediatric evaluations.

ALTERNATIVES

The larynx can be studied with standard radiography, tomography, contrast radiography, sonography, and computerized tomography (CT) as well as other special studies such as electroglottography, echoglottography, and electromyography. These tests may all be helpful, but none provide the ability to visualize the structures and to obtain tissue for diagnosis.

POSSIBILITY OF FAILURE

In most cases of laryngeal disease, laryngoscopy coupled with the history will lead to the correct diagnosis. Submucosal abnormalities may require further evaluation with a CT scan or magnetic resonance imaging (MRI).

CONTRAINDICATIONS

Laryngoscopy is relatively contraindicated for patients who have acute epiglottitis, because trauma can cause edema and airway obstruction. If the examination is essential, it may be performed in the operating room with the appropriate resuscitative equipment available. Other upper airway infections may cause increased secretion production and irritable airways causing an increased probability of laryngospasm. The presence of asthma or bronchospasm also should be noted and the patient managed carefully.

Patients who cannot or will not cooperate are poor candidates for laryngoscopy unless the procedure is done directly and with general anesthesia.

PREPROCEDURE PREPARATION

The patient should not eat for 6 to 8 hours before the test. A thorough history should be done to evaluate prior history of hypersensitivity to anesthetics. No anesthesia is needed in the indirect laryngoscopic evaluation on a calm, cooperative patient. Generally, prior to direct laryngoscopy, the patient is given a sedative and atropine. Dentures should be removed as well as contact lenses and the patient should be instructed to void.

PATIENT EDUCATION

The patient should understand the reason for the procedure and how it is performed. The use of sedating medications should be discussed and reassurance that the test will not obstruct the airway is important. The patient will feel that his/her swallowing mechanism will be impaired and will have a sense of uneasiness. This can rapidly become a state of panic unless a patient is warned about the sensation.

PROCEDURE

Indirect laryngoscopy is a simple office procedure performed with the patient sitting erect in a chair with the tongue stuck out as far as possible (figure 34–1). The operator grasps the tongue with a piece of gauze and holds it in place using a tongue depressor if needed. A warm laryngeal miror is positioned at the back of the throat and the larynx is visualized during rest and during phonation. Asking the patient to "pant like a puppy" helps to form a space between the tongue and the palate and allows better positioning of the mirror. Small polyps can be removed using this procedure. The development of inexpensive right-angle telescopes recently has begun to allow direct visualization with a procedure similar to that of indirect laryngoscopy. Minimal anesthesia is needed during procedures utilizing these newer scopes.

Direct laryngoscopy is generally done with the patient in a supine position with arms relaxed at the side. A general anesthetic may be administered or local anesthesia is sprayed into the patient's mouth and throat. Ventilation is maintained by the use of a small endotracheal tube. The lubricated laryngoscope is positioned in the patient's mouth down to the larynx. Examination and removal of specimens is done and any minor surgery such as removal of polyps or nodules can be accomplished. The technique of microlaryngoscopy has been adequately perfected to allow the operator to use both hands for the manipulation of other instruments. Carbon dioxide lasers have been used for both ablative and excisional surgery of the larynx during laryngoscopy.

Flexible laryngoscopy can be performed through the patient's nose, and a thorough examination can be performed. Instrumentation, however, is difficult through the flexible scope so this procedure is used mainly for diagnostic examination.

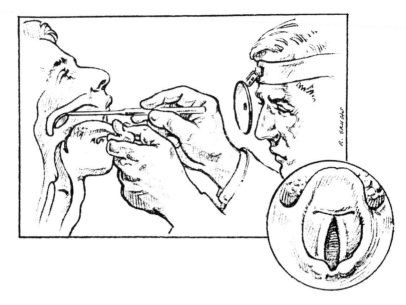

Figure 34–1. Indirect laryngscopy.

Following direct laryngoscopy, the patient is observed carefully, especially if general anesthesia has been administered.

POSTPROCEDURE INFORMATION

The patient should avoid clearing his throat or coughing since this may dislodge a clot at a biopsy site. Foods and fluids should be restricted until the gag reflex returns. Usually, the patient can begin to take sips of water within 2 to 8 hours. Smoking should be avoided for 24 to 48 hours. The sputum should be observed for blood and, if any is noted, the physician should be informed. Significant amounts of bleeding may require repeat examination. Any subcutaneous air or crepitations around the neck as indicated by swelling should be reported immediately because this may indicate trachea perforation.

COMPLICATIONS

Complications of laryngoscopy are rare when the operator has appropriate experience with the procedure. During the procedure, problems with laryngospasm or with hypersensitivity to the anesthesia can occur. These are more common in children. Laceration of the ventral surface of the tongue may occur as a result of extending the tongue over the teeth. This can be avoided by using sufficient gauze to insulate the tongue from the surface of the teeth.

PATIENT QUESTIONS

Will this test affect my voice?

Voice loss, hoarseness, and sore throat are all temporary. These symptoms can be relieved with throat lozenges or a soothing gargle initiated after the gag reflex returns.

I am a nervous and anxious patient—what about sedation?

Generally, no anesthesia or sedation is needed. If the patient has a sensitive gag reflex, a topical anesthetic can be applied to the pharynx and severe anxiety can be relieved by intravenous diazepam.

How can I breathe during the procedure?

If the patient is cooperative and takes regular breaths, adequate air intake will occur around the scope. If the patient panics and moves, the larynx will collapse on the scope and hinder respiratory efforts. It is essential that the patient remain relaxed.

CONSENT

Informed consent is required for direct laryngoscopy.

SELECTED BIBIOGRAPHY

Fried MP: A survey of the complications of laser laryngoscopy. *Arch Otolaryngol* 984;Jan:110:1:31.

Geyman JP, Kirkwod R: Telescope laryngoscopy. *J Fam Pract* 1983;Apr:16:4:789.

Hawkins DB, Clark RW: Flexible laryngoscopy in neonates, infants, and young children. *Ann Otol Rhino Laryngol* 1987;Jan–Feb:96:1:81.

White JF, Knight RE: Office videofiberoptic laryngoscopy. *Laryngoscope* 1984;Sep:94:9:1166.

35

Myringotomy

RICHARD SADOVSKY

Myringotomy is the incision of the tympanic membrane of the ear for the purpose of drainage of a fluid-filled cavity and the obtaining of a sample of the fluid for culture.

INDICATIONS

Buildup of fluid in the middle ear is the major indication for myringotomy. These fluid accumulations most commonly arise from otitis media. Serious otitis media is the accumulation of middle-ear fluid caused by repeated ear infections, allergy, enlarged adenoids, or infections of the mastoid. The frequency of serious otitis in children is well defined as is the clinical presentation. Adults can develop serious otitis and the examination will demonstrate a thickened and retracted tympanic membrane with decreased motility. Tympanometry can define this condition with high precision.

Bacteria are involved in a majority of the cases of acute otitis media. The variety of causes of fluid accumulation in the middle ear make the determination of successful treatment modalities somewhat more complex. It is not clear that routine myringotomy when used with or without antibiotics for the treatment of routine acute ofitis media is any better than antibiotics alone.

Specific indications for myringotomy include (1) persistence of a bulging tympanic membrane after adequate antimicrobial therapy, (2) persistent mucoid middle-ear infections, (3) continued pain even after 48 hours of antimicrobial therapy, (4) evidence of high toxicity at time of diagnosis of otitis media, (5) otitis media accompanied by severe facial pain or other cranial nerve complications, (6) a neonate with concomitant signs of sepsis, and (7) a host who is immunocompromised.

ALTERNATIVES

A myringotomy generally will not hasten the resolution of the typical case of otitis media although it may be helpful in alleviating pain. In most cases it is not necessary as it will not prevent the development of a middle-ear effusion. Otitis media will resolve spontaneously in most cases with antihistamine therapy with or without antibiotics and careful observation.

If the otitis is caused by obstruction of the eustachian tubes secondary to enlargement of the adenoid, adenoidectomy can be performed and is effective in resolving the problem. Any allergies contributing to the development of middle-ear fluid secondary to eustachian tube obstruction also require resolution and treatment.

CONTRAINDICATIONS

There are no contraindications to myringotomy.

PREPROCEDURE PREPARATION

No preprocedure preparation is necessary.

PATIENT EDUCATION

The patient should understand the procedure and, if a tube is to remain in place for drainage, that activity will be restricted for several days. If a ventilation tube is used for several months, the patient must avoid getting water into the tube. It is helpful to use visual aids to demonstrate the procedure. If a tube is going to be placed, show the tube to the patient.

If the patent is a child, care must be taken to explain the procedure in language appropriate for the child's age using visual aids when appropriate.

PROCEDURE

The entire procedure can be done in about 3 minutes for each ear by an experienced operator. Myringotomy is an office procedure requiring an unobstructed view of the entire tympanic membrane. The use of antiseptic solutions or anesthetics are usually not needed for very young children, but may be used by the operator if desired for older children or adults where immobilization may be a problem. All debris and cerumen must be removed from the canal and the largest speculum that will enter the ear should be used.

The site for the procedure may be obscured because of bulging and inflammation. The perforation of the tympanic membrane should be made in the lower half below the head of the malleolus. The incision is made with either a needle (tympanocentesis) or a myringotomy knife. In order to permit the release of thick, purulent material an adequate size puncture is necessary.

Any purulent material should be collected for examination and culture. A cotton wick may be placed in the external canal to aid drainage or a tube can be paced into the perforation allowing optimal drainage for several days. A ventilation tube may be placed to allow for free exchange of air between the outer ear and the middle ear, functioning like an accessory eustachian tube. The ventilation tube usually remains in the ear drum for 2 to 9 months. It is designed to slowly work its way out and fall into the external ear rather than into the middle ear (figure 35–1).

Heat myringotomy has been used recently to treat chronic otitis media. Based on the theory that 2 to 3 weeks of drainage are needed for resolution of chronic otitis media, burn perforations of the tympanic membrane have been used since they tend to resist closure. This technique is successfully being used to avoid the necessity for the placement of a ventilating tube.

POSTPROCEDURE INFORMATION

Bleeding and drainage of pus should stop with 1 to 2 days after the procedure. The physician should be notified if the discharge continues beyond the third day. If a cotton wick has been placed into the ear canal, it should be removed or replaced within 1 or 2 hours. The patient should not shampoo the hair or go swimming until the tympanic membrane has healed. If a ventilation tube has been placed through the membrane, the patient must use protection such as earplugs over the ear when swimming or showering, although recent studies have demonstrated that the instillation of a topical antibiotic solution in the ears after swimming can significantly reduce the risk of infection in patients with tympanotomy tubes. A reexamination should be performed within 7 to 14 days following the procedure to assess the middle ear status. Repeat hearing tests may be helpful in following middle ear drainage and resolution of infection or inflammation.

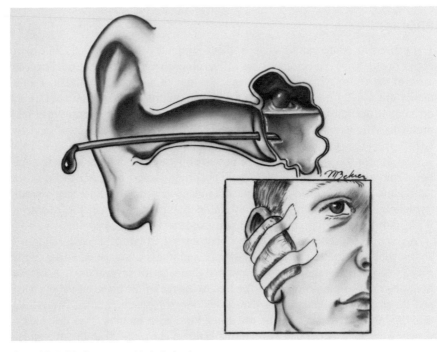

Figure 35–1. Myringotomy with drain in place.

COMPLICATIONS

Complications of myringotomy are extremely rare if the procedure is carried out carefully. The most frequent complication is laceration of the canal wall, which generally does not cause any significant problems. Injury to the facial nerve or middle ear structures is rare if the operator avoids making the incision in the superior quadrant of the tympanic membrane.

Other rare complications can include bleeding, persistent perforation of the tympanic membrane (more common when a tympanotomy tube is used), the formation of a cholesteatoma, disarticulation of the middle ear bony structures, and facial nerve injury.

PATIENT QUESTIONS

What is the possibility that the procedure will need to be repeated?

Some patients require repeat myringotomies because the tube involuntarily is extruded and the fluid reaccumulates. If the tube remains in place for an adequate amount of time, complete drainage of the middle ear should be achieved. It is possible that recurrent pathology within the middle ear or its drainage components may necessitate another myringotomy in the future.

Can myringotomy and drainage improve my hearing?

In both adults and children, the accumulation of fluid in the middle ear can impair the conduction of sound to the auditory nerve. Myringotomy and drainage can significantly improve hearing in these situations. Recent studies in adults with middle ear fluid accumulations demonstrated hearing improvement in approximately 75% of the cases. Even if a perforation persists after the myringotomy, little loss of hearing would be expected, since a small hole in the ear drum does not appreciably affect hearing.

Will I be given anesthesia prior to the procedure?

Infiltration of an anesthetic can be performed by infiltration of the external auditory meatus but this is generally more painful than the myringotomy itself. Sedation or intravenous analgesia can be given when absolutely necessary. In certain cases, general anesthesia may be utilized.

Will the procedure damage my hearing?

The small incision made in myringotomy will not impair hearing or weaken the tympanic membrane. Generally the membrane will heal competely within several days and almost invariably within 1 month.

CONSENT

Informed consent is required for this procedure.

SELECTED BIBLIOGRAPHY

Arcand P, Gauthier P, Biodeau G, Chapados G, Abea A, Desjardins R, Gagnon PP, Gueguerian AJ: Post-myringotomy care: a prospective study. *J Otoarynol* 1984;Oct:13:5:305.

Black B: Acute myringotomy. *Aust Fam Physician* 1987;May:16:5:617.

Brenman AK, Metzer CR, Miner RM: Myringotomy and tube ventilation in adults. *Am Fam Physician* 1982;Oct:26:4:181.

Gates GA: The role of myringotomy in acute otitis media. *Pediatr Ann* 1984;May:13:5:391.

van Buchem F, Dunk JH, vant Hof MA: Therapy of acute otitis media: myringotomy, antibiotics, or neither? *Lancet* 1981;Oct 24:2:8252:883.

36

Nasal Packing for Epistaxis

RICHARD SADOVSKY

Nasal bleeding, or epistaxis, rarely requires the assistance of a physician. A persistent nosebleed may require more aggressive therapy with consideration of nasal packing. The area of the nose on the anterior portion of the nasal septum is the most common site of anterior nose bleeds. Posterior nose bleeds most often occur behind the middle turbinate. Epistaxis in children and young adults occurs more often from an anterior site while epistaxis in the older adult with hypertension or atherosclerosis comes more often from a posterior source.

INDICATIONS

When a patient presents with persistent epistaxis and a bleeding site cannot be identified, an anterior nasal pack is needed. If the anterior packing fails to stop the hemorrhage it must be removed and a posterior nasal packing inserted. The posterior packing will act as a support against which more effective anterior packing can be positioned.

ALTERNATIVES

If a precise site of bleeding can be identified, cautery with silver nitrate sticks or an electrocautery unit may be performed. Care should be taken not to use the silver nitrate sticks over a large surface area because the resultant chemical burn can cause further beeding.

Surgical treatments, including vessel ligation, can be performed. Comparative studies have demonstrated fewer side effects with medical management than with surgical procedures.

POSSIBILITY OF FAILURE

The rare nose bleed that does not respond to nasal cauterization or packing may require selective arterial ligation of the blood supply of the nose or selective embolization of these same vessels.

CONTRAINDICATIONS

There are no absolute contraindications to nasal packing although there are some conditions that are relative contraindications. If some other etiology for exacerbation of bleeding has been discovered, nasal packing may be relatively contraindicated. Patients with evidence of a bleeding disorder may bleed more extensively if packing is inserted. This is especially true for posterior packing. If packing remains essential, lighter materials made of cellulose are preferred.

Patients with chronic obstructive pulmonary disease may have a significant decrease in their oxygen levels if posterior packing is placed. These patients require very close observation and monitoring.

PREPROCEDURE PREPARATION

A thorough history and medical examination is essential to evaluate for trauma, foreign body, allergy, bleeding disorders, or neoplasm. Once this is done, a good rapport with the patient is essential to permit nasal manipulation. A hematocrit, type match and cross match, prothrombin time, partial thromboplastin time, and a platelet count shoud be obtained. Arterial blood gas determination is appropriate if posterior packing is being considered. An intravenous line is appropriate if the patient is hypotensive or has lost a significant amount of blood.

PATIENT EDUCATION

Patients should be made as comfortable and calm as possible, and reassured that people do not die from nose bleeds. Information about the discomfort accompanying nasal packing should be given in a relaxed manner and the methods for dealing with the discomfort should be discussed. Removal of the packing will be easy and painless because the packing is well greased. It is generally only necessary to pack one side of the nose because bleeding bilaterally is rare unless a severe fracture has been sustained or a systemic disorder such as leukemia is present. Some physicians, however, do advocate packing both nostrils to maximize locaization of packing pressure. Packing will at least partially obstruct nasal breathing and may obstruct air passage totally.

PROCEDURE

Intramuscular or intravenous sedation is advisable to obtain optimal patient cooperation. The nose is anesthetized, generally with a topical cocaine or xylocaine solution, followed by insertion of cotton saturated with vasoconstrictive medication. The cotton is left in place for about 5 minutes and then removed. A careful examination follows, looking for sites of persistent oozing of blood or an irritated patch of nasal mucosa. Nasal packing, well lubricated with antibiotic ointment, is inserted through the nose with closed loops of gauze directed posteriorly. The packing material is applied sequentially from inferior to superior with pressure being directed at the bleeding area (figure 36–1). If unilaterial anterior packing is not sufficient, packing the opposite side may prevent movement of the septum, which might result in decreased pressure in the bleeding area.

The use of absorbable packing materials is being evaluated. These swell and form an artificial clot, which undergoes enzymatic degradation in 1 to 2 days and completely liquifies shortly after. Alternate techniques of nasal packing for both anterior and posterior nasal bleeding are under study. As yet, none have proved superior to the classical methods.

Posterior packing consists of a roll of gauze pads tightly tied with a silk suture. The ends of the suture are left long to permit movement of the pack on insertion and removal. Placement of the posterior pack involves passage of a catheter through the nose into the hypopharynx and retrieving it through the mouth with a clamp or forceps. The strings of the posterior pack are then tied to the catheter, the catheter is then retracted, and the posterior pack moves into the nasopharynx. An anterior pack is usually then placed in the same side as the posterior pack. Care should be taken to secure the trail suture material someplace where it will be easily accessible when it is time to remove the posterior packing material. Formal anterior and posterior nasal packing indicates the need for hospitalization and close observation of the patient.

Commercially manufactured posterior packs consisting of single or multiple balloons are available. These balloons are inflated with saline and can control epistaxis. However, these commercial preparations do not permit the localization of pressure and may cause pressure necrosis of adjoining tissue.

Both anterior and posterior packing are generally left in pace for about 5 days. The packs may be removed as early as day 3 if it is certain that bleeding

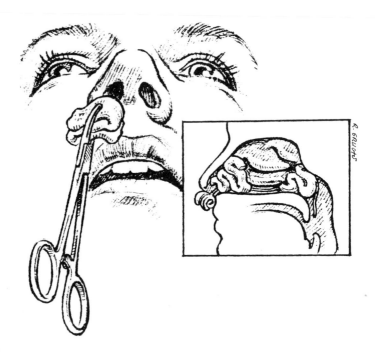

Figure 36–1. Nasal packing for epistaxis.

has stopped. Removal of the anterior packing material is done easily through the nose by wiggling the packing from the nasal chamber with a forceps. Posterior packing is delivered through the mouth by drawing on the single suture. Patients who have been hospitalized for observation should generally be monitored for additional bleeding for 24 hours following removal of the posterior packing.

POSTPROCEDURE INFORMATION

Patients with anterior packing can be cared for at home. The administration of a decongestant helps to decrease the volume of nasal secretions. The patient should be encouraged to remain in bed or at least at home while the packing is in place. A mild sedative might help to decrease the discomfort.

If the patient is hospitalized following nasal packing, close monitoring of the hemoglobin and hematocrit are needed. Systemic antibiotics are often administered to prevent the onset of sinusitis. Analgesia may be needed because of the discomfort of the packing material.

After removal of the packing material, the nasal mucosa will be irritated. The use of a normal saline nasal spray and antibiotic ointment will help heal and improve humidification of the affected tissue. If bleeding recurs, the patient should keep the head up and tilted slightly backward, applying steady pressure to both nostrils with the fingers for at least 5 minutes, and trying not to blow the nose. If the bleeding does not stop, the physician should be contacted.

COMPLICATIONS

The possibility of complications from nasal packing require that the patient be observed carefully. Pressure necrosis of the nasal ala may occur as can sinusitis resulting from obstruction of the natural ostia with secondary infection. Hypoxia can occur, particularly in older patients, and must be recognized as a possible cause of agitation in patients with nasal packing. Rare middle-ear problems such as otitis media and accumulations of blood can occur with blockage of the eustachian tube.

Technical errors can have serious consequences. A postnasal pack that is not anchored to a role of gauze anteriorly can become dislodged posteriorly and aspirated, with potentially fatal results. With posterior packing, a posterior pull string must be readily accessible so that the packing can be pulled out if dislodgment does occur.

Toxic shock syndrome from nasal packing has been reported. It is caused by absorption of an endotoxin produced by certain stains of *Staphylococcus aureus*. This is used as one of the bases for giving patients with nasal packing systemic antibiotics. Occasional cocaine reactions have been seen among patients who are sensitive or who have received an overdose during anesthesia. Since these reactions are potentially lethal, patients should be intubated and given cardiorespiratory support until the drug leaves the body.

PATIENT QUESTIONS

Will I require a transfusion?

Blood loss might not be readily apparent in the acute stage of epistaxis because hemodilution may not yet have occurred. It is possible that, with serial blood counts, severe blood loss will be detected and a transfusion might be advisable.

Will I be able to get enough air through the packing material?

Anterior packing alone rarely hinders air intake, especially when the packing is unilateral. Posterior packing may result in hypoxia and respiratory depression. Humidified oxygen should be administered by face mask while the packs are in place.

Will I be able to eat normally?

Eating is difficult for patients with nasal packing and food should be provided in as tempting a manner as possible. The use of a straw makes drinking easier. Plenty of fluids should be administered to avoid constipation and straining to defecate, which may raise the blood pressure in the nose and cause recurrence of epistaxis. Mouth washes can be used to keep the mouth moist and the patient should be encouraged to brush the teeth.

CONSENT

The control of epistaxis can be an emergency, life-saving procedure. In these cases, informed consent is not necessary. It is wise, however, to discuss the procedure with the patient and any relatives or friends available before proceeding. Under less threatening circumstances, it is a good idea to obtain consent for nasal packing.

SELECTED BIBIOGRAPHY

Fairbanks DN: Complications of nasal packing. *Otoaryngo Head Neck Surg* 1986Mar:94:3:412.

McDonad TJ: Nosebleed in children. Background and techniques to stop the flow. *Postgrad Med* 1987;Jan:81:1:217.

Perretta J, Denslow B, Brown CG: Emergency evaluation and management of epistaxis. *Emerg Med Cin North Am* 1987;May:5:2:265.

Schaitkin B, Strauss M, Houck, JR: Epistaxis: medica versus surgical therapy: a comparison of efficacy, complications, and economic considerations. *Laryngoscope* 1987;97:12:1388.

37

Vestibular Function Testing

RICHARD SADOVSKY

Vestibular function testing is performed as part of a neuro-otologic examination to screen for cerebellar or vestibular dysfunction in a patient complaining of dizziness, equilibrium problems, or nystagmus. The tests should follow a complete physical examination including patient performance of a variety of tasks with the eyes open and closed.

Evaluation of the interactions of the vestibular system and the muscles responsible for eye movement is performed by electronystagmography. Specific stimuli and tests, such as gaze, pendulum tracking, optokinetics, positional methods, and caloric testing are used to gauge this interaction in what is known as the vestibulo-ocular reflex.

Nystagmus, which is the involuntary right-left eye movement caused by the vestibulo-ocular reflex, occurs with the vestibular system's attempt to keep visual fixation while the head is moving. Nystagmus has two components. First, there is slow deviation in the opposite direction from the head movement. This is the slow phase and is mediated by the vestibular system. The fast phase, or rapid return to center, is controlled by the central nervous system. The description of nystagmus is in the direction of the fast phase.

Electronystagmography uses the measurement of the corneoretina potential, the difference between the positive charge of the cornea and the negative charge of the retina, to record nystagmus through electrodes located close to the eyes. A recorder is used to pick up the eye movements and it charts them on paper. This type of recording can be done in a dark room with the patient's eyes open or closed.

Reports have appeared in the literature that question the value of electronystagmography as a diagnostic test. The value of the procedure appears to depend upon the expertise of the examiners.

INDICATIONS FOR PROCEDURE

Electronystagmography is helpful in the identification of the causes of dizziness, vertigo, or tinnitus. In addition, unilateral hearing losses can be better diagnosed, and the presence and location (central, peripheral, or both) of a lesion can be determined.

Nystagmus is normal during a head turn; it is prolonged nystagmus that is found to be abnormal. Results are generally reported as normal, borderline, or abnormal. If abnormal, there is further description about the possibility of a peripheral, central, or undetermined lesion. These abnormalities can result from peripheral disease (end organ or labyrinth) resulting from conditions such as ototoxicity. Central disorders (cerebellar, cerebral, or brain-stem involvement) can result from demyelinating diseases, tumors, and circulatory disorders. Disorders of the eighth nerve are considered either peripheral or central depending on the examiner and may be caused by tumors.

The results of electronystagmography depend on the care taken during testing, patient cooperation, and the accuracy of the recordings. The persistence, direction, and intensity of nystagmus is used to localize the lesion.

ALTERNATIVES

If it is assumed that the major function of electronystagmography is to determine whether a lesion is peripheral or central, then the test performs a diagnostic function that cannot be otherwise accomplished. Computerized tomography (CT) scan appears to be the best way to localize retrolabyrinthine lesions, once the general location has been determined.

POSSIBILITY OF FAILURE

Debate is currently in progress about the productivity of vestibular evaluations. Promoters of this examination feel that nonproductivity occurs under conditions of inadequately trained personnel, the use of older techniques, and the poor standardization of terms used to report results. Electronystagmography is of specific value when performed by trained personnel.

CONTRAINDICATIONS

Electronystagmography is contraindicated in patients with pacemakers because the equipment may interfere with pacemaker function. The presence of back or neck abnormalities may limit the types of testing that can be accomplished because of range of motion difficulties.

A perforated ear drum is not a contraindication as an ear cot can be placed within the ear to avoid water entry into the middle ear during caloric testing. If this is done, finger cots must be used bilaterally and equidistant from the tympanic membrane.

PREPROCEDURE PREPARATION

The patient should be advised to avoid stimulants, antianxiety medications, sedatives, antivertigo drugs, and alcohol for 24 to 48 hours before the test. Tobacco should also be avoided as well as caffeinated beverages on the day of the examination. A light meal should be eaten since caloric testing may cause transient nausea. Emotional support is essential since the tests can be uncomfortable.

Immediately prior to the procedure, an otoscopic examination should be done. All cerumen should be cleared from the ear canals.

PATIENT EDUCATION

The procedure should be described to the patient and the ability of the test to evaluate visual-control and balance-control mechanisms related. The patient's cooperation throughout the test is essential.

PROCEDURE

To insure accurate results, the electrodes must be positioned properly. The skin is prepared with alcohol and a small amount of electrode paste is applied to each contact point. The flat electrode along with an adhesive collar is then pressed to the skin. If lateral nystagmus is being recorded, two lateral electrodes are placed as close to the outer canthus of each eye as possible. If vertical nystagmus is being recorded, two additional electrodes are placed above and below the center of one eye (figure 37–1).

The electronystagmography battery of tests can be done in a variety of sequences, although caloric testing is generally done last. The battery of tests generally takes about 60 to 90 minutes. The **calibration test** involves holding

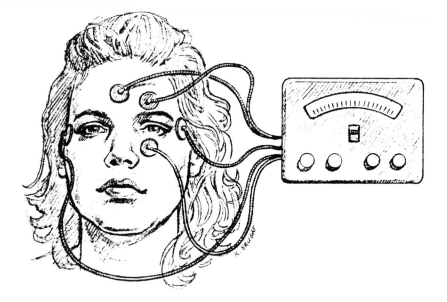

Figure 37–1. Monitoring eye movements during vestibular function testing.

the patient's head straight with his eyes directed at a light 6 to 10 feet away. The light is moved causing deviation of the patient's eyes allowing calibration of the stylus sensitivity on the recorder.

The **gaze nystagmus test** measures eye movements with the patient looking straight ahead. This is done with eyes open and then closed. This measures center-gaze nystagmus. Right-gaze and left-gaze nystagmus are also measured with the eyes open and closed. The **pendulum tracking test** involves having the patient follow a pendulum movement with eyes open and closed. **Optokinetics testing** involves having the patient follow a moving target until it disappears from view and then snapping the eyes back to catch the next moving object appearing in view. This is done both to the right and left. **Positional testing** requires that the patient move into various positions involving movement of the head and the body. **Water caloric testing** involves the introduction of water into the ear so that it hits the tympanic membrane directly. This is done with cool (30°C) and warm (44°C) water. If the patient does not respond to standard caloric stimulation, ice water calorics can be done. Caloric stimulation produces a convection motion of endolymph in the horizontal canals when these canals are placed in the vertical plane by an appropriate head tilt.

POSTPROCEDURE INFORMATION

The patient may complain of weakness, dizziness, or nausea following the examination. It is helpful if someone can accompany the patient to the examination and provide safe transportation home. The patient should simply relax until he recovers.

COMPLICATIONS

Vestibular function testing has no morbidity or mortality. The only complications to be reported occurred when perforations of the tympanic membrane were either not noted prior to caloric testing or were caused by overzealous instillation of water into the external auditory canal.

PATIENT QUESTIONS

Will this testing make me dizzy?

Vestibular function testing is generally performed for undiagnosed symptoms of dizziness and vertigo. There is a possibility that the positional changes and caloric testing required for the performance of the test will cause dizziness. The patient should be reassured that the discomfort will be temporary.

Will electronystagmography provide a diagnosis for my symptoms?

Electronystagmographic testing is helpful in localizing a disorder of the peripheral or central nerve system. With this localization, further testing is generally needed to pinpoint the problem, although syndromes like Meniere's are being diagnosed solely by the symptom complex and the test finding. In order to rule out the likelihood of a tumor or perhaps even demyelinating disorders when central disorders are noted, a CT scan or magnetic resonance imaging (MRI) will often be indicated.

CONSENT

These tests do not require any invasive procedures and oral informed consent is generally felt to be sufficient.

SELECTED BIBIOGRAPHY

Kumar A, Sutton DL: Diagnostic value of vestibular function tests: an analysis of 200 consecutive cases. *Laryngoscope* 1984;November:94:11:1435.

Norre ME: Screening methods for caloric testing. *Clin Otoaryngo* 1987;Jun:12:3:161.

Rubin W: Site of lesion vestibular function testing. *Laryngoscope* 1985;Feb:95:4:386.

VIII
Urologic Procedures

38

Dialysis

RICHARD SADOVSKY

Dialysis involves the movement of solutes across a semipermeable membrane when blood and a physiologic salt solution are perfused on opposite sides of the membrane. Waste products of protein metabolism pass from the blood to the dialysate while substances in greater concentrate in the dialysate move into the blood. The extent and rate of this passage depends on the surface area and permeability of the dialyzing membrane and on the rate of flow of blood and dialysate.

The newer technique of hemofiltration relies on ultrafiltration rather than on diffusion for the movement of solutes. This provides an improved clearance of larger molecules than can be obtained with hemodialysis. Difficulties do exist, however, in this newer procedure, and its place in routine management of chronic renal failure needs further review.

INDICATIONS

Dialysis should be initiated at an appropriate time to prevent further deterioration or complications from the accumulation of renally excreted chemicals in the body. The causative factor for the accumulation could be acute or chronic renal failure. Urgent indications include coma, pericarditis and/or pericardial effusion, symptomatic peripheral neuropathy, uncontrollable hyperkalemia, malignant hypertension, uncontrollable fluid overload or pulmonary edema. Prophylactic dialysis is probably indicated in patients with significant uremic symptoms such as nausea, vomiting, poor mentation, or reversal of sleep pattern. Severe acidosis, azotemia with creatinine levels over 8 mg%, blood urea nitrogen (BUN) levels over 100 mg%, and creatinine clearance less than 5 cc per minute indicate the likelihood of severe renal failure requiring prophylactic treatment.

ALTERNATIVES

Acute and chronic renal failure can be managed with peritoneal dialysis. Dialysis consisting of diffusion and ultrafiltration can occur through the peritoneal membrane. Diffusion occurs from blood to dialysate (for substances such as urea and creatinine) and from the dialysate to the blood (for substances such as calcium, acetate, and lactate). The rate of diffusion is critically influenced by the thickness of the peritoneal membrane, the surface area exposed to the dialysate, the peritoneal capillary flow rate, and several other factors.

Peritoneal dialysis might be chosen by the patient for a variety of reasons. This procedure can be performed independently without a partner and avoids the use of heparin. In addition, this procedure is a suitable substitute for patients who have no access remaining to the blood system. Being a slower process, peritoneal diagnosis may also offer a lessening of symptomatic metabolic disturbances. Insulin can be infused into the intraperitoneal space by being combined with the dialysate. This is desirable in therapy for insulin dependent diabetics. Standard intermittent peritoneal dialysis is much less effective than hemodialysis in controlling disturbances in urea, but it may be preferable when anticoagulation (as required for hemodialysis) would be hazardous, or while waiting for maturation of vascular access.

Continuous ambulatory peritoneal dialysis is becoming a more widely accepted method for treating patients with end-stage renal disease. This treatment is particularly suitable to patients capable of self-care at home, patients with diabetes, and those with unstable cardiovascular systems.

The option of transplantation is also available and considerations of cost and long-term survival are important in choosing the appropriate form of therapy for end-stage renal disease. Transplantation, generally advocated in the young, uncomplicated patient is becoming more applicable to other populations because of improved results with new immunosuppressive agents such as cyclosporine.

CONTRAINDICATIONS

There are no specific contraindications to hemodialysis although complications are more frequent in patients with metastatic disease, cerebrovascular disease with severe hemiparesis, hepatorenal syndrome, and advanced organic brain disease.

Contraindications to ambulatory peritoneal dialysis include severe chronic obstructive pulmonary disease, malnutrition, or chronic back problems. Hemodialysis is generally preferred to peritoneal dialysis in severe uremia, poisonings known to benefit from hemodialysis, disorders compromising the efficiency of peritoneal dialysis such as vasculitis, scleroderma, and aortic aneurysm, and respiratory failure.

PREPROCEDURE PREPARATION

Early placement of an arteriovenous access is needed if chronic hemodialysis is to be the method of treatment because a period of 1 to 10 weeks is often needed before it can be used. In patients who receive peritoneal dialysis, or in early transplantation, prophylactic fistula preparation is not necessary.

The hepatitis B vaccine should be administered to all patients beginning hemodialysis.

PATIENT EDUCATION

Introduction to patients currently on dialysis who have positive attitudes about the treatment is very encouraging. This communication can help reinforce the concept that a normally active life is still possible while on dialysis.

Patients should actively participate in all decisions about the reason for dialysis and the type of dialysis to be performed. Proper and early preparation of the patient is important in reducing emotional and psychological stresses and in preventing physiologic complications.

PROCEDURE

Access to the blood stream is necessary initially. This can be done temporarily by placement of a catheter into the femoral, subclavian, or other large vein and, optimally, an additional catheter in the contralateral vein or some other superficial vein to return blood to the body. Permanent blood access involves an internal device known as a fistula, or, if the patient does not have adequate veins for access, an arterio-venous graft usually made of synthetic material.

The choice of dialyzer depends largely on the patient's size, endogenous creatinine clearance, and weight gain. For older, more infirm patients with medical problems such as cardiac instability, a dialyzer with a lower ultrafiltration rate may be more appropriate.

The procedure involves pumping the patient's heparinized blood through the blood compartment of the machine at a rate of 200 to 300 ml per minute (figure 38–1). Blood is taken to test for hematocrit, BUN, potassium level, and clotting-time evaluations. Monitoring systems watch for changes in pressure, the presence of blood in the dialysate, and other changes that might indicate malfunction, obstruction, or line separation.

Peritoneal dialysis requires that a catheter be inserted into the peritoneal cavity either temporarily or semipermanently depending on the clinical situation. The volume of dialysate generally instilled for peritoneal dialysis is 2 liters, but enhanced clearances can be obtained with 3 liters. The flow rate of the dialysate and the splanchnic blood system and other factors affect the efficacy of this procedure.

The choice of dialysis method requires cooperative thought between the patient, the physician, and the patient's family. Home dialysis is clearly the method of choice for patients able to perform this technique. If peritoneal dialysis is required because of patient preference, cardiovascular instability during hemodialysis, lack of a blood access, or inadequate facilities for home hemodialysis, the question becomes: How much can the patient do alone and how much family support is available? Chronic ambulatory dialysis is ideal for the patient with the manual dexterity who has the ability to learn and comply with a relatively demanding schedule. There are even devices available that permit peritoneal dialysis by the visually impaired.

POSTPROCEDURE INFORMATION

Dialysis requires the cooperation of family members and friends in both management of the procedure and in the interim support of the patient. The extent to which the family can participate may determine the ability of the patient to have ambulatory dialysis. Access to a nurse or physician 24 hours a day diminishes the anxiety of the family and the patient. Major areas of emphasis in the educational program should include dietary and fluid restrictions, rationale, purpose, and side effects of each of the prescribed medications, which over-the-counter medications should be avoided, and pertinent observations and emergency care of the access.

Peritonitis as a result of peritoneal dialysis can be diminished by aseptic technique. Showering must be done to avoid submersion of the catheter tip although the patient can go swimming with the catheter tip appropriately covered. Betadine may be used around the catheter and the exit site. Antibiotic ointments are generally not recommended.

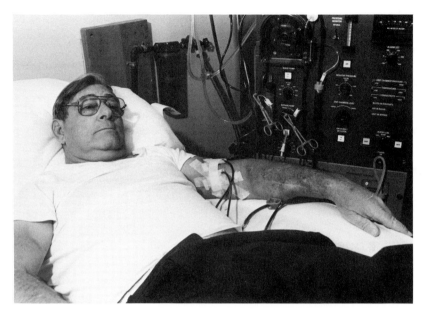

Figure 38–1. Hemodialysis using a fistula.

COMPLICATIONS

Complications of dialytic therapy can occur from access problems, the dialysis procedure itself, and other general medical problems not directly related to the procedure. Hemodialysis access-related complications may include clotting, infection, aneurysm and pseudoaneurysm, ischemia and gangrene, or highoutput congestive heart failure. In peritoneal dialysis, one may have malfunction causing pain or obstruction, fluid leakage, catheter cuff erosion, or exit-site and tunnel infections. These access-related complications are the most common cause of admission of these patients to the hospital and the struggle to maintain a patent access can be a severe psychologic stress on the patient.

Complications related to the dialysis process include hypotension, which is the most common complication occurring in about 10% of all dialysis procedures, disequilibrium syndrome, cardiac arrhythmias, electrolyte imbalances, fever, air embolism, hemorrhage, muscle cramps, pruritus, and hepatitis. Older patients have a diminished response in heart rate to the clinical shock induced during dialysis and are more likely to develop hypotension. Anemia is also a constant problem. With the discovery that dialysis patients can tolerate very low hematocrit, the transfusion rate for dialysis patients has dropped significantly. Transfusions are now reserved for patients who are symptomatic from their anemia or who are being prepared for surgery. Decreasing laboratory studies in stable patients to once every 3 months eliminates a very real source of blood loss. The recent use of recombinant erythropoietin has generally corrected the anemia in almost all the patients in whom it was used.

Complications specific to peritoneal dialysis include peritonitis, hydrothorax, bowel perforation, pain, ascites, abdominal wall hernias, and backache.

The most common causes of death in centers performing dialysis have been cardiovascular and sepsis. Long-term morbidity is probably more dependent on risk factors at the time of initiation of dialysis than on the type of treatment chosen for the patient.

Suicide or withdrawal from dialysis represents a substantial psychiatric morbidity. Dialysis patients may halt treatment, eat foods high in potassium content, or take overdoses of drugs. Suicide by these methods, particularly the incidence of hyperkalemia, is probably underestimated.

PATIENT QUESTIONS

Should I use an internal or an external access device?

This question depends on the chronicity of the hemodialysis planned. External shunts are almost never used in chronic dialysis. Internal devices are cosmetically more acceptable, but may require 1 to 6 weeks to mature sufficiently for use. The choice of the vascular access to be used depends on the urgency of initiation of hemodialysis, the length of time it is anticipated that hemodialysis will be needed, and the feelings of the patient.

What diet is appropriate for the patient on dialysis?

Dietary management of the patient must include an adequate intake of protein needed to replace amino acid and protein losses during dialysis. Protein intake should approximate 1.5 grams per kilogram of body weight. The caloric intake is also important and unless the patient is obese, an intake of 25 to 35 calories per kilogram of body weight per day will help to maximize protein utilization. Dairy products should be restricted to reduce the phosphate content of the diet. Sodium intake should be limited to 2 to 4 grams daily. Potassium intake should be restricted, limiting the selection of fruits and vegetables. The diet for the diabetic is essentially the same as that for the nondiabetic with the exception of the need for more careful structuring of the meals to conform with insulin administration. Supplementation with vitamin B complex, ascorbic acid, and folic acid are used to offset any deficiency introduced by the combined dietary restriction and dialysis loss. Aluminum hydroxide administration may be necessary to bind phosphorus in the stomach and diminish absorption although the description of aluminum-related osteomalacia has been well described. Foods with high phosphorus content, such as dairy products, should be limited. Vitamin D preparations are often administered to reverse osteomalacia and hypocalcemia.

Will my diabetes alter the success of treatment of end-stage renal disease with dialysis?

Diabetics with end-stage renal disease die earlier than nondiabetic renal failure patients. The average survival at 1 year is around 75% to 80% and 40% to 50% at 3 years. This contrasts with nondiabetics on hemodialysis who show a 1-year survival rate of over 80% and a 3-year survival rate of 50% to 60%. Survival rates with transplanted kidneys appears better, especially when a living, related renal transplant is used.

Is dialysis painful?

Dialysis involves multiple steps and a certain amount of discomfort is unavoidable. The preparation of an access for peritoneal or hemodialysis requires a minor surgical procedure. The patient on peritoneal dialysis may initially note some intraperitoneal irritation. This should disappear as the patient adjusts to the sensation of the dialysate flow. Occasionally the pain will be aggravated if the catheter pokes against the rectum or bladder. Pain between the shoulder blades during peritoneal dialysis may be referred pain caused by stretching and irritation of the diaphragm.

Will I need to alter my medication dosages when I begin dialysis?

The dialyzability of drugs being used by the patient is an important fact and should be evaluated. The dialyzability of a drug depends on the amount of protein binding, its molecular weight, and tissue binding. All three factors must be considered. Dosages of medications may need to be increased.

CONSENT

Informed consent is required for placement of a permanent or temporary access as these are invasive procedures. Individual consents for each dialysis session are not required.

SELECTED BIBLIOGRAPHY

Baldree KS, Murphy SP, Powers MJ: Stress identification and coping patterns in patients on hemodialysis. *Nurs Res* 1982;Mar–Apr:31:2:107.

Charytan C, Spinowitz BS, Galler M: A comparative study of continuous ambulatory peritoneal dialysis and center hemodialysis. Efficacy, complications, and outcome in the treatment of endstage renal disease. *Arch Int Med* 1986;Jun:146:6:1138.

Comty CM, Collins AJ: Dialytic therapy in the management of chronic renal failure. *Med Clin North Am* 1984;Mar:68:2:399.

Khanna R, Oreopoulos DG: Dialysis: continuous ambulatory peritoneal dialysis and hemodialysis. *Clin Endocrinol Metab* 1986;Nov:15:4:823.

Wise TN, Levine DJ, Johnson RW: The decision to discontinue hemodialysis. *Gen Hosp Psychiatry* 1985;Oct:7:4:377.

39

Lithotripsy

RICHARD M. STILLMAN AND RICHARD SADOVSKY

Extracorporeal shock wave lithotripsy (ESWL) uses high-energy sound waves, generated by a spark plug and focused by a hemielliptic reflector to a focal point where maximal energy is concentrated. The early machines required the patient to be placed in a water tank to facilitate passage of the sound wave with minimal energy loss. Newer machines no longer require the water bath. The energy is focused on a calculus, which is fragmented into sand-like particles. Lithotripsy has been used successfully for 8 years in the treatment of urinary tract calculi.

Laboratory studies of the use of lithotripsy for fragmentation of biliary tract calculi have confirmed the existence of several potential problems that have only recently begun to be solved. Therefore, this chapter deals mainly with the use of extracorporeal shock wave lithotripsy to treat urinary tract calculi.

Early reports describe the use of lithotripsy in clearing pancreatic stones from the main pancreatic duct in patients with chronic pancreatitis. At present, lithotripsy for this indication is limited to reducing the size of the stone fragments and making removal by endoscopy easier.

INDICATIONS

Shock wave therapy is useful for removing the majority of kidney stones, either single or multiple, with an aggregate diameter of under 2 cm or under 1 cm if located in the lower portions of the kidney. Several medical panels have recommended shock-wave therapy and percutaneous nephrolithotomy for stones larger than 2 cm. Stones located in the kidney, ureter, or in a transplanted kidney can be treated. Any stone in the lower ureter, below the level of the pelvic bones, cannot be treated by lithotripsy because the shock wave cannot be transmitted through the bony structures. Calcium phosphate and calcium oxalate stones appear to be easier to treat than cystine and struvite stones. Stone formation in children can be managed by ESWL.

Kidney stones are fragmented into sand-like particles. These pulverized fragments will be passed spontaneously in the urine. All of the fragments are passed in the urine within 3 months in about 75% of patients.

The lithoptriptic destruction of gall stones is a newer topic with different issues. The tortuosity of the cystic duct, the chemical make-up of the stones, the lack of inherent peristaltic capability of the common bile duct, and the seriousness of the potential complications all pose dilemmas different from lithotriptic therapy for renal stones. Results in Europe are promising, and further studies have recently begun in the United States.

ALTERNATIVES

Multiple forms of lithotripsy include lasers and microexplosives. Detailed discussions of these experimental alternatives is beyond the scope of this book. There are 4 alternatives to lithotripsy. The first is conservative management with hydration and dietary manipulation to prevent growth of new calcium stones or existing ones, or pharmacotherapy to prevent the progression of metabolic stones (e.g., allopurinol for uric acid stones, penicillamine for cystine stones, phosphate or thiazide diuretic for oxalate stones). Conservative management is best limited to asymptomatic patients with relatively small stones.

The second alternative is percutaneous intervention (endourology). A percutaneous nephrostomy from the flank into the renal pelvis allows passage of instruments for stone extraction. Although these endourologic methods approach a high degree of success, multiple treatments may be required, and there is a risk of substantial bleeding. Endourologic methods are used for stones exceeding 3 cm in diameter and for staghorn calculi. These latter stones may be crushed by endourologic methods into smaller fragments that are then subjected to extracorporeal shock wave lithotripsy.

The third alternative is ureteroscopy. Stones in the lower third of the ureter are best removed by ureteroscopy. Stones in the middle or upper third of the ureter are usually treated by manipulation back into the renal pelvis, followed by extracorporeal shock wave lithotripsy. The fourth alternative is open surgical removal of the stones. Surgical removal is best reserved for patients not amenable to the other methods described or when the other methods of stone removal fail.

The development of chemical dissolution treatments for stones is beginning to make progress. Dissolution and flushing techniques for gallstone treatments have been used fairly widely, but newer drugs such as ursodeoxychlic acid, a naturally occurring bile acid, are currently available as an oral drug for dissolution of cholesterol gallbladder stones. There are no equivalent drugs yet available for treatment of kidney stones.

CONTRAINDICATIONS

Contraindications to extracorporeal shock wave lithotripsy include anticoagulation, bleeding diathesis, sepsis, pregnancy, and renal malignancy. Additional technical contraindications include gross obesity or obstruction distal to the target stone. Although shock-wave generation is coordinated with the R-wave of the electrocardiogram (ECG) to minimize the chances for arrhythmia, lithotripsy is frequently avoided in patients with cardiac pacemakers.

PREPROCEDURE PREPARATION

The patient was usually admitted for an overnight hospital stay in the early days of lithotripsy, but now the procedure is being performed more frequently on an outpatient basis. Routine blood tests are performed to assure the absence of coagulation abnormalities. An electrocardiogram and chest x-rays are obtained to confirm the absence of medical problems that might contraindicate or change the method of anesthesia. Frequently, other urologic procedures may be required prior to extracorporeal-shock-wave lithotripsy. Such procedures might include placement of a percutaneous nephrostomy tube if the ureter is obstructed, or placement of a ureteral catheter to help localize or manipulate the stones. Antibiotics may be started prior to the procedure.

PATIENT EDUCATION

The patient should be made aware that the procedure will require epidural or general anesthesia, that shock waves will be used to fragment (not to remove) the stones, and that the stones should pass spontaneously in the urine over the next several months. A Foley catheter will be placed. There will be blood in the urine, and the passage of the stones may be accompanied by pain. It is possible that urologic instrumentation will be required for the patient in the future.

PROCEDURE

Ambulatory ESWL is becoming more common, although patients with urinary tract obstruction, sepsis, intractable pain, or nausea and vomiting should probably be hospitalized. The total procedure time is 60 to 90 minutes. Using the early machines, the patient was placed on the gantry chair of the lithotripter and maneuvered into the appropriate position in the water tank (figure 39–1). With the newer machines, the patient simply lies flat on a special procedure table. The patient is anesthetized most frequently with epidural anesthesia, and much less often by local or general techniques.

Ultrasound or x-ray is used to pinpoint the stone to be fragmented. Radiopaque stones are easiest to treat by lithotripsy because biplanar fluoroscopy can locate them precisely. Stones that are radiolucent but not visible to ultrasound examination require retrograde urography for precise location. Shock waves focused on the stone are generated by the lithotripter and travel through the patient's soft tissues to be focused on the stone. When the waves hit the stone, energy dissipation causes fragmentation of the stone. Bone is not affected. In order to fragment the stone into sand-like particles, approximately 1,000 to 2,000 shock waves of approximately 1 millisecond duration each are required.

COMPLICATIONS

Blood in the urine is expected following extracorporeal shock wave lithotripsy. Many patients complain of discomfort during passage of the pulverized stone fragments. In about 75% of patents, all fragments are passed within 3 months. However, in some cases, some fragments will not pass, or a column of fragments will line up in the distal ureter requiring endoscopic or endourologic procedures for their removal. Acute complications can include ileus, infection, or pain.

Postlithotripsy kidney changes on magnetic resonance imaging (MRI) imply that the procedure is not totally benign. Studies are being done to evaluate the extent of renal dysfunction and increased rate of stone growth following the procedure. Enzyme changes including elevations of serum bilirubin, creatine phosphokinase, (CPK), and serum glutamicoxaloacetic transaminase (SGOT) can occur as can a rise in serum amylase.

Mortality is minimal, related mostly to the required anesthesia. Morbidity includes bleeding (nearly all patients have hematuria), discomfort during passage of the fragments (in 25% of patients) and the need for subsequent endoscopic or endourologic procedures (in less than 10% of patients). Pulmonary contusions and perirenal hematomas have been reported. Urosepsis is the complication with the greatest potential for serious consequence and prophylactic antibiotics are often administered before and after the procedure.

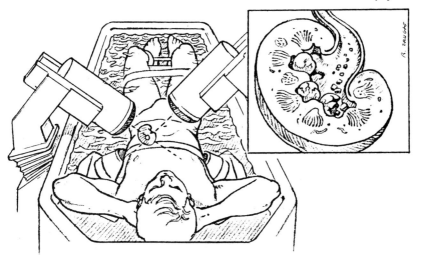

Figure 39–1. Lithotripsy using a water immersion tank. Newer lithotripters are now available that do not require water immersion.

Long-term complications have hinted at a decrease in renal function that may be permanent as represented by a fall in the effective renal plasma flow to the treated kidney. Sustained hypertension occurring immediately after treatment or developing several months later may be permanent. Further study is required into the long-term complications of renal stone lithotripsy.

POSTPROCEDURE INFORMATION

Family members should be advised that postprocedure bleeding and discomfort may occur intermittently for up to 3 months. Patients should remain well hydrated and may require antibiotics, antiemetics, or antispasmodics.

Once the chemistry of the stones is determined, dietary management, medications, and increased fluid intake can all be used to decrease the likelihood of recurrence.

PATIENT QUESTIONS

Is there any alternative to lithotripsy?

There are 4 alternatives to extracorporeal shock wave lithotripsy that are described above. The decision of which alternative to pursue depends on many factors and should be a mutual decision between the physician and the patient.

Will there be any pain?

Every patient who undergoes ESWL requires some form of anesthesia. The repeated discharges needed to break up the stone can be quite painful. Local infiltration or intercostal nerve blocks are helpful, but are often inadequate to ablate deep visceral pain. Adequate analgesia can best be provided by a combination of somatic and visceral nerve blocks or by general anesthesia, although local infiltration may suffice when a single stone in the renal pelvis is being treated. In pediatric patients, general anesthesia is preferred. There may be some residual pain after the procedure, but that can be treated with oral analgesics.

What are the chances that lithotripsy won't work and that another procedure will be needed?

Approximately 10% of patients will fail to pass some of the stone fragments spontaneously. In these cases, one of the alternative methods discussed will be required. Approximately one-third of these will require an endourologic procedure.

In addition, lithotripsy does not alter the likelihood of recurrence, and, without medical prevention, recurrent stone formation can be anticipated.

How much radiation is involved?

This is variable between different lithotripters, but, with appropriate safeguards, the total radiation is generally less than that of a routine barium enema study. Radiation exposure is proportional to the size and total number of stones, as well as the number of shocks required to break up the stone and it is a danger when fluoroscopy is used to localize the stone. Ultrasound localization of the stone eliminates the need for ionizing radiation completely.

Can lithotripsy be used for removal of gallstones?

Currently, there remain some questions about the potential use of extracorporeal shock wave lithotripsy for treatment of gallstones. The body's ability to pass fragments of gallstones is limited. This is because the gallbladder's contractility is diminished by stone disease. It is also because the common bile duct narrows as it enters the duodenum. If a stone fragment moves from the gallbladder and lodges at the distal end of the common bile duct, it may cause jaundice and pancreatitis.

It is also unclear whether lithotriptic treatment of gallstones provides any advantages to surgery in terms of risk, cost, convenience, and efficacy. The major disadvantage of lithotriptic gallstone treatment is the possibility of recurrence of stones. However, factors such as reduced need for general anesthesia, postoperative pain, number of days of hospitalization, and possibility of outpatient treatment make further work on gallstone lithotripsy valuable. More study on lithotripter treatment of gallstones will clarify its value in the future.

CONSENT

Signed informed consent is required explaining in detail the risks, benefits, and alternatives to this procedure.

SELECTED BIBLIOGRAPHY

Alkem P: Percutaneous ultrasonic destruction of renal calculi. *Urol Clin N America* 1982;9:145.

Chaussy C, Schmidt E: Extracorporeal shock wave lithotripsy: An alternative to surgery for kidney stones. *Urol Radiol* 1984;6:80.

Ferrucci JT: Biliary lithotripsy: what will the issues be? *AJR* 1987;149:2:227.

O'Brien WM, Rotolo JE, Pahira JJ: New approaches in the treatment of renal calculi. *Am Fam Physician* 1987;36:5:181.

Sackmann M, Delius M, Sauerbruch T: Shock-wave lithotripsy of gallbladder stones; the first 175 patients. *N Eng J Med* 1988;318:393.

40

Urethral Catheterization and the Urologic System

RICHARD SADOVSKY

The use of urinary catheters has become an essential part of modern medicine. There are many types of catheters that vary in size and formula depending on the purpose for use. The passage of a urethral catheter into the bladder is performed for diagnostic and therapeutic purposes and can be removed immediately after urine is obtained, left in for a brief period, be repeated intermittently, or be permanent. The names for these different procedures are spike catheterization, clean intermittent catheterization, and indwelling catheterization.

INDICATIONS

Insertion of a catheter is the simplest way to empty the bladder when there is obstruction or urinary retention. This can be done in an acute situation or to help maintain proper hygiene in a comatose or obtunded patient. Urinary incontinence can be controlled using an indwelling catheter, but is generally not a long-term indication. An additional, although rare, therapeutic indication for catheterization is balloon dilatation of a urethral stricture. In the hospital, the urinary spike catheterization is used to accurately measure urine output when indicated in patients who cannot reliably collect their own urinary output. Clean intermittent catheterization is also used in the management of incontinence caused by neurogenic bladder or some obstructive problem that cannot be resolved.

Diagnostic indications for spike catheterization include obtaining specimens for culture, chemical analysis, and cytology, and for the performance of special laboratory studies such as voiding **cystourethrograms**, **urodynamic studies**, and the **determination of post-voiding residual volume** in the bladder.

Voiding cystourethrograms (VCU) involve the injection of contrast material into the bladder to evaluate urethral function during voiding and to diagnose vesicoureteral reflux. This is generally done in males and allows good visualization of the anterior half of the urethra, but is also used in females to evaluate incontinence, reflux, and other urethral problems.

Cystometrograms involves measuring pressures to evaluate bladder dysfunction, bladder outlet obstruction, or lack of coordination (dyssynergia) in the lower urinary tract function. This test is helpful in evaluating for neurogenic bladder with uninhibited contractions secondary to the neurologic defect. This is important because of the usually poor surgical outcome in patients with this type of stress incontinence. The patient's response to thermal sensation is tested with instillation of warm fluid. Then using gas or normal saline instillation, sensations of fullness are noted along with any other reflexes. The residual volume is also calculated.

Urodynamic flow studies evaluate urine flow allowing the detection of lower urinary tract dysfunction or obstruction. Urodynamics performed with a video can offer flow studies, electromyography, a urethral pressure profile, and information about sensation.

Post-voiding residual volume determinations assist in the diagnosis of poor emptying of the bladder as a result of bladder wall dysfunction or outlet obstruction.

ALTERNATIVES

Noninvasive test such as x-ray and computerized tomagraphy (CT) scan can be used to look at urogenital structures, but the resolution of the interiors of the structures is poor unless the lesion is large and there is some displacement of the structures. Non-invasive tests give minimal information about the function of the segments of the urinary tract, although scanning techniques can help to localize obstructions or asymmetric urine flow.

Cystoscopy and ureteroscopy allow direct visualization of urinary structures, but require anesthesia and have a higher morbidity.

CONTRAINDICATIONS

The presence of an anatomic abnormality that prevents the smooth passage of the urinary catheter is an absolute contraindication. Relative contraindications would include (1) the presence of a urinary tract infection, (2) an immunocompromised host, and (3) diabetes mellitus.

PREPROCEDURE PREPARATION

If at all possible a urinalysis should be done prior to catheterization. Patients who are having a radiologic examination performed may receive a laxative since overlying gas or feces in the lumen of the bowel can obscure the urologic tract on x-ray. If contrast material is going to be instilled, any prior history of hypersensitivity should be obtained although new "hypoallergenic" material is now available at a much higher cost. A sedative can be administered prior to the lengthier diagnostic procedure if needed.

PATIENT EDUCATION

The patient should understand the reason for the procedure as well as how the procedure will be done. Since the procedure may be somewhat embarrassing to the patient, the method should be explained carefully and in a manner that allays anxiety and encourages questions. The possibility of some discomfort during the passage of the catheter should be discussed. If contrast is going to be instilled through the catheter, a sensation of heat and/or pain may be noted. During some segments of the procedures, the patient may feel the need to urinate. This is normal. The patient should be told that removal of the catheter is less uncomfortable.

PROCEDURE

The technique in males differs from that in females as would be anticipated by the difference in anatomy. The patient should be in a supine position with the legs spread apart. An antiseptic is used to thoroughly clean the urethral meatus and the surrounding area. Using sterile technique, the well-lubricated catheter tip is passes into the urethra applying steady pressure (figure 40–1). Copious amounts of lubricating gel should be used to permit easy passage. If there is minor resistance from the urethral sphincter or the prostate, a smaller catheter can be used. If the catheter cannot be passed, it must not be forced. If indicated, a urologist should be consulted to assist in the catheter insertion.

The catheter is in the bladder when urine begins to flow through it. Flushing the catheter easily with saline can also aid in determining the location of the catheter tip within the bladder, but the only sure way to know that the catheter is

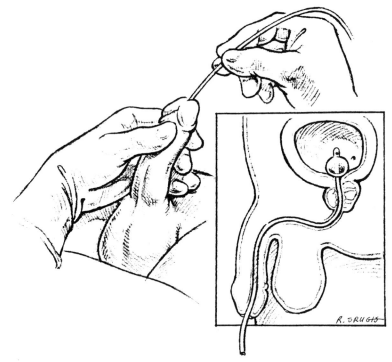

Figure 40–1. Urethral catheterization.

in the bladder is to see urine. If the catheter is meant to remain in place to drain the bladder, the balloon at the tip is inflated with sterile water (not saline) and the distal end of the catheter should be preconnected to a closed collecting system. If the placement of the catheter is for a diagnostic procedure, the appropriate test is performed, such as the instillation of contrast material or the connection of the catheter to a pressure measuring device.

During radiologic procedures, the catheter can be pushed into the bladder and contrast material instilled at that level, or even higher, into the ureter, allowing visualization of one or both of the ureteral collecting systems. The renal calyces can be opacified in this manner.

It is advisable to obtain a urine culture when an indwelling catheter is removed.

POSTPROCEDURE INFORMATION

Patients who have gone through a procedure utilizing contrast material should receive adequate fluids to flush out all contrast medium. Gross hematuria after the third or fourth urination is abnormal and the physician should be informed.

Chills or fever related to extravasation of contrast material or sepsis should be seen within 24 hours.

Patients who are on a clean intermittent catheterization regimen require support and encouragement. Noncompliance to proper technique can predispose to infection and increase the frequency of incontinence.

The family of the patient with an indwelling catheter should be taught the general steps of the procedure, how the system should be cared for after the catheter insertion, and how the patient can move around with the catheter. Attention should be paid to any complaints of the patient, the color and odor of the urine, and the presence of sediment or encrusting along the collection tube external to the urethra. Vitamin C supplements and fluids are helpful in preventing infection. Antibiotics should be reserved for episodes of acute infection or for prophylaxis in the patient with frequent recurrences of infection.

COMPLICATIONS

The most common complication is infection that can occur in as many as 1% to 2% of patients who are spike catheterized. This incidence rises in more susceptible patients such as diabetics, the elderly, and the immunocompromised. Indwelling catheters have an even higher incidence of infection with virtually 100% of the patients developing bacteriuria after 3 days but fewer than 1% developing symptomatic infections.

Indwelling catheters can also cause urethritis, prostatitis, sepsis, local erosion, stricture, urethral abscess, urinary retention and epididymitis in men, and vaginal infections in women. Painful urination may occur during early urination following removal of the catheter, but this symptom is usually transient.

Clean intermittent catheterization for relief of storage and emptying problems of the urinary tract can cause incontinence, asymptomatic bacteriuria and overt urinary tract infections, mechanical problems due to the catheterization such as edema or erythema, trauma causing minor lacerations, and bladder calculi.

Patients with lesions of the cervical cord may have an autonomic reflex associated with bladder distension, especially during cystometric studies. This may cause a rise in blood pressure, severe headaches, a decrease in the pulse rate, flushing, and perspiration, but this can be relieved by propantheline bromide given parenterally.

PATIENT QUESTIONS

Once I begin intermittent catheterization, will I have to continue doing it forever?

This is a complex question and the answer is uncertain. The indication for catheterizations must be reviewed. Pharmacologic agents that decrease the intravesicular pressure, such as anticholinergic agents or increase bladder outflow resistance such as alpha sympathomimetics can be used to manage incontinence. Adjunctive surgery can be considered to increase bladder outflow resistance if the intravesicular pressures are low. Urodynamic testing prior to the institution of intermittent catheterization is helpful to distinguish patients who are more likely to remain incontinent. Catheters are rarely used for incontinence longer than 1 week except perhaps in bed-ridden patients who are at higher risk for skin breakdown.

How can infections secondary to indwelling catheters be minimized?

The development of the closed catheter system has decreased the incidence of bacteriuria significantly. Entry of bacteria still can occur at the most proximal site, i.e., the mucous sheath between the catheter and the urethral mucosa. Local antibiotic usage appears not to be effective except possibly when antibiotic-impregnated gauze is used to encircle the catheter and contacting the periurethral area. Irrigation of the catheter with antibacterial formulas has been used without any proof of efficacy. Systemic antibiotics have been used in patients who require catheterization for relatively short periods, but the development of bacterial resistance must be considered. There is no clear formula for infection prevention in the patient with the long-term indwelling catheter, but some reports indicate that bacteriuria may be prevented with the use of intermittent catheterization rather than an indwelling catheter.

What are the indications for long term catheterization?

The indications for long-term urethral catheterization include (1) management of decubiti and other skin wounds, (2) inability to change clothes and bed linens because of painful physical movement, (3) a decision by the family and the patient that the need for dryness is greater than the risk of catheterization, and (4) overflow incontinence secondary to obstruction that cannot be relieved.

Will catheterization affect my sexual functioning?

Patients should be assured that catheterization will not affect their sex lives.

How often should the catheter and drainage bag be changed?

There is no uniform policy for the changing of catheters and collection bags. In general, if the urine is flowing freely, the catheter is not caked with debris, then there is no evidence of sepsis or pus in samples, and the bag is functioning well, then there is no reason to change the system. This can be for as long as 6 to 8 weeks. A schedule for change must be designed to match individual needs.

Will my activities be restricted with an indwelling catheter or with intermittent catheterization?

Patient and family education should clarify these questions. The patient with the indwelling catheter will be able to move around, travel, and socialize with the catheter attached to a portable and virtually invisible collecting system, usually a leg bag collection attachment. Patients who are intermittently catheterizing themselves can do this in any bathroom using clean technique. The only limitation to activities for these patients is their own imagination.

CONSENT

Although a consent form is not considered necessary for the placement of a urethral catheter, the concurrent use of contrast material does require an informed consent.

SELECTED BIBLIOGRAPHY

Burkitt D, Randall J: Catheterization: urethral trauma. *Nurs Times* 1987;Oct:28–Nov 4:83(43):59.

Freeman S, Chapman J: Urologic procedures *Emerg Med Clin North Am* 1986;Aug:4(3):543.

Gregory JG, Purcell MH: Urinary incontinence in the elderly. Ways to relieve it without surgery. *Postgrad Med* 1986;Aug:80(2):253.

Schaeffer AJ: Catheter-associated bacteriuria. *Urol Clin North Am* 1986;Nov:13(4):735.

Warren JW: Catheters and catheter care. *Clin Geriatr Med* 1986;Nov:2(4):857.

IX

Male and Female Reproductive System Procedures

41

Amniocentesis

RICHARD SADOVSKY

The origin of amniotic fluid is unclear, but it is known that its original composition is very close to that of interstitial fluid. Amniotic fluid exhibits metabolic changes in the fetus, protects the fetus from external trauma, and maintains a constant body temperature. As the fetus matures, the fluid becomes more diluted with hypotonic fetal urine. Amniocentesis is the needle aspiration through the abdominal wall of 10 to 30 ml of this fluid for analysis. These procedures should be performed only if the risks of an abnormality are greater than the risks of the procedure. Amniocentesis is appropriate in situations where the parents would not choose a therapeutic abortion in order to either allay anxiety or to allow the family to prepare and adjust to the future family situation.

INDICATIONS

Analysis of amniotic fluid can detect several birth defects including Down's syndrome and spina bifida. In addition, hemolytic diseases of the newborn, certain metabolic disorders, pulmonary immaturity, and chromosomal abnormalities can be detected. Gender and sex-linked disorders such as hemophilia can also be determined as can fetal age. Amniocentesis is not indicated solely because the parents want to know the sex of the fetus. Specific indications for this procedure include pregnancy associated with advanced age (maternal age over 35), family history of genetic, chromosomal, or neural tube defects, or previous miscarriage. Because of possible complications, amniocentesis is contraindicated as a general screening test.

Analysis of the amniotic fluid includes a variety of tests, some of which can be done instantly, while others require a laboratory capable of employing sophisticated techniques. Tests that can be done instantly include evaluation for meconium, blood, and a foam test to look for the presence of surface-active material (surfactant). Chemical tests include quantitation of bilirubin, creatinine, uric acid, glucose, estriol, fetal thyroid hormones, alpha-fetoprotein, acetylcholinesterase, the lecithin-sphingomyelin ratio, and the presence of phosphatidylglycerol. Other tests include bacterial cultures and chromosome analysis.

Blood in the amniotic fluid usually comes from the mother and does not indicate any abnormality. It may, however, be fetal in origin and be a sign of damage to the fetal, placental, or umbilical cord vessels by the amniocentesis needle and may affect the quantitations of other amniotic chemical contents. The determination of whether the blood present is of fetal or maternal origin can be done rapidly using the Apt test, which is based on the fact that fetal hemoglobin is alkali resistant and adult hemoglobin will change to hematin after the addition of alkali.

The presence of significant amounts of bilirubin may represent hemolytic disease of the newborn. Meconium, which is a semisolid material found in the fetal gastrointestinal tract, may enter the amniotic fluid during periods of fetal distress. Creatinine levels should correspond to the maturity of the fetal kidneys. Alpha-fetoprotein is produced in the liver and the gastrointestinal tract. High quantities may represent neural tube defects, multiple pregnancies, esophageal or duodenal atresia, cystic fibrosis, impending fetal death, or other abnormalities. Since the results and interpretation of the alpha-fetoprotein level may sometimes be difficult to evaluate, the presence of a high level of alpha-fetoprotein should indicate the need for a high-resolution ultrasound examination to help detect the presence of an anatomical abnormality.

Uric acid in the amniotic fluid increases as the fetus matures. Elevated levels may represent erythroblastosis fetalis, familial hyperuricemia, or other metabolic problems. Estriol and its conjugates can appear in varying amounts. This is decreased in erythroblastosis fetalis. The lecithin-sphingomyelin ratio verifies fetal pulmonary maturity. Phosphatidylglycerol levels aid in the determination of fetal pulmonary maturity. Glucose levels can aid in assessing the presence of poor glucose control in the patient with diabetes.

Many other enzymes are present in the amniotic fluid and in cell cultures from the amniotic fluid. The presence or absence of these enzymes have few known clinical implications, although the presence of increased levels of acetyl-cholinesterase may occur with neural tube defects and other serious malformations. Amniocentesis may also be used for therapeutic purposes, such as inducing mid-trimester abortion by intraamniotic injection of prostaglandins, or decompressing the uterus overdistended by polyhydramnios late in pregnancy.

ALTERNATIVES

Ultrasonography can be used to verify fetal viability, determine gestational age by measurement of the biparietal diameter, determine placenta and fetal position, diagnose multiple gestations, and detect gross fetal abnormalities. The use of ultrasonography in the detection of congenital heart defects is currently under study. It is believed that at the levels used in obstetrical ultrasonography, high-frequency sound waves present no risk to the mother or the fetus, but recently questions have been raised about the risks of this procedure and studies are currently under way to clarify this question.

Chorionic villi sampling is a relatively new technique used to diagnose chromosomal abnormalities during the first trimester. This procedure is performed between the weeks 9 and 12 of pregnancy and can be an earlier alternative to the genetic amniocentesis. The procedure is done under ultrasound visualization using a transvaginal approach. The placental tissue obtained can be used for chromosomal analysis and, because this is composed of rapidly dividing cells, results are often available within 2 to 10 days. Risks from this procedure have not been clearly quantified and the inability to obtain alpha-fetoprotein levels from this procedure is a limitation. Patients with risk for neural tube defects should have amniocentesis. As the technique of chorionic villi sampling becomes more developed, it may replace amniocentesis because of its decreased risk and its ability to make earlier diagnoses.

High concentrations of alpha-fetoprotein in the maternal serum indicate an increased risk of neural tube disorders, but the specificity of this test is much lower than that of ultrasound alone or ultrasound combined with amniocentesis. A low concentration of maternal alpha-fetoprotein has recently been recognized to reflect an increased possibility of Down's syndrome.

POTENTIAL FOR FAILURE

A variety of interfering factors can affect the ability of the amniocentesis to provide the desired information. Placing the fluid in a clear tube will result in abnormally low bilirubin levels. Blood or meconium in the fluid will affect the lecithin-sphingomyelin ratio. Maternal blood in the specimen may lower the creatinine level. The presence of fetal blood will alter the alpha-fetoprotein result. Maternal diseases unrelated to pregnancy such as cirrhosis, teratoma, gastric carcinoma, and others can cause increased alpha-fetoprotein levels, and plastic disposable syringes can destroy amniotic fluid cells.

CONTRAINDICATIONS

There are no contraindications to amniocentesis.

PREPROCEDURE PREPARATION

There is no need for restriction of food or fluids. The bladder should be emptied prior to the procedure.

PATIENT EDUCATION

The patient should understand that the test detects fetal abnormalities, but that a normal test result does not guarantee a normal fetus since some fetal diseases are not detectable. Test results will not be available for approximately 2 to 6 weeks. The stinging sensation of the local anesthesia should be anticipated and reassurance should be provided about who will perform the test and the rarity of adverse affects.

The patient should understand the need not to touch the sterile field during the procedure. Hands should be placed over the head or in some appropriate position.

PROCEDURE

Amniocentesis can be done only after the week 16 by which time the quantity of amniotic fluid reaches approximately 150 ml. With the woman lying flat on her back, the position of the fetus is determined by palpation and ultrasound permitting location of a pool of amniotic fluid. The skin is prepared with an antiseptic solution; local anesthesia is injected intradermally and then subcutaneously. The procedure can be performed either transabdominally or suprapubically. Generally a 20 gauge needle with stylet is used to puncture the abdominal wall and uterus and enter the amniotic cavity (figure 41–1). Fluid is aspirated into a syringe and deposited into an amber or foil-covered test tube. The needle is then withdrawn, and a small dressing or bandage is placed over the needle insertion site. The sample of amniotic fluid is centrifuged, allowing the supernatant to be sent to the laboratory for chemical studies, and the precipitated cells sent for biochemical analysis and culture.

Many physicians feel that Rh-negative women without Rh antibodies should be treated with anti-D immunoglobulin after third trimester amniocentesis.

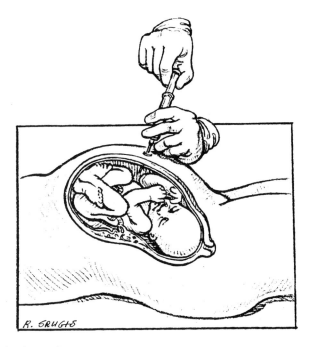

Figure 41–1. Amniocentesis.

POSTPROCEDURE INFORMATION

Post-test care should routinely include the monitoring of fetal and maternal vital signs regularly for at least 30 minutes.

The doctor should be notified if the patient feels any abdominal cramping or pain, chills, fever, shows any vaginal discharge or bleeding, leakage of serous fluid, or if there is any abnormal fetal activity or lack of activity. Emotional support may be necessary during the period of waiting for results since anxiety can increase greatly during several weeks needed to determine the results of the amniocentesis.

COMPLICATIONS

Fetal loss, the major risk of amniocentesis, occurs in less than 0.5% of those pregnancies having amniocentesis. Repeat amniocentesis is needed in less than 0.1% of cases. Fetal injury from puncture has been found to be minimal.

Other maternal risks include sepsis, hemorrhage, and Rh sensitization. This latter complication can be avoided by carefully avoiding the placenta because trauma may increase fetal-maternal transfusion and worsens the immunization.

Counselling-communication problems can occur, and parents must realize that prenatal diagnosing is not infallible. Errors in karyotyping and biochemical analysis are possible. Error rates of 0.2% to 0.3% have been reported in large series of amniocenteses. Careful counselling is essential so that decisions can be made with proper information and consideration.

PATIENT QUESTIONS

Is amniocentesis painful?

The injection of local anesthetic involves a pin-prick that will be felt by the patient. After that, the pain from amniocentesis should be minimal. Many patients have described the pain as being equivalent to that felt while having blood withdrawn from the arm. In addition, a pulling sensation may be felt during the aspiration of fluid.

Will I have any other discomfort during the procedure?

The supine position required for the procedure is often uncomfortable, especially as the uterus grows heavier during the latter stages of pregnancy. The woman may experience postural hypotension that, combined with anxiety, may cause symptoms of dizziness, nausea, and occasional vomiting. This can be eased by raising the head slightly.

Should I have ultrasonography prior to or during amniocentesis?

Most medical centers are doing ultrasound immediately prior to amniocentesis or even accompanying amniocentesis with real-time ultrasonography. This is advantageous to allow more accurate location of the placenta avoiding accidental needle punctures of this structure. In addition, information can be obtained about the presence of multiple gestations, allowing the collection of amniotic fluid from both fetuses. Another advantage of ultrasound is the ability to recognize the small percentage of pregnancies that are missed abortions and unnecessary amniocentesis can be avoided.

What is the likelihood of having the procedure repeated because of inadequate sample size or laboratory problems?

Occasionally insufficient fluid is obtained or amniotic fluid cells cannot be successfully cultured and a second amniocentesis is required. This is less likely to occur when the procedure is performed by an experienced operator. If the procedure is performed at 16 weeks by a capable operator, failure to obtain amniotic fluid can be reduced to less than 1%, and culture failure to 2% or less.

CONSENT

Amniocentesis requires informed consent.

The decision for amniocentesis should be made by both parents. Many families in high-risk categories do not wish to have a prenatal diagnosis. A request for an amniocentesis should not be considered a commitment for abortion of an affected fetus. Parents should be asked, if they would not want to terminate an affected fetus, is the risk of amniocentesis truly appropriate? If the decision of the family is an informed one and they wish to have knowledge prenatally about the health of their baby, the physician should abide by their wishes.

SELECTED BIBLIOGRAPHY

Hanson FW, Zorn EM, Tennant FR, Marianos S, Samuels S: Amniocentesis before 15 weeks gestation: outcome, risks, and technical problems. *Am J Obstet Gynecol* 1987;Jun:156(6)1524.

Lorenz RP, Willard D, Botti JJ: Role of prenatal genetic counseling before amniocentesis. A survey of genetics centers. *J Reprod Med* 1986;Jan:31(1):1.

O'Brien WF: Midtrimester genetic amniocentesis. A review of the fetal risks. *J Reprod Med* 1984;Jan:29(1):59.

Robinson A, Henry GP: Prenatal diagnosis by amniocentesis. *Annu Rev Med* 1985;36:13.

Williamson RA, Varner MW, Grant SS: Reduction in amniocentesis risks using a real-time needle guide procedure. *Obstet Gynecol* 1985;May:65(5):751.

Zorn EM: Amniocentesis: its uses and abuses, and how to prepare patients. *Consultant* 1985;Nov 30:25(17):69.

42

Colposcopy and Colpocentesis

RICHARD SADOVSKY

Colposcopy is the visual examination of the cervix and the vagina using an instrument (colposcope) containing a light source and a magnifying lens. Biopsies can performed on suspicious looking areas. This, in combination with endocervical curettage, makes colposcopy a valuable diagnostic tool. The procedure is also used therapeutically in the treatment of carcinoma in situ (CIS) in combination with destructive modalities such as cryotherapy, laser, electrocauterization, and surgical ablation.

INDICATIONS

Colposcopy is used to visually evaluate (1) cervical neoplasias following a positive Pap test, (2) vaginal or cervical lesions, (3) conservatively treated cervical intraepithelial neoplasias, (4) patients whose mothers received diethylstilbestrol during pregnancy, and (5) women with clinically suspicious cervices, especially with contact bleeding even in the presence of a negative Pap smear. Abnormal colposcopy findings include a variety of patterns that may indicate underlying cervical intraepithelial neoplasia (CIN) or invasive carcinoma. Other visible abnormalities include inflammatory changes caused by infection, atrophic changes from old age or the use of oral contraceptives, erosion usually caused by changes in vaginal flora, and papillomas and condylomas usually caused by viruses.

Patients who are undergoing colposcopy for positive Pap smears should be referred for the procedure as soon as possible. In over 90% of patients with abnormal Pap smears, colposcopy and the appropriate biopsies can either confirm or exclude the presence of invasive carcinoma. Other diagnostic uses of colposcopy include the evaluation of postcoital bleeding and the collection of cervical mucus in the infertile patient.

Therapeutic uses of colposcopy include cryosurgical eradication of cervical intraepithelial neoplasia done in the office without anesthesia or analgesia and electrocautery. Carbon dioxide lasers are being used with great precision and minimal hazards.

ALTERNATIVES

Diagnostic cytology using a variety of methods to obtain samples is the easiest and least expensive way to screen the cervix for abnormalities. There is general agreement, however, that cytologic examination and colposcopy together complement each other and diagnostic accuracy is increased. For routine screening, cytology is the method of choice, with the cells being collected by a properly performed Pap smear.

Diagnostic conization has been the most frequently used procedure to exclude invasive cancer. Although there is some variation in opinion, when the endocervical canal curettings do not contain neoplastic tissue, the colposcopically directed biopsies are sufficiently accurate in determining the cause of abnormal smears, without the need for conization. It is desirable to avoid conization because of the possibilities of such surgical complications as hemorrhage, infection, cervical stenosis, and infertility, and to reduce medical expenses.

POTENTIAL FOR FAILURE

Interfering factors may impair visualization by colposcopy. These can include failure to adequately clean the cervix of materials such as creams and medications. An unsatisfactory examination occurs when the limits of the squamocolumnar junction cannot be completely visualized. However, if invasive cancer has been recognized and confirmed by biopsy, then the patient has had the appropriate evaluation. In cases where the entire junction cannot be visualized and preinvasive cancer is suspected, further examination must be done, such as endocervical curettage during colposcopy or diagnostic conization. Diagnostic cone biopsies are indicated when (1) there is extension out of sight into the cervical canal, (2) multiple abnormal smears with negative colposcopic results, (3) lesions in which the level of invasion implied by the smear is greater than that noted from the biopsies, (4) extension of a lesion to an area greater than half of the cervix, and (5) endocervical curettage abnormalities. The accuracy of the colposcopic examination is highly dependable if there is correlation between the colposcopic and histological appearance of the tissue.

In pregnant patients, colposcopic patterns are exaggerated because of increased vascularity of the cervix. This, in addition to the thick, tenacious mucus during pregnancy and the inflammatory component present, makes examination more difficult. A shallow cone biopsy may be performed, but the risks are increased.

The recent introduction of the cervicograph, an optical instrument with which a picture of the entire cervix can be obtained, allows evaluation using a projector in a darkened room. This permanent recording of cervical surface changes would allow a more objective evaluation and a temporal recording of cervical changes. The cervicogram cannot replace colposcopy in making clinical decisions since histologic examination is not performed.

CONTRAINDICATIONS

None.

PREPROCEDURE PREPARATION

None.

PATIENT EDUCATION

The patient should understand fully the purpose of the procedure and that it provides more information than a routine vaginal examination. The patient can eat or drink freely prior to the test, and told that the procedure will require 10 to 15 minutes. The possibility of a biopsy should also be explained.

PROCEDURE

Colposcopy can be performed in the operator's office in approximately 15 to 30 minutes. The patient is assisted in assuming lithotomy position, advised to breathe through the mouth, and to relax the abdominal muscles. The cervix is swabbed with acetic acid or vinegar to remove mucus. A careful examination of the cervix and the vagina is performed, and the squamocolumnar junction (the transformation zone) is thoroughly evaluated using the colposcope. Endocervical curettage and biopsy of any abnormal site that appears can be done. (figure 42–1). Transformation zone abnormalities can include one of several patterns: white

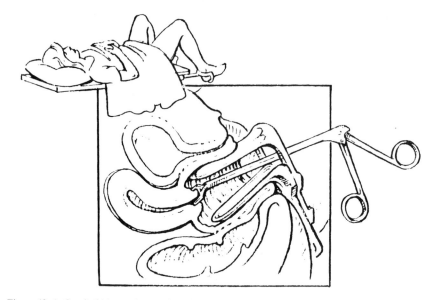

Figure 42–1. Cervical biopsy done under colposcopic visualization.

epithelium, mosaic structure, punctation, leukoplakia, or abnormal vascular patterns. Each of these patterns appears to have a histologic correlate, but biopsy is essential to confirm the diagnosis. Bleeding is stopped by cautery, pressure, or hemostatic solutions.

Endocervical curettage can be performed during colposcopic examination. This procedure detects disease in the canal and probably should be done with every examination. Negative curettage seems to correlate closely with the absence of invasive carcinoma.

POSTPROCEDURE INFORMATION

The biopsy may cause mild cramping, spot bleeding, or a vaginal discharge for a few days. The patient should be advised to refrain from intercourse and to avoid inserting anything into the vagina (except a tampon) until biopsy site healing is complete. This generally requires a 1 to 2 week period of abstention. Excessive bleeding should be reported to the physician.

COMPLICATIONS

The biopsies may cause some minimal bleeding. Otherwise, there are no complications or problems following colposcopy.

PATIENT QUESTIONS

Will the procedure hurt?

Generally, colposcopy is done without any anesthesia or analgesic. The biopsies may cause a slight sensation, but the procedure is minimally uncomfortable.

Will the procedure interfere with my ability to get pregnant?

The statistics are that colposcopy does not interfere with fertility or the ability to carry a baby to term.

Why have I been asked to have repeat colposcopy?

If the Pap smear indicates severe dysplasia and the colposcopically obtained biopsy indicates mild dysplasia, the procedure may need to be repeated with additional biopsies. If the discrepancy persists, conization may be required. If the Pap smear suggests a lesser dysplasia than the biopsy, the patient should be treated on the basis of the biopsy histology since Pap smears can be underread.

CONSENT

Consent is required for colposcopy and biopsy.

SELECTED BIBLIOGRAPHY

Benedet JL, Anderson GH, Boyes DA: Colposcopic accuracy in the diagnosis of microinvasive and occult invasive carcinoma of the cervix. *Obstet Gynecol* 1985;Apr:65(4):557.

Hall JB, McGee JA, Marroum MC, Dee L: Evaluation of the cerviscope as a screening instrument. *Gynecol Oncol* 1985;Jan:20(1):17.

Mosely KR, Dinh T, Hannigan EV, Dillard EA, Yandell RB: Necessity of endocervical curettage in colposcopy. *Am J Obstet Gynecol* 1986;May:154(5):992.

Rodney WM, Felmar E, Morrison J, Richards E, Cousin L: Colposcopy and cervical cryotherapy. Feasible additions to the primary care physician's office practice. *Postgrad Med* 1987;Jun:81(8):79–82.

Walker P, Singer A: Colposcopy: who, when, where, and by whom? *Br J Obstet Gyn* 1987;Nov:94(11):1011.

43

Cone Biopsy and Conization

RICHARD SADOVSKY

Conization is the removal of the diseased part of the cervix by taking a cone-shaped wedge of the organ. The terms *cone biopsy* and *conization* are often used synonymously for a variety of surgical procedures from standardized biopsies to large cone-shaped amputations of the uterine cervix.

INDICATIONS

Cone biopsy and conization are considered therapeutic tools as well as diagnostic procedures. When colposcopy is not possible, cone biopsy of the cervix offers a good method of diagnosing cervical neoplasia in the patient with an abnormal cytology and no visible lesion. Random punch biopsies are insufficient to rule out invasive cancer.

When colposcopy is available, cone biopsy may still be necessary in patients whose lesions extend deep into the cervical canal, when an invasive lesion is suspected, or when technical problems prevent an accurate colposcopic diagnosis. The greatest possible precision is obtained from the cone biopsy. Cone biopsy also helps if there is a significant lesion and a lack of correlation between cytology, colposcopy, and the directed biopsy. A positive endocervical curettage requires a cone biopsy because of the need to grade the severity of the intraepithelial lesion or to eliminate the possibility of an invasive lesion.

Therapeutic indication for conization include cervical intraepithelial neoplasms that have progressed to carcinoma in situ. These include lesions occupying more than 2 quadrants of the cervix. Cone is considered a true therapeutic method only when it is clear that all abnormal tissue has been removed.

The advent of hysteroscopic techniques will allow more accurate measurements of endocervical extension of neoplasia. This will increase the ability to perform more tailormade cone biopsies suitable to each specific situation and, by decreasing the size of the cone biopsy needed, decrease the likelihood of complications.

Diagnostic cone biopsy allows evaluation of the transitional zone and the endocervical tissue as a search for dysplastic or neoplastic cells. The depth and extent of disease can be determined.

ALTERNATIVES

Colposcopy, when available, has become a popular method by which to evaluate the patient with a positive Pap smear. Lesions that are visible should be biopsied using a punch technique in order to prevent an unnecessary cone biopsy. Iodine solutions are being used to help identify potentially abnormal areas that can then be biopsied.

Destructive forms of therapy for cervical intraepithelial neoplasia include electrocoagulation, cryotherapy, and laser techniques. The disadvantage of these alternatives is that no tissue is obtained for microscopic confirmation of the diagnosis. These destructive techniques are more successful when the lesion occupies 2 or fewer quadrants of the cervix and are probably adequate when preceded by colposcopy and followed by regular Pap tests and repeat colposcopy.

Hysterectomy is another alternative form of therapy and is imperative in invasive forms of carcinoma. In the case of incomplete conization or when neoplastic tissue remains beyond the range of the conization procedure, then hysterectomy may be indicated. The risks and expense of this procedure need to be carefully evaluated.

POTENTIAL FOR FAILURE

Occasionally, if the cone biopsy is not properly performed, additional tissue must be obtained by repeating the procedure. A cone biopsy is the most valuable and anatomically accurate way of evaluating endocervical abnormalities.

CONTRAINDICATIONS

Patients with evidence of cervical infections should be treated with an antibiotic, and the procedure should be postponed until the infection is resolved. Cone biopsy in pregnancy is associated with a high risk of complications related to bleeding and premature labor. Cytology, colposcopy, and biopsy should be performed and, then if these are all inconclusive, only should cone biopsy be considered during pregnancy. If the procedure must be done, bleeding and premature labor can be minimized by performing a wedge biopsy under colposcopic guidance and by doing the procedure during the second trimester.

PREPROCEDURE PREPARATION

Patients are advised not to eat or drink from the midnight before the procedure. The bladder should be emptied so that proper manual examination of the pelvic organs can be performed. If an intrauterine device (IUD) is in place, it should be removed and the procedure should be postponed until after the next menses. A urinalysis and a hematocrit are performed on the patient. Some operators also do a bleeding profile.

PATIENT EDUCATION

A discussion about alternatives should be held, especially when therapeutic conization is being done for neoplasia. The patient often has specific concerns that may affect the decision about method of treatment. A thorough discussion will gain patient compliance in the total therapeutic plan.

The patient should understand the procedure and its indication. Terminology should be explained so that the patient feels at ease during the procedure.

PROCEDURE

Cone biopsy is generally performed in the hospital under general anesthesia with most patients able to go home the next day. Recent experience with short-stay procedures has shown that this procedure can be done on an outpatient basis under local anesthesia with a paracervical block. The patient is placed in the lithotomy position following anesthesia. A scalpel or laser is used to remove the cone being guided by colposcopy and/or application of an iodine solution to determine the location of the squamocolumnar junction. The cone, being removed must contain the junction area. This may be shallow in younger women, or deep in older, nulliparous women.

A local injection of epinephrine or vasopressin solution may help to reduce the bleeding, but this is contraindicated when cardiac effects may be dangerous to the patient. An intracervical injection of 50 to 100 ml of normal saline may help to decrease bleeding by volume effect on the surrounding tissue. The extent of the tissue removed is in accordance with the colposcopically visible lesion. If the lesion is not visible, then about two–thirds of the cervical canal should be removed (figure 43–1). Iodine solutions are also used to determine the extent of lesions.

The cervical defect remaining after the procedure can be left open or can be stitched closed. Superficial cauterization is done to stop punctate bleeding spots. The wound and the vagina are generally packed for 48 hours with a gauze material.

Endocervical and uterine curettage are generally performed with a cone biopsy, but the indications for this are unclear and, in the patient who has not had any abnormal uterine bleeding, the yield of this procedure is very low.

Conization has recently been performed with the CO_2 laser. These are also usually done in the operating room with general anesthesia although the use of laser conization on an outpatient basis is gaining popularity. This eliminates the need for general anesthesia since many operators using laser are anesthetizing patients with paracervical blocks. Laser conization appears to permit preservation of tissue structure for adequate histologic examination. In addition, vaporization can be performed in surrounding peripheral areas where tissue evaluation is not needed. Some operators have reported a lower postprocedure bleeding rate as well as a lower frequency of stenosis, and decreased infections.

Some operators recommend insertion of an antibiotic vaginal cream for 1 to 2 weeks following the procedure.

POSTPROCEDURE INFORMATION

Bleeding may begin immediately following the procedure or a week or more after surgery. If significant bleeding occurs, the physician should be contacted. The patient can return to full activity within 2 days after the procedure, but should abstain from coitus until after the 4-week follow-up visit. Douching should also be avoided until advised by the physician.

Long-term follow up is an essential feature when cone biopsy is used to treat intraepithelial neoplasms. The majority of recurrences take place within 2 to 3 years, but cases in which recurrence have happened as long as ten years later have been recorded.

COMPLICATIONS

Bleeding is the major complication of cone biopsy and occurs in 5% to 10% of all cases. This is more common when the conization is performed during the menstrual and post-partum periods. Cervical stenosis, which may present as menstrual dysfunction or dysmenhorea, infection, uterine perforation, or injury

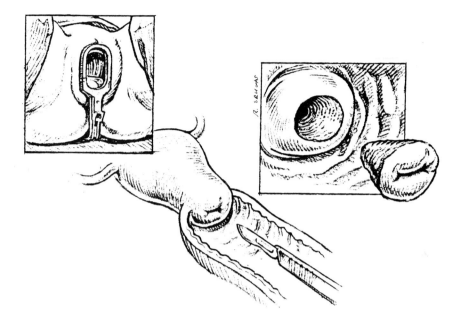

Figure 43–1. Conization.

to the rectum or bladder, occur much more rarely. Cervical stenosis, more common in post-menopausal patients, can be easily resolved by dilation with paracervical block infiltration.

PATIENT QUESTIONS

Will conization prevent recurrences of cervical intraepithelial carcinoma better than destructive techniques?

When patients make themselves available for close follow up, the destructive techniques can be as effective as conization in preventing recurrences of neoplasm. In situations in which patient follow up is poor, cone biopsy does have the lower recurrence rate. The actual rate depends on complete removal of the entire lesion. Most medical studies have found a 30% incidence of positive margins. Positive margins occur more frequently in patients with more severe lesions and in older patients. Even patients with negative margins require close follow up. A repeat cone biopsy or hysterectomy is indicated in patients with positive margins or who develop a positive cytology during the follow up stage.

Will I be able to have sexual intercourse after the procedure?

Patients are advised to refrain from intravaginal intercourse for several weeks, that is, until after the first follow-up visit. It is possible that coitus will be accompanied by some discomfort and mild bleeding. These symptoms should disappear with time, and the ability to have sexual intercourse should return to normal. Any severe pain or significant bleeding should be reported to the physician.

What form of anesthesia should I have?

A cone biopsy can be done under local anesthesia with a paracervical block. Regional or general anesthesia, however, does provide better anesthesia and allows more cervical manipulation giving the surgeon greater ability to evaluate the proximal organs and to do biopsies when necessary.

Will this procedure affect my ability to have a baby?

Menstrual cycles will not be significantly affected by the procedure although the two or three periods following the procedure may be heavy and prolonged. The question of fertility following cone biopsy is a controversial one. Some researchers have concluded that there is no evidence to suggest that fertility or the rate of spontaneous abortion is affected by cone biopsy. It does seem pretty clear, however, that the fertility rate of the woman remains unchanged. Data on premature delivery are less conclusive with some researchers asserting that there is a higher risk of premature delivery following cone biopsy. The answer to this might lie in the type of cone biopsy that is performed. A "large" therapeutic biopsy may weaken the cervix to a greater degree.

CONSENT

Informed consent is required for the anesthesia and the procedure.

SELECTED BIBLIOGRAPHY

Iverson T: Outpatient cervical conization with the CO_2 laser. *J Reprod Med* 1985;Aug:30(8):607.

Killackey MA, Jones WB, Lewis JL Jr.: Diagnostic conization of the cervix: review of 460 consecutive cases. *Obstet Gynec* 1986;Jun:67(6):766.

Kuoppala T, Saarikoski S: Pregnancy and delivery after cone biopsy of the cervix. *Arch Gynecol* 1986:237(3):149.

Larsson G, Gullberg B, Grundsell H: A comparison of complications of laser and cold knife conization. *Obstet Gynecol* 1983;Aug:62(2):213.

Sharp F, Cordiner JW: The treatment of CIN: cone biopsy and hysterectomy. *Clin Obstet Gynaecol* 1985;Mar:12(1):133.

Zbella EA, Deppe G, Gleicher N: Outpatient versus inpatient cone biopsy of the cervix. *Mt. Sinai J Med (NY)* 1986;Feb:53(2):80.

44

Culdoscopy and Culdocentesis

RICHARD SADOVSKY

Culdoscopy is a relatively simple procedure allowing a close, clear view of the ovaries and tubes. The procedure is used primarily for diagnosis, but operative culdoscopy is also performed. The procedure can be accompanied by curettage.

Culdocentesis refers to cul-de-sac needling by which the presence of blood in the peritoneum can be used as evidence of pregnancy.

INDICATIONS

The categories of indications for culdoscopy include (1) unexplained sterility, (2) unexplained pelvic pain, (3) menstrual abnormalities, and (4) indefinite pelvic mass. Patients with infertility who have been completely evaluated with noninvasive tests or in whom there is evidence of possible tubal adhesions should have culdoscopy or laparoscopy. Unexplained pelvic pain can also be evaluated with this procedure as can pelvic masses. Menstrual abnormalities can be clarified by evaluation for ovarian abnormalities, endometriosis, and tubal pregnancy. Any question that can be resolved with inspection of the tubes and ovaries within the pelvic cavity may be an indication for culdoscopy.

Indications for culdocentesis include suspected tubal pregnancy. If rupture of the tube or tubal abortion has taken pace, there will be sufficient blood in the cul-de-sac for identification by aspiration. Culdocentesis is positive in 70% to 95% of cases of proved ectopic pregnancies. The most common nonpregnancy treated cause of a positive culdocentesis is a ruptured ovarian cyst. Most important, the patient with hemoperitoneum may be asymptomatic and may escape detection unless culdocentesis is performed.

Other possible outcomes from culdocentesis include clear or straw-colored serous fluid in small amounts that would indicate normal peritoneal fluid. Cloudy exudative or purulent fluid indicates an infective process. Blood that clots rapidly may have been obtained from a vein in the region and not from the peritoneal cavity. A dry tap, in which no fluid is aspirated, has no diagnostic value.

The procedure is simple and can be performed in the office. In addition, serous fluid can be removed from the peritoneal cavity allowing the avoidance of an abdominal puncture. This may be desirable in the presence of abdominal scars or when skin infections contraindicate a transabdominal route.

ALTERNATIVES

Operative and diagnostic culdoscopy is being replaced in many centers by the laparoscopic approach. The indications for culdoscopy and laparoscopy are almost identical. Many physicians fee that laparoscopy is easier to learn, visualizes the anterior pelvic areas more easily, and permits greater visualization of the total extent of the tubes. Another advantage of laparoscopy is the greater comfort of the prone position required for this procedure. A decision as to whether laparotomy is needed can be done rapidly and the procedure can be done immediately if appropriate. Minor procedures may also be easier through the laparoscope. Other advantages of laparoscopy include a lower failure rate, decreased postoperative discomfort, and greater feasibility of laparoscopy when culdoscopy is contraindicated. However, supporters of culdoscopic techniques claim that the procedure is simpler and can be performed without anesthesia. More information may be obtained by culdoscopy in the infertility work-up because of clear viewing of the pelvic organs when performed by experts. In addition, newer culdocentesis techniques are making examinations and fluid accumulations by this technique simper, safer, and less painful. These can be done on an outpatient basis and at lower cost.

Culdocentesis should be done with expertise and some caution. False negatives may be common especially when the needle point fails to enter the peritoneal cavity. False positives may occur when blood is obtained from a vein or extraperitoneal hematoma.

Ultrasonography is also being used to detect ectopic pregnancy. This procedure is still somewhat imprecise and depends greatly on the expertise of the ultrasonographer. Many pathologic conditions can hinder the ability of the ultrasonographer to detect ectopic pregnancy including adhesions, ovarian cysts and neoplasms, hydrosalpinx, and leiomyomas. Recent advances in ultrasonography have made it more effective as a tool in the diagnosis of ectopic pregnancy.

POSSIBILITY OF FAILURE

It has been found that, if tenting of the vaginal vault cannot be achieved, the procedure should not be attempted because of the likelihood of pelvic adhesions that make insertion of the trocar difficult or impossible. About 5% of culdoscopic procedures are unsatisfactory because of thick adhesions or adherent loops of bowel.

CONTRAINDICATIONS

Contraindications to culdoscopy include the inability of the patient to assume the appropriate knee-chest position, obliteration of the cul-de-sac, and evidence of pelvic inflammatory disease. Patients who have physical deformities or decompensated heart disease preventing the knee-chest position should not undergo culdoscopy. In addition, the cul-de-sac puncture cannot be performed through the intact hymen or when the vagina opening is inadequate due to prior surgery or disease.

Examination is often unsatisfactory in the presence of a markedly enlarged uterus because of insufficient space for maneuvering the scope. A preliminary examination of the patient should always be performed to avoid the performance of an unsuccessful procedure.

PREPROCEDURE PREPARATION

The patient should give a compete history and undergo a physical examination, including pelvic examination, prior to the procedure. The pelvic examination is essential to indicate any possible contraindications to culdoscopy or any cues that the procedure will not permit adequate visualization of the pelvic organs. The cervix must be freely moveable and the posterior fornix should be able to be stretched into a dome configuration.

Before culdoscopy, a patients should have a compete blood count, blood chemistry analysis, and a chest roentenogram.

PATIENT EDUCATION

The patient should understand the procedure and that the operative time will probably be approximately 15 minutes. A Fleet's enema should be self-administered by the patient the night before the test. The patient should take nothing by mouth after the midnight before the examination and a friend or family member should accompany the patient to the test location.

PROCEDURE

The patient is usually placed under heavy sedation. Proper position involves a tight knee-chest position with the back swayed and the abdomen hanging free. A careful vagina cleaning is performed and the posterior lip of the cervix grasped with a tenaculum. Infiltrative anesthesia using an epinephrine-containing solution may be used to further reduce local discomfort. With the cervix pressed forward and downward, a trocar in its sheath is inserted at the apex of the vagina vault directly in the midline. Steady pressure is placed on the trocar aligning it with the spinal cord. As the trocar penetrates the peritoneum, a "spring" is felt. Air can be added to the intraperitoneal cavity to help separate the pelvic organs from the intestines.

The culdoscope is then inserted through the sheath of the trocar while the operator is looking through the scope. A light source is connected and the ovary and tubes should be in view. If needed, the uterus can be moved using the tenaculum attached to the cervix allowing, with rotating movement of the scope, a full view of the cul-de-sac. Tubal patency can be evaluated by injection of dye into the uterine cavity and watching for spillage into the peritoneal cavity.

Operative culdoscopy involves the same procedure up to the operation. The incision is widened laterally and the operation is performed in place or with the tubes and ovaries brought into the vagina with a clamp. This type of vaginal wound will require postoperative suturing. The most common procedure being performed in this manner is tubal ligation.

The procedure for culdocentesis begins in the same manner with a cannula being inserted through the trocar. A syringe is attached to the cannula and aspiration is performed (figure 44+1).

POSTPROCEDURE INFORMATION

Postprocedure instructions should include the prohibition of douching and intercourse for a full week. Strain of the abdominal muscles should be avoided as severe coughing or vomiting may increase intraabdominal pressure and force air through the diaphragmatic space causing subcutaneous emphysema. The patient should be observed for signs of brisk bleeding more than 24 hours after the procedure, abdominal pain or fever, or any other unusual symptoms.

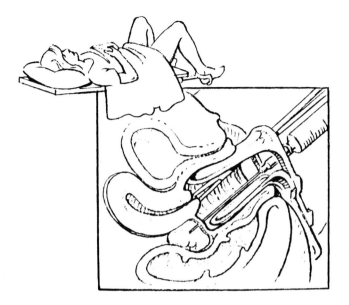

Figure 44–1. Following initial puncture in the knee-chest position, the cannula is left in place and the patient is turned on her back for fluid aspiration.

COMPLICATIONS

Complications of culdoscopy are rare. Possible problems include inability to enter the peritoneal cavity, rectal perforation, or bleeding from the vaginal cuff. Extraperitoneal perforations on the rectum are generally associated with endometriosis and pelvic adhesions. These complications are usually benign if they occur and are discovered before the peritoneum is penetrated, and the procedure is immediately halted. Patients should be given several days of systemic antibiotics. Later complications, such as peritonitis and abcess formation, may require more extensive therapy.

Excessive bleeding from the trocar puncture is usually caused by improper placement techniques and can be controlled with vaginal packing. Bleeding may occur in a delayed manner several days following the procedure and immediately after sexual intercourse or some other cause of increased intravaginal pressure.

An unusual complication is subcutaneous emphysema evidenced by shortness of breath and crepitus. This requires bedrest and can be avoided by carefully expelling air from the peritoneal cavity prior to removal of the cul-de-sac sheath.

PATIENT QUESTIONS

Should I have culdoscopy or laparoscopy?

Both of these procedures have supporters for many overlapping indications. Laparoscopy appears to be easier to learn, and the performance of the procedure in the prone position as well as other factors make it more desirable. If a follow-up procedure is contemplated that can be performed by laparotomy, then laparoscopy would probably be the preferred diagnostic procedure. The most important factor, however, is the skill of the physician performing the examination. A significant minority of gynecologic physicians feels that the avoidance of anesthesia and the relative ease of performing culdoscopy make it the procedure of choice. This decision should be carefully discussed with the physician, keeping in mind the medical indications and contraindications, and the skill of the examiner.

Should I consider culdoscopy for female sterilization?

Inability to complete the procedure as planned and technical failure appear to occur more frequently in tubal sterilization when the procedure is done using culdoscopy. The need to carefully select patients who can undergo this culdoscopic procedure also speaks against its widespread use for this indication. The somewhat undignified knee-chest position also lessens the attraction of culdoscopy. However, culdoscopy has the advantage of leaving no scar, appearing to be less invasive, and requiring only outpatient facilities and local anesthesia.

Should culdoscopy be done initially to determine the presence of ectopic pregnancy?

Recent advances in ultrasound have made it possible for sonography to be very sensitive to the presence of ectopic pregnancy. When performed in conjunction with a qualitative serum pregnancy test, a higher degree of accuracy is achieved in the diagnosis and exclusion of ectopic pregnancy in patients presenting with pelvic pain than with any other single test. The value of culdocentesis in this specific situation occurs when the symptoms are more puzzling or absent, when the sonography and serum examinations are inconclusive, or when rupture of a tubal pregnancy is suspected and the patient may require hospitalization.

CONSENT

Culdoscopy and culdocentesis are invasive procedures that require informed consent.

SELECTED BIBLIOGRAPHY

Diamond E: Diagnostic culdoscopy in infertility: a study of 4000 outpatient procedures. *J Reprod Med* 1978;21:1:23.

Eisinger SH: Culdocentesis. *J Fam Pract* 1981;Jul:13(1)95.

Mansi ML: The role of culdocentesis in evaluating pelvic pain in women. *J Am Osteopath Assoc* 1984;Apr:83(8):576.

Romero R, Copel JA, Kadar N, Jeanty P, Decherney A, Hobbins JC: Value of culdocentesis in the diagnosis of ectopic pregnancy. *Obstet Gynecol* 1985;Feb:25(1):54.

Trott A: Diagnostic modalities in gynecologic and obstetrical emergencies. *Emer Med Clinics of North Am* 1987;5(3):405.

Weckstein LN, Boucher AR, Tucker H, Gibson D, Trettenmaier MA: Accurate diagnosis of early ectopic pregnancy. *Obstet Gynecol* 1985;65(3):393.

45

Laparoscopic Tubal Ligation

RICHARD SADOVSKY

Tubal sterilization is a safe and reliable procedure for female sterilization. This procedure is probably the most commonly performed laparoscopic surgical procedure in the United States. Tubal procedures can be performed on outpatients with minimal side effects. The reversibility of tubal ligation depends on the procedure used to interrupt the fallopian tubes and the skill of the operator performing the repair.

INDICATIONS

Female patients requesting permanent sterilization should be considered for laparoscopic tubal ligation. The decision should be made carefully with the understanding that reversibility may not be possible. Patients should be asked to consider this at some length and to understand that the most common reason for requesting reversal of the procedure is remarriage. The patient and her partner should fully understand the implications of the procedure and be asked to consider settings in which regret and misgivings are likely to occur.

If the patient is part of a couple, then the couple should work out any ambivalence about sterilization together. There should be a real commitment to ending fertility.

ALTERNATIVES

Minilaparotomy using local anesthesia has been used for tubal sterilization. Surgical entry into the peritoneal cavity is made under direct vision. The complication rate is low and major complications have only rarely been reported. Comparisons of this procedure with the laparoscopic route have resulted in various opinions as to which procedure is preferable.

Hysteroscopic tubal sterilization techniques are under investigation. These would be advantageous because they would avoid entry into the peritoneal cavity and could be done in the outpatient setting. Procedures currently being evaluated include the blind transcervical instillation of tubal occlusive solutions such as quinacrine and methyl cyanoacrylate; both sclerose the tubes completely making reversal impossible.

Visualization by the hysteroscope allows destruction of the interstitial portion of the tube by electrocautery or the injection of occlusive substances or solid inert devices to produce sterilization. The use of silicone plugs is demonstrating some promise. At present, these hysteroscopic alternatives are relatively unavailable to practicing physicians.

Hysterectomy performed for sterilization is generally thought to be unjustifiable because of its unacceptable morbidity rates.

For technical reasons such as inoperative complications, adhesions, obesity, or pelvic masses, laparoscopic sterilization cannot be completed in about 0.5% of patients. Many of these patients can undergo laparotomy for the desired tubal sterilization.

Success rates for tubal sterilization vary depending on the type of technique and the expertise of the surgeon performing the procedure. Using electrocoagulation, either unipolar or bipolar, the failure rate is approximately 2 to 3 per 1000 with the greatest likelihood of an unwanted pregnancy occurring during the first year following the procedure. This failure rate appears to be the best achievable with mechanical ligation also.

CONTRAINDICATIONS

There are no contraindications to laparoscopic tubal ligation although factors such as obesity and prior abdominal and pelvic surgery make the procedure more difficult. In addition, the likelihood of noncompletion because of technical factors is more probable.

PREPROCEDURE PREPARATION

The patient should not eat for 8 to 12 hours prior to the procedure. The bladder should be completely emptied before laparoscopy.

PATIENT EDUCATION

The patient should be well informed about all aspects of the procedure. The emotional stress of the procedure should be addressed in early counselling sessions. Women using intrauterine devices (IUD) should probably remove them, and women using oral contraceptives should stop one month prior to surgery. Patients should be advised to use some other form of contraception in the interim.

PROCEDURE

The entire procedure requires approximately 45 to 60 minutes (figure 45–1). With the patient in the proper position, either lying flat on the table or in the lithotomy position, anesthesia is administered using either general or local techniques. Local infiltration of anesthetic is used in the skin of the infraumbilical region and continuing deeper into the fascia and the peritoneum along the projected trocar course. If the surgeon is using a second site for insertion of operative tools, similar anesthesia is provided to that site.

The abdomen is inflated with carbon dioxide or nitrous oxide. The initial incision is made between the umbilicus and the pubic hairline and the laparoscope, an instrument with the diameter of a pencil and having a hollow shaft and a light source is inserted.

It is technically possible to perform the procedure through a single puncture. This involves insertion of the operating tools through the appropriate laparoscopic channel. Many gynecologists prefer a double puncture technique permitting separation of the operating portion from the visual portion of the procedure.

The fallopian tubes must be anesthetized independently, and this is done by dripping an appropriate agent over the sterilization site of each tube once visualization has been achieved.

Various electrical and mechanical procedures have been developed for laparoscopic sterilization. Electrical methods may employ unipolar or bipolar modes. The unipolar mode, in which the tube is grasped by a forceps and electrocoagulation is performed alone or with ligation, has recently lost favor because of the greater likelihood of inadvertent burns. Bipolar coagulation is performed with a forceps that carries both the active and the return electrode. The current travels only from one pole to the other instead of travelling throughout the body. The danger of sparking is eliminated, decreasing the risk of burns.

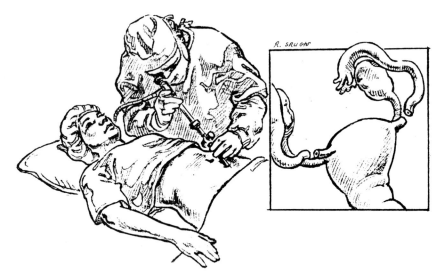

Figure 45–1. Laparoscopic tubal ligation.

Care must be taken to ensure that the mucosa is completely destroyed in order to eliminate the possibility of an inadvertent pregnancy.

Thermocoagulation uses localized heat generated at the forceps tip. After two contiguous burns are created, the tubes are transected in the center of the destroyed areas. Since heat transmission is limited to 2 mm depth, the cut edges must be recoagulated to ensure tubal occlusion.

Mechanical techniques involve occlusion using clips or rings. Special clips such as the Hulka clip and the Filshie clip have been developed. These are applied with special tools and are relatively simple. Falope rings made of nonreactive silicone rubber can be applied relatively easily.

POSTPROCEDURE INFORMATION

Several days of abdominal soreness are to be expected after the procedure. All temperatures above 100°, fainting, bleeding, or persistent or increasing pain should be reported to the physician. The patient should avoid intercourse, lifting, and other strenuous exercise for 1 to 2 weeks following the surgery. There may be some changes in menstrual flow and perhaps some minor feelings of stress and anxiety. These should be managed appropriately.

COMPLICATIONS

Laparoscopic sterilization requires careful attention to detail. The overall rate of intraoperative or postoperative complications is felt to be around 2%. Unintended laparotomy is the most frequent of these complications and was most often needed to complete the procedure because of inadequate visualization. Laparotomy for technical reasons is more likely to be necessary in women with prior history of pelvic or abdominal surgery or obesity greater than 120% of ideal body weight. A small percentage of laparotomies are performed because of operative complications including bleeding. The choice of procedure, band versus electrocoagulation, does not seem to affect the risk of complications.

The use of general anesthesia seems to be associated with more complications than the use of local anesthesia, but this may be explained by the fact that the surgeons using local anesthetic techniques may have had more skill or more experience with the procedure.

Other rare complications include bowel injuries due to burns or trocar perforation. Occasionally, thermal bowel injuries are not recognized until the patient presents with signs and symptoms of peritonitis. Infections occur in a small percentage of cases (approximately 0.15%) and present as cellulitis or pelvic inflammatory disease as long as 2 weeks after the procedure. A Centers for Disease Control (CDC) surveillance study estimated the death rate for tubal sterilization (all techniques) to be 3.6 in 100,000 women.

The amount of postoperative discomfort may depend on the procedure used. The Falope rings cause somewhat more discomfort than do the other procedures.

PATIENT QUESTIONS

What type of anesthesia will be used?

General anesthesia is usually employed for laparoscopic tubal ligations although the properly trained surgeon working with a well-prepared patient can use local anesthesia.

Is the tubal sterilization procedure reversible?

Sterilization should be offered only as a permanent form of contraception, although some women may request reversal some time in the future. This is generally more common among younger women, women who are having poor relationships, or during a period of voluntary termination of pregnancy when the patient appears particularly unsettled. Other psychological tragedies can lead to the request for reversal of sterilization. Procedures that have involved limited amount of tissue destruction may permit a limited possibility of reversal. The clip and ring methods probably have the greatest rate of reversal success.

I currently have an IUD in place. Should I remove it prior to tubal sterilization?

Anecdotal data suggest an increase in the rate of postoperative infection in cases in which the IUD is removed simultaneously with tubal sterilization. Large multicentered trials in many centers, however, have not borne this out and revealed no increased incidence of infection or other complications when an IUD was in place within 1 month prior to sterilization. Additional data are needed to make a definitive recommendation about the timing of the IUD removal.

What is the post-tubal ligation syndrome?

Post-tubal ligation syndrome is a symptom complex that has been described differently by different authorities. In some studies, the symptoms are described as abnormal bleeding and pain, while in others it includes subsequent events such as hysterectomy. This syndrome, being so ill-defined, probably has no meaning and may not even exist. The development of postprocedure bleeding abnormalities and pain may be related to prior use of oral contraceptives.

What is the likelihood of an ectopic pregnancy following tubal ligation?

Ectopic pregnancies occur at a slightly higher rate following tubal ligation, depending largely on the type of procedure done and the frequency of the woman's sexual activity.

Can I have tubal ligation immediately following the delivery of my baby?

Laparoscopic tubal ligation cannot be performed during the immediate postpartum period because the uterus and the fallopian tubes have not descended to their normal positions. Sterilization by minilaparotomy can be done with 72 hours after childbirth avoiding an additional hospital stay.

Will sterilization decrease my sex drive?

Sterilization has no effect on the sex drive nor does the procedure cause weight gain. Physicians have been unable to distinguish any hormonal changes occurring with any consistency following tubal ligation.

Consent

Federal regulations require that, when the procedure is federally funded, candidates for sterilization must be 21 years old and mentally competent. A woman cannot choose to be sterilized while she is undergoing labor nor while requesting an abortion. Consent cannot be given while the patient is intoxicated or impaired in any way. Surgery cannot be performed until 30 days after the consent has been signed to allow the patient to reconsider. The consent automatically expires after 180 days.

The practicing physician is well advised to follow these federal guidelines in handling patients requesting tubal sterilization procedures.

SELECTED BIBLIOGRAPHY

Bhiwandiwala PP, Mumford SD, Kennedy KI: Comparison of the safety of open and conventional laparoscopic sterilization. *Obstet Gynecol* 1985;Sep:66(3):391.

Chick PH, Frances M, Paterson PJ: A comprehensive review of female sterilization—tubal occlusion methods. *Clin Reprod Fertil*. 1985;Jun:(2):81.

Huggins GR, Sondheimer SJ: Complications of female sterilization: immediate and delayed. *Fertil Steril* 1984;Mar:41(3):337.

Pool F, Kohn I: What to tell patients about sterilization. *RN* 1986;May:49(5):55.

Siegler AM, Hulka J, Peretz A: Reversibility of female sterilization. *Fertil Steril* 1985;Apr:43(4):499.

Taylor PJ, Freedman B, Wonnacott T, Brown S: Female sterilization: can the woman who will seek reversal be identified prospectively? *Clin Reprod Fertil* 1986;Jun:4(3):207.

46

Mammography

DAVID H. GORDON

Mammography was first used in 1913 when radiographs of a large number of breasts were performed with correlation of the gross and microscopic anatomy. Early studies were able to distinguish infiltrating from circumscribed carcinoma and a nonpalpable breast carcinoma was recognized on the radiograph. Stereoscopic techniques of mammography began in the early 1930s and classified normal and abnormal findings. The next advances came in the 1950s with reports about mammography and duct injection, and the reporting of carcinomatous microcalcifications resembling fine grains of salt in approximately 30% of breast cancers.

Benign and malignant mammographic findings were better defined in the 1950s. These were correlated with histologic sections and reliable mammographic criteria for the diagnosis of carcinoma were established.

In the 1960s mammography was made more clinically applicable by the introduction of a high milliamperage (MA) low kilovoltage (KV) technique using industrial film, and excellent results were reported. In 1965 the American College of Radiology produced a series of standard recommendations on techniques, radiation dosages, and applications of mammography. The ability of mammography to reveal breast cancer has steadily improved, and there is little doubt about its ability to detect malignant disease before it becomes palpable.

INDICATIONS

Indications for mammography have been evolving over the past several years. In general, mammography is applied to the evaluation of palpable masses in the breast, evaluation of patients with nodular or lumpy breasts (fibrocystic disease), and as a screening modality for women with a strong family history of breast carcinoma and for women in general. The American College of Physicians, the American College of Obstetrics and Gynecology, and the Canadian Task Force on the Periodic Health Examination endorse screening mammograms for all women beginning at age 50. Newer recommendations from the American College of Radiology, the American Medical Association, and the American Cancer Society advocate baseline mammogram at age 40, screening mammography every 1 to 2 years between the ages of 40 and 50, and annual mammography after age 50. Various experts have recommended routine annual mammography as early as age 30. The established guidelines are not widely recognized. Great variation exists in different geographic areas and even from one physician to another.

It is commonly felt that women who have a family history of breast cancer should have mammography more frequently than the above guidelines indicate. The risk factor of excess dietary fat intake has not been found to correlate with increased frequency of breast carcinoma, although there does appear in some studies to be an increase in breast cancer incidence in women who drink moderate amounts of alcohol compared to those who drink no alcohol. Alcohol as a risk factor for breast carcinoma is still being studied. The role of birth control pills in breast cancer development is unclear, but estrogen replacement therapy does appear to cause breast cancer. According to many researchers, the major risk factors that appear to count most are age and family history.

Mammography is accurate in evaluating a palpable mass. When combined with ultrasound for masses that suggest cysts and followed by aspiration, accuracy is in the range of 80% to 90% depending on the quality of the mammography and the expertise of the reviewer. Once a mass is palpated, it is unlikely that mammography alone will be able to assign a definite diagnosis to the mass. However, there are criteria for the identity of fibroadenomatous masses that include clear margination around a 360° circumference, umbilication of the mass, a lucent halo, and typical popcorn calcification. Round, well-circumscribed masses that are homogeneous in appearance may be defined as cystic. Ultrasound and aspiration are still recommended for increased accuracy.

If the mass fails to meet any of the above criteria, and, in addition, has any of the so-called malignant criteria of breast masses, it must be biopsied. The criteria for malignancy include large vessels going to and exiting the mass, skin thickening or retraction, nipple retraction, irregular outline with tentacles of soft tissue density extending into the surrounding fatty parenchyma, and the typical sand-like calcifications that are suggestive of carcinoma. The latter criteria of calcifications is not specific for carcinoma as only about one quarter to one-third of masses with this criteria will turn out to be malignant on biopsy.

In screening mammography, when no mass is palpable, typical fine, sand-like microcalcifications may be seen (figure 46–1). Once the surgeon knows these are present, he may be able to palpate the mass. When the lesion is thus defined, a biopsy is required by fine needle under mammographic guidance. Histology is then done to look for malignancy. Excisional biopsy may be necessary. If the lesion is not palpable, a needle localization must be done with removal of the mass.

In women with fibrocystic disease of the breast, or so called mammary dysplasia, mammography can be difficult to interpret. The mammographic appearance of the breast will vary with the stage of the menstrual cycle, and a suspicious mass can be reevaluated at another time of the menstrual cycle. Women with this condition will often have multiple biopsies.

Note: ANY MASS WHICH CANNOT BE SPECIFICALLY DEFINED AS BENIGN SHOULD BE BIOPSIED.

ALTERNATIVES

Xeroradiography, or xeromammography, is no longer considered to be as good a modality as mammography in evaluation of the breast. Although it may be even more sensitive to calcifications than standard mammography, it does not yield as good tissue contrast and definition as does the standard technique.

Thermography and breast transillumination are of historical interest only and should not be relied upon for any diagnostic information. Magnetic resonance imaging (MRI) of the breast is in a primitive state at present. Preliminary articles state that MRI is not as effective in defining breast masses as is standard mammography with compression. The lack of the ability of MRI to image calcifications is a serious limitation of this technique.

Clinical breast examinations by the physician appears to be finding fewer and fewer of cancerous lesions, with a recent study demonstrating that only 8% of breast lesions are discovered on physical examination with 90% being found with mammography. The ability of the clinician to distinguish true breast cancers on manual examination is a skill that is essential for every physician to develop.

Self-examination is important, but there are no statistics that show that this procedure really saves lives. Most self-detected lesions are large and have a poor

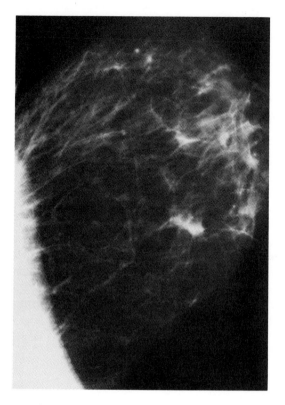

Figure 46–1. Mammography (Courtesy of AFP Imaging and Sorodex).

prognosis. Women can be taught to discover lesions as small as 1.5 cm, and they should be encouraged to learn and continue self-examination.

POSSIBILITY OF FAILURE

Mammography is the most sensitive test available to diagnose breast carcinoma early in its development. Failure will occur only if the examiner uses poor radiographic or interpretive technique or if the mammography results are not properly followed up. When a mass is found on mammography that does not meet absolute criteria for benignity, a biopsy must be done. Cystic masses require confirmation by ultrasound with possible aspiration of the fluid. The ultimate proof of benignity or malignancy is biopsy, and if there is any question about the nature of the mass, this should always be done. Nonpalpable calcifications must always be biopsied with needle localization.

CONTRAINDICATIONS

There are no absolute contraindications to mammography. One must balance the risk of radiation, which is fairly substantial since high MA and low KV x-rays are needed to produce high contrast examination of the breast.

PREPROCEDURE PREPARATION

No preprocedure preparation is necessary. No coagulation studies are required prior to needle localization because the breast is a relatively avascular area and the needle is small.

PATIENT EDUCATION

The patient should be reassured that the procedure will involve minimal discomfort. She will be required to disrobe and have a breast examination performed by the supervising radiologist. Most radiology offices utilize female technicians so as to minimize the embarrassment and anxiety that a female patient may have by being undressed in front of a male technician.

PROCEDURE

After a manual breast examination is performed, the breast is placed on a holder and various views are taken (figure 46–2). Both breasts are examined in both cephalocaudal (top to bottom) and mediolateral projections. Axillary projections may be obtained as well as spot films with compression views when indicated.

A needle localization is a more invasive procedure and is usually done after a screening mammogram has defined the presence of suspicious calcifications. This procedure involves identifying the lesion in two views at mammography and then transfixing the lesion with either a needle or a spring-wire device that is injected into the lesion (figure 46–3). The patient then goes immediately from the mammography room to the operating room where the lesion is removed using the needle or the spring-wire as a guide. The specimen is then x-rayed to make sure that the calcified lesion has been removed.

POSTPROCEDURE INFORMATION

The patient may want someone to accompany her to the mammogram procedure, but this is not necessary. The emotional impact of the procedure may require support. If a biopsy is done, warm compresses can be used to relieve tenderness and minimal swelling that may result.

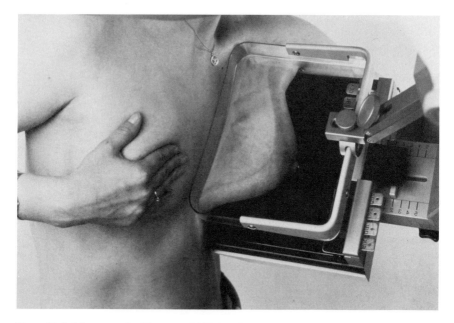

Figure 46–2. Mammography (Courtesy of AFP Imaging and Sorodex).

COMPLICATIONS

After effects of mammography are related to the potential of carcinogenesis due to exposure to radiation. The procedure should be performed only when appropriately indicated. Surgical removal of a nonpalpable, mammographically discovered mass depends on the age of the patient and whether general or local anesthesia is used to perform the excision. A relatively superficial lesion removed under local anesthesia has virtually no associated morbidity. A deeper lesion that may require general anesthesia and dissection carries a small incidence of morbidity and mortality due to the anesthesia and the operative procedure.

PATIENT QUESTIONS

What is the risk of radiation to the breast?

It is currently felt that the risk of the radiation to the breast is less than the potential value of mammography when the procedure is done with appropriate indications and proper techniques.

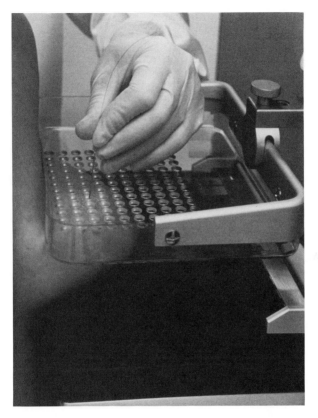

Figure 46–3. Needle localization of suspicious microcalcifications (Courtesy of AFP Imaging and Sorodex).

Is the procedure painful?

Compression of the breast is required during the mammographic procedure. This pressure is usually gentle and should not cause a significant amount of pain. Needle localization, when needed, is minimally painful. Local lidocaine placed in the skin may burn on injection, but the needles used for localization are very fine and should not cause pain.

What happens if a nonpalpable lump is found on mammography?

Nonpalpable lesions noted on mammography should be evaluated by ultrasound to determine whether the lesion is solid or cystic. If the lesion is sharply defined and there is no evidence of anything else inside it, probably nothing needs to be done. If the lesion turns out not to be a cyst, the next step is either open biopsy or fine needle biopsy. Nonpalpable lesions detected on mammography are malignant 20% to 30% of the time.

If I have a palpable breast lesion, is mammography helpful?

For a palpable lesion, needle aspiration remains the simplest and cheapest way to determine whether it is a cyst. Mammography is not needed if the aspiration demonstrates a cystic lesion, or if malignant cells are obtained. Clinical correlation with the pathology results is always necessary to determine the need for further study, since cells cannot be aspirated from a small percentage of malignant lesions that are too dense. An open biopsy may be needed in these cases and certain clinicians feel that mammography may be a useful adjunct in equivocal cases.

CONSENT

Consent is not required for routine mammography. Consent is routinely obtained for needle localization.

SELECTED BIBLIOGRAPHY

Bassett LW, Gold RH: The evolution of mammography. *Amer J Radio* 1988;March 150:493.

Feig SA: Radiation risk from mammography: is it clinically significant? *Amer J Radio* 1984;143:469.

Hall FM, Storella JM, Silverstone DZ, Wyshak G: Nonpalpable breast lesions: recommendations for biopsy based on suspicion of carcinoma at mammography. *Radio* 1988;167:353.

Moskowitz M: Mammography to screen asymptomatic women for breast cancer. *Amer J Radio* 1984;143:457.

Thomas P: The muddle over screening breast cancer. *Med World News* 1988;May 9:34.

47

Vasectomy

RICHARD SADOVSKY

The term *vasectomy* is actually a misnomer currently used to describe the surgical procedure of interrupting the flow of sperm through the vas deferens. Painful epididymal infections can be significantly reduced by this procedure. Normal sexual activity can be permitted following the procedure without the concern of pregnancy.

INDICATIONS

Indications for vasectomy are facilitation of family planning by blocking the passage of sperm into the ejaculate and to prevent the ascending infections that can cause epididymitis.

Some physicians perform vasectomy prior to the removal of a diseased prostate gland in order to prevent the movement of infected material from the prostate duct into the epididymis, although this is rarely done.

ALTERNATIVES

Tubal ligation as a method of permanent contraception is discussed in detail in another chapter. Oral contraceptives are associated with a measurable and significant morbidity. Condoms used with spermicidal cream can yield good birth-control results.

POSSIBILITIES OF FAILURE

Studies throughout the world indicate a failure rate for vasectomy of 0.15 per 100 person-years. This is slightly higher than the rate for sterilization of the woman by tubal ligation. There is no way of predicting the man who will be fertile even after vasectomy. The chances of this occurring are decreased by care and precision on the part of the physician.

CONTRAINDICATIONS

The major contraindication to vasectomy is the desire for temporary sterilization only, when the man does not understand the results of the procedure, or when there is some reluctance to the sterilization. The resolution of marital problems is also not a good basis for the procedure. Emotional complications postoperatively are likely to occur in men who present with hypochondriasis, a delicate image of their masculinity, or incomplete understanding of the procedure.

Other physical contraindications include allergic reactions to anesthetic agents, a bleeding tendency, inability to palpate the vas, intrascrotal scarring or hernia, and an uncooperative patient.

PREPROCEDURE PREPARATION

A sperm evaluation is generally done initially to be certain the patient is not azospermic, in which case the vasectomy would not be necessary.

The patient is advised to practice good hygiene prior to the procedure cleaning the genital area with a good antibacterial soap. Occasionally preoperative sedation is provided, but most physicians find they can use verbal anesthesia effectively.

PATIENT EDUCATION

All alternative forms of contraception should be discussed with the patient and his partner prior to consideration of vasectomy. The procedure should be considered permanent although microsurgical techniques are allowing reanastomosis, which restores fertility in less than 50% of the patients on whom it is performed.

Every man must be aware of the difference between this procedure and castration. Vasectomy will not affect "manhood" and virility, only the transport of sperm. The patient must understand that sterility is not immediate and all other questions should be appropriately answered. Total patient confidence is important and a relaxed man will be a better surgical candidate.

The patient should bring an athletic supporter to the procedure and should be accompanied by another person who can assist with transportation home. The patient will probably be able to return to normal activities the next day, but this depends on the individual's recuperative powers.

PROCEDURE

Vasectomy is usually an office procedure and usually requires about 30 minutes (figure 49–1). The testes and vas are completely examined. Congenital unilateral absence of the vas occurs in about 1 man in 500. If the vas cannot be palpated on careful examination, then the operation is performed only on the contralateral side and subsequent absence of sperm in the semen will prove unilateral absence of the vas.

Anesthesia involves infiltration of the skin where the incision is to be made and blocking the spermatic nerve with a deeper injection. The nerve accompanies the vas in its sheath so the anesthetic must be injected into the sheath.

The operative procedure involves division and removal of a section of the vas, the sealing of its urethral end (at minimum), and the closing of the sheath over the urethral end of the vas to create a barrier of fascia between the two cut ends. The most common procedures involve ligation, clipping, or cauterization of the ends of the vas. The fascia sheath, when closed properly, acts as a good barrier to recanalization of the vas. A few sutures are used to close the incision and the patient can then leave the physician's office.

Percutaneous obstruction of the vas using electrical or chemical means has been attempted. These techniques have not yet been found to be as successful as incisional procedures.

POSTPROCEDURE INFORMATION

The patient can apply an icebag over the scrotal bandages for the initial several hours with the scrotum immobilized if the pain and swelling are disturbing. There may be some swelling and discoloration (black-and-blue marks), which should slowly recede. An athletic supporter worn for the first 24 hours following the procedure will help to relieve discomfort.

Abstention from all sexual activity for 2 days is advisable. Sterility, however, may not occur immediately after surgery, and some form of birth control should be continued until the absence of sperm in the ejaculate is confirmed. Prophylac-

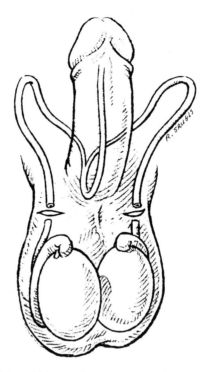

Figure 47–1. Vasectomy incisions with interruption of the vas deferens.

tic antibiotics are generally prescribed in the United States. Patients may develop a variety of anxiety symptoms, therefore they should have ready access to their physicians.

There may be sperm left above the area where the vas deferens has been cut and fertility may still exist until all these sperm have been ejaculated. This may take 12 to 20 ejaculations. To confirm sterility, semen specimens should be analyzed regularly looking for the total absence of sperm.

COMPLICATIONS

Specific physical complications include spermatic granulomas of the vas and the epididymis resulting from extravasation of sperm through the end of the vas or from a rupture in the epididymal wall. This may occur a week to several years following the procedure. Granulomas of the vas appear to be common following the use of clips or ligation, and rare with fulguration techniques. Granulomas can be painful and should be evacuated when cystic. Painless granulomas do not require treatment. No deaths have been reported following vasectomy.

The formation of antisperm antibodies occurs in approximately 50% of men following vasectomy. These have no effect on the health of the man, but can be important if the patient seeks return of fertility.

Good preoperative counselling will prevent most of the psychological complications that occur following vasectomy.

PATIENT QUESTIONS

Is a vasectomy reversible?

Anastomosis following vasectomy is possible using microsurgical techniques. This procedure may require general anesthesia and an overnight stay in the hospital. Patients should be advised that the restoration of fertility is not guaranteed and pregnancy rates following microsurgery have not been well studied. Although as many as 80% to 90% of reversal procedures are successful in restoring the presence of sperm in the ejaculate, a much lower percentage of pregnancy, approximately 30% is actually achieved. The likelihood of subfertility in the face of repair appears to be higher in men who have high titers of antisperm antibodies.

Will I change in any other way following the vasectomy?

There is no evidence that vasectomy in any way changes the endocrine status of the man. The quantity of ejaculate is not perceptibly changed, and the patient will probably not notice any difference. There is no evidence of change in sexual functioning following the procedure and most patients report no change in sexual satisfaction. The only known physical effects are postoperative pain, and the slim possibility of hematomas or infection. Only anecdotal reports have discussed long-term effects of vasectomy, and these are limited to delayed thrombophlebitis and the presence of circulating antibodies to sperm. There is no documentation of harm caused by this latter condition.

Should I store sperm in a sperm bank for future use?

Frozen semen banks have made it possible for a man to retain a form of sterility. Frozen sperm has been used with success up to 5 to 10 years after storage although there are cost and legal barriers to widespread sperm storage.

Is vasectomy painful?

In the rare instance when general anesthesia is used, there is no pain at all. If local anesthetic is used, the only pain will be the injection of anesthesia. After the operation there is a little discomfort that can be relieved by aspirin and codeine compounds. There may also be the discomfort of feeling like being sexually aroused but unable to ejaculate. This discomfort usually resolves after 1 to 2 days depending on the individual. The stitches are generally removed in about 5 days. There are no reported cases of painful ejaculation following vasectomy.

What happens to the sperm following vasectomy?

Following vasectomy, the amount of sperm in the ejaculate decreases steadily to zero by approximately the tenth ejaculation. Prostatic fluid will continue to be produced and ejaculated. Sperm production continues in the body for some time with the sperm being destroyed by macrophages and other body defense mechanisms. Most physiologists theorize that eventually the cells that produce sperm will atrophy and die in vasectomized men.

CONSENT

Vasectomy for sterilization is generally legal in the United States. The patient should sign a written consent that includes the following considerations: (1) that the patient requests the operation for the purpose of permanent prevention of bearing further children, (2) that the operation may fail to cause sterility, and (3) that the patient understands that sterilization may not be immediately produced and that achievement of sterilization can only be determined by future semen analysis. Contraception must be advised postoperatively until the semen analysis clearly indicates sterility.

Although it is not a legal requirement, it is wise to obtain agreement from both partners and to be certain that the procedure is clearly understood.

SELECTED BIBLIOGRAPHY

Babayan RK, Krane RJ: Vasectomy: what are community standards? *Urology* 1986;Apr:27(4):328.

Kendrick JS, Gonzales B, Huber DH, Grubb GS, Rubin GL: Complications of vasectomies in the United States. *J Fam Pract* 1987;Sep:25(3)245.

Newton JR: Sterilization. *Clin Obstet Gynecol* 1984;Dec:11(3):603.

Pfenninger JL: Preparation for vasectomy. *Amer Fam Phys* 1984;Oct:30(4):177.

Schmidt SS: Vasectomy. *Urol Clin North Am* 1987; Feb:14(1):149.

X
Dermatologic Procedures

48

Dermabrasion

RICHARD SADOVSKY

Dermabrasion, or skin planing, has both cosmetic and therapeutic uses. Dermabrasion of facial skin is a procedure for reducing facial scarring caused by acne or other traumatic accidents and reducing evidence of actinically damaged skin. Facial dermabrasion is a reliable procedure with dependable results when performed properly. Dermabrasion can be performed on many parts of the body where malignant and premalignant changes are found. The dorsum of the hand seems to be a particularly responsive area to this procedure. Spot "dermasanding" with an abrasive fabric can be performed by hand to remove a variety of superficial lesions and has recently been used to remove wrinkle lines in older women.

INDICATIONS

The most common indication for dermabrasion is postacne scarring and the treatment of chronic facial acne. Patients chosen for dermabrasion are generally those in whom both treatment with systemic or topical antibiotics and isoretinoin have failed.

Actinically damaged skin is the second most common indication for this procedure. More recently, dermabrasion has been used on patients with neurofibromatosis and scarring following chicken pox, tattoos, and a variety of other superficial dermatologic conditions.

ALTERNATIVES

There are no ideal alternatives to dermabrasion. Some procedures that have been attempted include collagen injections, scar excision, chemical peeling, and punch grafting. These are actually adjunctive procedures rather than alternatives, although chemical peeling has its advocates among dermatologists. Chemical peeling done with trichloroacetic acid or other exfoliant has been successful in light peeling with minimal complications. Light peeling solutions can be used repeatedly and are available in beauty salons. Chemical intermediate peeling should be done by a physician and seems to be reasonably safe. Deep peeling, or chemabrasion, can cause all the complications seen with dermabrasion. A full-face chemical peel can be used prior to dermabrasion when appropriate. These therapeutic decisions are individualized depending on the patient's needs and the physician's experience. The recent use of 5 fluorouracil preparations has decreased the use of dermabrasion in solar-damaged skin treatment, but planing appears to have a much greater prophylactic effect.

When used for treatment of malignant and premalignant lesions, dermabrasion may not be as good a procedure as radiotherapy, chemosurgery, or scalpel excision. Its value appears to be its ability to prevent further development of keratoses or epitheliomas.

Recent use of lasers to remove deep tattoos has been promising.

POSSIBILITY OF FAILURE

An appropriate level of experience and a high grade of skill are needed to obtain reliable results. Too often, the procedure is done by surgeons who are inadequately prepared and the results may not be satisfactory. When the procedure is performed by a skilled surgeon, a 65% to 85% cosmetic improvement can be anticipated.

CONTRAINDICATIONS

The procedure is contraindicated in patients who have unrealistic goals. They may need to be refused treatment if they are unwilling to understand that some scarring may remain following the procedure.

Another contraindication is the patient who has severe acne that is actively forming thick scars. When the scarring process spontaneously diminishes, careful dermabrasion can be attempted, with the patient having complete understanding of the risk of postoperative serious scarring. Corticosteroids, used topically or intralesionally, may reduce scarring in these patients.

Radiodermatitis caused by prior radiation therapy for acne may alter the epidermal structures and lead to unsatisfactory healing.

Patients using isoretinoin during the prior 6 months should be treated with great care. Isoretinoin can alter the dermatologic structures thereby affecting the healing process following dermabrasion. Some dermatologic surgeons recommend a skin biopsy on patients receiving isoretinoin treatment in order to assess the status of the sebaceous glands, and that a small spot dermabrasion be done in a low-profile area in order to ascertain the quality of healing of the facial skin following the procedure.

Other contraindications include (1) cryoglobulinemia, which mitigates against the use of topical refrigerant dermabrasion techniques; (2) vitiligo, which may worsen with dermabrasion but which can be tested by doing a spot dermabrasion; (3) presence of herpetic scarring; (4) evidence of cold allergy or cryoglobulinemia; and (5) history of poor scarring.

PREPROCEDURE PREPARATION

Men are asked to be clean shaven when they come for dermabrasion. The patient's face should be carefully examined and defects should be recorded on the chart. Laboratory examination should include a complete blood count and an evaluation of cryoglobulins and cryoprecipitates.

Some patients may benefit from surgery performed before the dermabrasion. These patients include those with deep scars and linear atrophic scars. These procedures should be performed at least 4 weeks before dermabrasion.

PATIENT EDUCATION

Patients should have a clear understanding of the nature of the procedure and its results. Before and after photographs are often helpful in this explanation, and a photographic summary of the procedure and postoperative period is useful. Therapeutic goals need to be realistically discussed. It is probably best to get the patient to agree that 50% cosmetic improvement is an acceptable goal, however, a less successful outcome is possible.

The patient should come to the procedure in light clothing that does not need to be pulled over the head to be removed. To minimize excessive bleeding during the procedure, ingestion of salicylates or birth control pills should be halted.

PROCEDURE

The patient is often premedicated with a small dose of barbiturates 60 minutes before the procedure. After this premedication, the procedure requires at least 1 hour. The face is cleaned with an appropriate cleansing solution and cotton is placed in the external auditory canal to prevent entry of the liquid refrigerant. Just before surgery, meperidine and hydroxyzine are given intramuscularly in order to have a relaxed patient during the procedure. Most surgeons use a "prechill" technique by having the patient hold an icebag against the face for 30 minutes.

Dermabrasion should be performed over the entire face in order to encourage blending of skin color. Tape may be applied to outline the borders of the procedure. The prechill makes the skin relatively solid allowing abrasion without distortion. Refrigerant spray is used to provide total anesthesia in the area being abraded. The skin is frozen in small segments until it becomes absolutely firm. Generally, infiltrative or regional anesthesia is not used.

As each segment of skin is treated, dermabrasion to the desired depth is performed without allowing complete thawing of the skin. Dermabrasion is performed using a rotating metal instrument, either solid or a brush, whose contour can be changed to match the needs of the specific patient (figure 48–1).

After dermabrasion, the surgeon may chemically peel the nonabraded areas of the face with trichloroacetic acid. This is particularly useful in patients with periorbital hyperpigmentation.

POSTPROCEDURE INFORMATION

The patient must be accompanied to the procedure by a friend or relative since it will not be possible to operate an automobile following the procedure. Postoperative care includes allowing the patient to sleep for several hours. Twenty-four hours after the procedure the dressings should be removed, and the patient applies wet compresses with a terry cloth facial mask. A half-strength boric acid solution is recommended by many surgeons. Initially, these wet packs should be applied for 10 to 12 hours daily. The duration of the wet packs decreases to 4 hours per day or less in the second week. When not using wet packs, the patient should apply petrolatum covered with Saran Wrap to avoid drying of the area. Medication should be provided for pain relief if needed. The patient should be discouraged from drinking alcohol as anecdotal reports have described more pain in these patients than those who avoid alcohol altogether.

Erythema, edema, crust formation, and some pain will be experienced by every patient. Reepithelialization is often complete after 14 days and the patient may return to work. Exposure to the sun should be avoided. Sunscreens can be used after the fourth week with trial exposure to the sun. Hydrocortisone creams and water-based cosmetics may be used for the next 2 to 3 months to

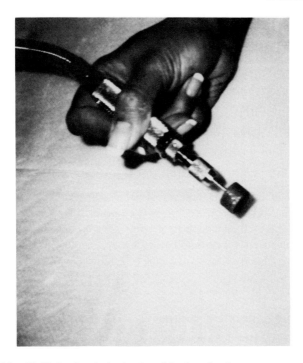

Figure 48–1. A hand-held abrasive planing head used for dermabrasion.

encourage erythema to subside. The skin color generally returns to normal by the end of the third month. Patients should be cautioned not to evaluate cosmetic improvement for at least 6 months following the procedure.

COMPLICATIONS

Anticipated side effects of dermabrasion include milia formation that are generally self-limiting. A slight flare of acne may occur, but this generally subsides within several weeks to several months. Purpura, hypopigmentation, and hyperpigmentation may occur, but generally recede. Permanent hypopigmentation may occur, and it most commonly seen in dark-skinned patients.

Complications include postoperative scar formation and infections. These are minimized by careful observation of postoperative care recommendations. Excessive crusting can allow bacterial and viral growth and should be treated by removal of the crust and systemic antibiotics. Herpes simplex infection can occur and are thought to be caused more frequently by primary infection rather than reactivation of old herpetic lesions. Acyclovir can be used systemically or topically to mitigate this complication. Patients with histories of prior herpetic lesions are frequently pretreated for 3 days with Zovirax® capsules, with the treatment being continued for 2 weeks following dermabrasion.

Other possible complications include hemorrhage, pain, erythema due to premature exposure to the sun, and scarring. These can be minimized by careful technique and good instructions.

PATIENT QUESTIONS

What is planing or dermabrasion good for?

The most popular use is the removal of acne scarring. Results are generally good, but not perfect. The procedure is not useful in the treatment of freckles and wrinkles because these tend to recur after the procedure. Prophylaxis of skin cancers and precancers (keratoses) caused by sun or other carcinogen exposure can be effective. Tattoos may or may not be removable depending on the depth of the dye.

What is the postoperative course?

The patient stays in bed for a day or two following major dermabrasion procedures. There is some bleeding and crusting early in the course of recovery. Crusting continues for about 10 days. The patient can return to work after crusting has decreased. The skin remains red for up to 12 weeks. During this time the patient must avoid the sun.

Is it painful?

Most patients, especially those who are highly motivated, report minimal pain or discomfort.

Is it possible that the procedure will have to be repeated?

Occasionally up to 3 dermabrasions may be required to treat particularly difficult areas. This may be true especially of tatoos that are deeply embedded in the skin. One dermabrasion, however, is the general rule.

CONSENT

Informed consent is needed for dermabrasion. It is also appropriate to record the patient's stated goal on the chart and, if it is unrealistic, it should be explained by the surgeon and the explanation recorded on the chart.

SELECTED BIBLIOGRAPHY

Farrior RT: Dermabrasion in facial surgery. *Laryngoscope* 1985;May:95:5:534.

Fulton JE: Modern dermabrasion techniques: a personal appraisal. *J Dermatol Surg Oncol* 1987;Jul:13:7:780.

Orentreich D, Orentreich N: Acne scar revision update. *Dermatol Clin* 1987;Apr:5:2:359.

Roenigk HH: Dermabrasion: state of the art. *J Dermatol Surg Oncol* 1985;Mar:11:3:306.

Stegman SJ, Tromovitch TA: Cosmetic dermatologic surgery. *Arch Dermatol* 1982;Dec:118:12:1013.

49

Phototherapy

RICHARD SADOVSKY

The use of sunlight in the treatment of many skin disorders began more than 200 years ago. More recently it was found that specific wavelengths of sunlight were of greatest therapeutic importance and that an artificial light source could produce these wavelengths and accomplish the desired effect within a reasonable and predictable amount of time.

The 2 major types of artificial light sources are (1) incandescent, and (2) arc. Incandescent light sources discharge visible and infrared radiation and, therefore, are used mainly to produce visible lighting and to give off heat. Arc light sources are best known for their ability to give off ultraviolet (UV) light, but they are also capable of emitting large amounts of visible and infrared radiation. Arcs are ordinarily used for phototherapy. These produce line spectrum, so named because emitted radiant energy is concentrated in relatively few wavelengths (bands) extending in the ultraviolet region.

Important factors in phototherapy include the optical properties of the skin (including the interaction of the radiation with the living components of the skin), the radiant energy spectrum utilized, and the penetration profile of radiation into the skin. Photochemistry takes place with absorption of electromagnetic radiation and results in a variety of reactions in the skin including DNA changes, melanogenesis, and photocarcinogenesis either with or without an inflammatory response. The overall effects of phototherapy relate to cellular damage, changes in cell function, changes in cell kinetics, and cell loss. These processes may affect cells in any layer of the dermis including cells in the blood and support tissues of the skin.

Photochemotherapy involves the use of ultraviolet light therapy following administration of oral or topical drugs. This is commonly used in treatment of psoriasis and other dermatologic disorders and is aimed at achieving higher therapeutic effectiveness and a lower toxicity than each of its elements alone. This form of treatment is still under investigation, but wider application is anticipated in the future.

INDICATIONS

A large number of skin conditions as well as organ diseases are reported to have benefited by ultraviolet therapy. The consensus is that ultraviolet therapy is helpful in the treatment of vitiligo, mycosis fungoides, psoriasis, acne vulgaris, herpes, seborrhea, and atopic conditions.

The repigmentation of vitiligo with photochemotherapy is currently being performed with a wide variety of therapies, however, an ideal regimen has yet to be determined. Mycosis fungoides has been treated with either ultraviolet light alone or by photochemotherapy. Generally, treatment of mycosis fungoides is only palliative and requires ongoing treatment. Psoriasis treatment with photochemotherapy has been found to have some efficacy and is better standardized than therapies for other dermatologic problems. Atopic dermatitis appears to improve with phototherapy alone, but amelioration is enhanced by photochemotherapy.

Visible light is used for treatment of neonatal jaundice caused by hyperbilirubinemia. Relative indications for visible light phototherapy include a bilirubin greater than 10 mg/100 ml in the premature infant, greater than 5 mg/100 ml in the high risk infant, and in situations of mild hemolytic anemia with elevated bilirubin. Phototherapy appears to increase the excretion of unconjugated bilirubin in the bile by converting it to water-soluble isomers. Phototherapy has also been used in the treatment of uremic and biliary pruritis.

ALTERNATIVES

Alternatives to phototherapy include topical or systemic chemical therapy. The precise role for phototherapy and photochemotherapy in common dermatologic disorders such as psoriasis and allergic-contact dermatitis has been established while in other disorders, questions still exist.

POSSIBILITY OF FAILURE

Problems occur with the standardization of light measurements in phototherapy treatments. The variation in the responses of meters that measure ultraviolet in terms of "irradiance" and "radiant exposure" causes inaccuracy in the interpretation of studies done at different locations. This has led many physicians to believe that effective quantities of ultraviolet light therapy based on action spectra are not sound or measurable. The development of thermophiles for the quantitation of extended source radiometry has recently improved the ability to measure true irradiance. With further standardization efforts, sensitive comparisons between photodermatologists may become possible.

CONTRAINDICATIONS

A careful history of the patient's reaction to sun exposure, including the tendency to develop erythema and the capacity to tan, allows an estimation of the relative risk of ultraviolet light therapy. Persons who develop marked erythema following short exposure to ultraviolet light have no inherent epidermal melanin and cannot tan. These patients are at the highest risk of acute and chronic complications of phototherapy.   Immunosuppressive disorders contraindicate phototherapy as does any prior evidence of dysplastic melanocytic nevi.

PREPROCEDURE PREPARATION

There is no specific preparation needed for phototherapy.

Preparation for photochemotherapy requires a careful history, physical examination, and laboratory evaluations of hematological, renal, and hepatic functions. A thorough slit-lamp examination should also be performed before and during photochemotherapy.

PATIENT EDUCATION

Patients should understand the treatment that they are to receive and the possibility of minor burning with erythema, blistering, and pain. Special eye glasses will be worn to protect the eyes from harmful ultraviolet light and exposure will be limited to the time prescribed. Special measures will be taken to protect extremely sensitive areas such as pendulous skin, chronic actinically exposed areas, and male genitalia.

PROCEDURE

The minimal erythema dose (MED) is the biologic standard used as the dosage unit in prescribing ultraviolet therapy. The abdomen is generally used as a test site with the MED measured by the production of a perceptible erythema 8 hours after exposure. In phototherapy, the result desired is rarely achieved by a single-light exposure. Decisions must be made about frequency of exposure, the radiation doses, and increments in dose, if any, for succeeding exposures. Smaller increments are used for patients with sensitive skin. Precise regimens have not been established and erythema of the skin is the major boundary condition on the regimen.

Frequency of radiation is somewhat limited by the course of the erythema reaction. Daily radiation is generally done only in the hospital and limited to less than 7 exposures weekly (figure 49–1). Two or three treatments per week can be given in the office. Phototherapy can be performed at home with the patient taking all the appropriate precautions.

The ultraviolet output of all mercury vapor lamps decreases with use. Tests to determine the exposure time needed to produce minimal erythema should be made every 3 to 6 months, depending on the hours of operation.

When combination therapy is planned, preparations can be used topically, orally, or intravenously. Substances that have been used include topical corticosteroids, tar preparations, psoralens, systemic retinoids, and methotrexate.

Neonatal phototherapy should be performed with a plexiglass shield between the infant and the light source. The eyes and gonads should be protected during periods of radiation. The infant's body temperature and weight should be closely monitored to prevent hyperthermia and dehydration.

POSTPROCEDURE INFORMATION

The patient can anticipate some reddening of the skin with a feeling of warmth. A cool compress may relieve this minimal discomfort as will a cream or ointment prescribed by the physician. The patient should not be exposed to natural sunlight for lengthy periods during phototherapy.

COMPLICATIONS

Acute side effects of phototherapy include edema, bulla formation, and painful inflammation of treated skin. These will generally subside if minimal treatment is given, as with acute sunburn. Chronic effects include the potential development of cataracts, and the enhancement of skin cancer development (mainly squamous cell cancers) especially in fair-skinned individuals and those receiving previous x-ray therapy. There are also some data demonstrating evidence of immunosuppressive effects of ultraviolet light therapy. The field of photoimmunology is widening rapidly.

Photoallergy may occur in certain sensitized individuals resulting from a cell-mediated immunological phenomenon in which a photoantigen with a carrier protein is formed. Photosensitization occurs when the ingestion or application

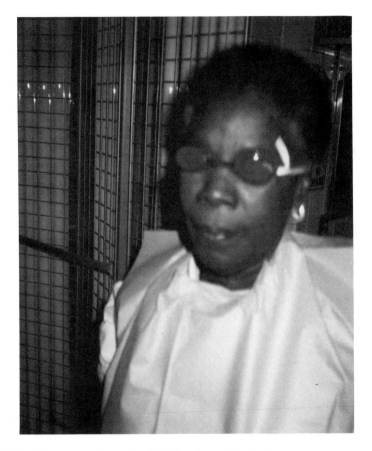

Figure 49–1. Patient prepared to reveive facial phototherapy treatment

of a drug followed by irradiation with ultraviolet light causes irritation or a sunburntype reaction. Examples of common photosensitizing medications include phenothiazines, oral hypoglycemic agents, and sulphonamides.

Treatment with visible light may cause transient diarrhea and skin rashes. There may be a prolonged grey-green discoloration of the skin, urine, and stool in children who have a component of obstructive jaundice (bronze baby syndrome).

Photochemotherapy may cause cutaneous aging, actinic damage, carcinogenic changes, and cataract formation.

PATIENT QUESTIONS

Does phototherapy cause cancer?

Since the exposure to UV light during phototherapy is approximately the same as the annual exposure for an outdoor worker in Scandinavia, the hazards are comparable. Although there may be a relationship between UV light exposure and squamous cell carcinoma, there is probably no increased risk of malignant melanoma. Close observation by the physician is recommended following completion of therapy.

Photochemotherapy, depending on the nature of the drug used, may have some carcinogenic effect. This is more true in patients who have a history of skin cancer or who sunburn easily and tan poorly.

Will phototherapy improve my psoriasis?

Treatment results with phototherapy in psoriasis are generally reported as good to excellent with some centers reporting as high as 95% clearing rate in appoximately 90% of patients. Generalization is difficult because solid data that are comparable between studies are not readily available. Phototherapy appears to be more valuable in treatment of seborrheic and eruptive types of psoriasis, but less effective in chronic plaque forms of the disease.

CONSENT

Consent is required when phototherapy is administered in the office or in the hospital.

SELECTED BIBLIOGRAPHY

Anderson TF: Pediatric phototherapy. *Pediatr Clin North Am* 1983;Aug:30:4:701.

Fitzpatrick TB: Ultraviolet-induced pigmentary changes: benefits and hazards. *Curr Probl Dermatol* 1986;15:25.

Fritsch P, Honigsmann H: Combination phototherapy—a critical appraisal. *Curr Probl Dermatol* 1986;15:238.

Morison WL: PUVA combination therapy. *Photodermatol* 1985;Aug:2:4:229.

Wolff K: Therapeutic photomedicine: History, state of the art, and perspectives. *Curr Probl Derm* 1986;15:1.

50

Skin Grafting

RICHARD M. STILLMAN

Skin grafting involves transplantation of a layer of human skin from one site to another. The skin graft is completely detached from its blood supply (donor site) and moved to another site from which blood supply will be obtained (recipient area). Skin grafts can be used to cover a variety of skin defects, for cosmetic or functional reasons. The site from which the skin is taken and its thickness determine its durability and its ability to withstand adverse conditions such as infection or poor blood supply in the recipient site.

INDICATIONS

Skin grafts have been used to cover defects resulting from major burns, venous or arterial ulcers of the extremities, defects resulting from the excision of malignant skin lesions, or traumatic defects. A split-thickness skin graft is a sheet of skin that contains epidermis and a partial thickness of dermis. Thin split-thickness grafts are the most reliable in surviving transplantation because minimal vascularity is required. Donor sites for split-thickness skin grafts heal more rapidly for the thinner grafts. On the other hand, thin grafts often have poor cosmetic results and minimal resistance to surface trauma.

Full-thickness skin grafts include the epidermis and all of the dermis (figure 50–1). They have superior cosmetic results, but require excellent vascularity of the recipient site for survival.

Composite grafts include skin, subcutaneous tissue, cartilage, and possibly other tissue. Composite grafts have the best cosmetic results, but require the maximal blood supply for any possibility of survival and "take."

Split-thickness grafts are used in areas where blood supply is marginal or where large amounts of denuded skin require coverage. Full-thickness grafts are used where blood supply is good and cosmetic result is important. Composite grafts are used where blood supply is excellent and where cosmetic results are vital such as on the face.

ALTERNATIVES

Xenografts (e.g. pig skin) are useful as a *temporary* skin replacement for large denuded areas, such as burn injury.

POSSIBILITY OF FAILURE

Graft take is variable. Where the skin graft is applied to a highly vascular area, graft take is usually successful. Where the graft is applied to an avascular area such as a distal extremity—especially in a patient with diabetes or peripheral vascular disease—skin graft take is more variable. The graft may take only partially, in which case further grafting may be required. Not all grafts are successful, and some are only partially successful. Subsequent repeat grafting may be needed in certain cases.

CONTRAINDICATIONS

Skin grafting is contraindicated where the recipient site is infected or poorly vascularized. However, where this underlying condition can be corrected, local wound care is essential for 3 weeks before infection is cleared and vascularity is improved.

PREPROCEDURE PREPARATION

The donor site is shaved and both donor and recipient sites are scrubbed with an antiseptic solution (e.g., Hibiclens®).

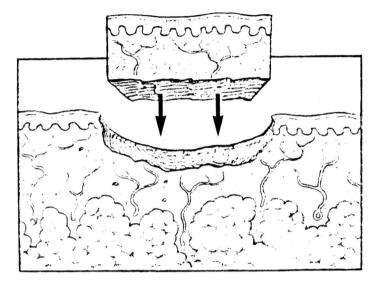

Figure 50–1. Full thickness skin graft applied to a wound.

PATIENT EDUCATION

The patient should be advised as to the anticipated donor site, the size of the graft necessary, the thickness of the graft necessary, the anticipated cosmetic deformity of the donor site, the anticipated duration of disability and immobilization required, and the approximate chances of nontake of the graft. The patient should be informed that the resulting cosmetic effect may never equal that of intact skin.

PROCEDURE

For small grafts, local anesthesia can be used. For more extensive grafts, regional or general anesthesia is required. The donor site and the recipient site are prepared using an appropriate antiseptic solution, the recipient site is debrided to insure viable blood supply at the base of the graft.

There are several methods for harvesting the skin graft. A simple tangential excision with a knife (e.g., Blair or Ferris-Smith knife) is possible but requires skill on the part of the operator to avoid a graft of irregular depth and appearance. A dermatome (e.g., Drum type or Brown type) when used by a skilled surgeon will reliably produce a graft of a uniform width and thickness. The dermatome will be set to 0.005 to 0.012 inches for a thin split-thickness graft, 0.012 to 0.018 inches for a medium-thickness graft, or 0.018 to 0.028 inches for a thick split-thickness skin graft. The graft is measured 20% to 30% larger than the anticipated recipient site to allow for shrinkage when the graft is removed. There are small battery-operated small-head dermatomes (e.g., Davol) that can be used under local anesthesia even at the bedside or in the office setting to obtain small split-thickness skin grafts. The availability of this instrument has made the widespread use of pinch grafts uncommon.

Pinch grafts, in which a small piece of skin is grabbed with a forceps, transected with a blade, and then secured to the recipient site, are rarely used today. This is because the newer dermatomes have overcome the adverse results of pinch grafts often leaving a pocket-mark donor area, irregular thickness, and poor coverage of the recipient area. In selected cases, however, pinch grafts may be acceptable.

To expand the limited coverage area that is possible with split-thickness skin grafting to accommodate the larger area needed for a sheet graft, a meshing instrument is available that will carve into the graft a pattern of multiple diamond-shaped, parallelograms in a lace-like pattern. To do this, the freshly harvested skin graft is placed with the dermal side down onto a plastic sheet that acts as a carrier. The carrier is manufactured with multiple transverse parallel incisions that will crosscut with the straight knives of the mesher. Expansion ratios are available of 1:1 to 1:3 up to 1:9. In most cases, the 1:3 expansion ratio is used.

Many different types of dressing have been used to cover the donor site. A commonly used material today is OpSite,® which is a semi-occlusive plastic membrane that will help contain exudate and minimize postoperative pain. It is transparent, allowing observation of the healing site. The recipient site requires more compulsive wound care. This is because graft survival depends directly on contact with the blood supply, fluid's not being allowed to collect beneath the graft, hematoma formation's or serous exudates' being recognized and removed. It also requires that there be no movement of the graft on the underlying recipient site for the first couple of days. This is to allow formation of neovascular connections.

In order to maintain good contact between the graft and the recipient site, a pressure dressing may be required. In many cases this pressure dressing is tied over the graft using sutures placed in the adjacent skin. In other cases a bulky dressing is taped in place.

A dilemma in the care of the recipient site is that, while frequent observation is necessary to detect fluid collection below the graft, the very process of removing the occlusive dressings to observe the graft may disrupt the neovascular connections. Many surgeons leave the dressing intact for 3 to 5 days unless there is overt evidence of infection or hematoma formation as manifested by increasing pain, surrounding cellulitis, fever, or a foul smelling exudate. Other surgeons risk possible disruption of the graft and carefully change the dressing daily. An underlying hematoma or seroma is gently evacuated through a cut in the graft or in the preexisting holes in a meshed graft.

POSTPROCEDURE INFORMATION

Family members should be aware that the patient may have difficulty walking if the graft is placed on the ankle, foot, or leg. There may be an immobilizing device such as a plaster or plastic splint and the use of crutches or a walker may be recommended. In some cases, strict bed rest will be recommended. The family should be aware of the warning signs of infection such as fever, red streaks or redness around the graft site, or a foul odor.

COMPLICATIONS

There is usually minimal pain in both donor and recipient areas. Of course, extremely large skin grafts such as those used for treatment of substantial burns may have significant associated pain. There may be bleeding from the donor site, which is treated with a compression dressing or with dressing change. The recipient site may need to be immobilized.

Systemic complications are very rarely encountered.

PATIENT QUESTIONS

Will I be able to fully use the area of the body on which the graft has been placed?

The recipient site often requires immobilization to permit adequate revascularization of the graft. This is especially true of grafts around joints in which a plastic or plaster splint may be used.

Will the graft procedure hurt?

When the procedure is performed under general or regional anesthesia, there should be minimal pain. When performed under local anesthesia, there is pain associated with the injection of the local anesthetic and there may be pain with cleansing of the recipient site. There is usually little postoperative pain.

Will there be a cosmetic deformity from the donor site?

There may be a small scar or discoloration of the skin at the donor site. The operator must weigh the cosmetic deformity that may be created by harvesting the graft against the potential good that the graft will do for the recipient site.

What happens if the graft fails to take?

The most common solution to this problem is additional skin grafting. However, an attempt is made to try to determine why the graft failed. Some of the reasons may relate to infection, or poor blood supply. In some cases, a further delay may allow local treatment of the recipient site in order to improve the likelihood of complete take of the next graft.

CONSENT

An informed consent is needed for this procedure.

SELECTED BIBLIOGRAPHY

Browne EZ, Jr.: Complications of skin grafts and pedicle flaps. *Hand Clin* 1986;May:2(2):353.

Davison PN, Batcheldor AG, Lewis-Smith PA: The properties and uses of non-expanded machine-meshed skin grafts. *Brit J Plast Surg* 1986;39:462.

Glogau RG, Stegman SJ, Tromovitch TA: Refinements in split-thickness skin grafting techniques. *J Dermat Surg Oncol* 1987;Aug:13(8):853.

Hill TG, The evolution of skin graft reconstruction. *J Dermat Surg Oncol* 1987;Aug:13(8):834.

Lesesne CV, Rosenthal R: A review of scalp split-thickness skin grafts and potential complications. *Plas Reconst Surg* 1988;May:757.

Silferskiold KL: A new pressure device for securing skin grafts. *Brit J Plast Surg* 1986;39:567.

Skouge JW: Techniques for split-thickness skin grafting. *J Dermat Surg Oncol* 1987;Aug:13(8):841.

XI
Immunologic and Lymphatic Procedures

51

Lymph Node Biopsy

RICHARD M. STILLMAN AND RICHARD SADOVSKY

Lymphatic channels, which parallel the venous drainage system in the body, are the blind origins of the lymphatic system. These channels begin peripherally and remove excess fluid from body tissues. The lymph moves centrally through the lymphatic vessels and collecting ducts that empty into the venous system at the base of the neck. Lymph is filtered throughout its passage by lymph nodes. Superficial nodes are accessible to examination and include those in the epitrochlear, axillary, infraclavicular, supraclavicular, popliteal, inguinal, and cervical areas. Peripheral lymphadenopathy may represent a benign pathological condition such as reactive hyperplasia or inflammation, a primary malignancy of the lymphoid system, or a metastatic lesion of a solid tumor originating elsewhere in the body. Biopsy of an abnormal superficial lymph node leads to a specific diagnosis in 40% to 60% of cases.

Lymph nodes in the paraaortic and the parailiac areas, while not palpable, may be determined to be abnormally large by imaging studies such as sonography, computerized tomagraphy (CT) scan, or magnetic resonance imaging (MRI). Enlargement of lymph nodes may be physiologic (common in children), or pathologic, caused by infection, neoplasm, or hematologic disease. Biopsy of an enlarged lymph node often determines a precise pathologic or microbiologic diagnosis.

INDICATIONS

Normal lymph nodes are generally palpable in the inguinal and cervical areas in children and in the inguinal areas of adults. Peripheral lymphadenopathy is a common developmental finding through young adulthood. Childhood significant lymphadenopathy is usually caused by infection but may represent some form of malignancy. During adulthood, significant lymphadenopathy more often represents tumor. A variety of local and systemic diseases may result in lymphadenopathy and a definitive diagnosis can be provided by a history, physical examination, and noninvasive studies. Where this is not possible, lymph node biopsy is indicated.

Determination of exact criteria for lymph node biopsy depends on multiple factors including patient's age, history and physical examination, size of the enlarged node, disease prevalence, and x-ray results implying significant pathology. The strong correlation between an abnormal chest roentenogram and granulomatous or malignant peripheral lymphadenopathy has been well established in both children and adults. The correlation between the size of the node and the likelihood of discovering significant pathology is less clear. Many clinicians omit lymph node size as a criteria for biopsy.

ALTERNATIVES

In most cases, a definitive diagnosis of the cause of lymphadenopathy can be made by a meticulous history, physical examination, and noninvasive studies. Localized lymphadenopathy is often a result of localized trauma, infection, or even minor scratches and bites from insects or household pets. Hepatomegaly or splenomegaly associated with lymphadenopathy suggests systemic lymphoproliferative disease. Enlargement of mediastinal lymph nodes or associated pulmonary pathology may be visible on chest roentenogram and be suggestive of tuberculosis, sarcoidosis, lymphoma, or metastatic disease. Addison's disease, hypopituitarism, hypothyroidism or hyperthyroidism, and other metabolic diseases may also be associated with painless lymph node hyperplasia.

Fine needle aspiration of lymph nodes using a simple needle and syringe have demonstrated as high as a 95% predictive rate of positive results. These results compare favorably with those of lymph node excisional biopsy. This procedure is convenient for the patient and the physician, can be done on an outpatient basis, is relatively painless, and provides good correlation between cytologic morphology and histopathology. The yield by fine-needle biopsy appears to be somewhat lower in situations in which intraabdominal or retroperitoneal sites are examined although improved imaging techniques and skill of the operators is improving these statistics. Suspicious or unclear situations should be determined by surgical biopsy.

POSSIBILITY OF FAILURE

In a minority of cases, lymph node specimens will reveal only reactive hyperplasia and a specific diagnosis can not be made by pathologic evaluation. The history and physical examination should be reassessed attempting to isolate local or systemic causes of lymph node disease. When this work up is nonproductive, a subsequent lymph node biopsy is performed 1 to 3 months later, and may provide a definitive diagnosis. Often in these cases nonspecific lymphoid hyperplasia is an early pathologic change of lymphoma and subsequent biopsies will show the characteristic pathologic findings.

CONTRAINDICATIONS

Lymph node biopsy is contraindicated in cases in which the etiology of the lymph node enlargement can be determined from noninvasive tests. Lymph node biopsy is relatively contraindicated in patients with coagulopathy. The distinction must be made between an inflamed lymph node and pathology of another nearby structure. For example, the acute onset of a tender inguinal mass accompanied by nausea, vomiting, or abdominal pain should suggest the possibility of incarcerated femoral hernia.

PREPROCEDURE PREPARATION

Prior to lymph node biopsy, the patient should clean the affected area with an appropriate antibacterial cleanser. Where cervical lymph node biopsy is to be performed in a male, the face and neck should be carefully shaved.

PATIENT EDUCATION

The patient should be advised of the reason for lymph node biopsy, the intended biopsy site, the type of anesthesia that will be used, and the expected postoperative incisional pain. Patients should be informed that there is no certainty that the lymph node biopsy will provide a diagnosis. If this occurs, further workup may be needed.

PROCEDURE

Diagnostic nodes are not always the most accessible ones. Superficial nodes may show only hyperplasia and, whenever possible, the largest lymph node in the region should be selected for biopsy. Following surgical preparation of the biopsy site, anesthesia, generally local, is administered. An incision is made through the skin and subcutaneous tissue directly overlying the suspected lymph node. Where there is diffuse lymphadenopathy the biopsy of cervical or axillary nodes is preferred to biopsy of inguinal nodes, because the former are more likely to provide a pathologic diagnosis. There is some value in multiple biopsies, particularly from the supradiaphragmatic and subdiaphragmatic areas, for the purpose of staging lymphomas or for recognizing different histology when present.

For an excisional biopsy, the lymph node is dissected free from surrounding tissue (figure 51–1) and lymphatic vessels are electrocauterized or tied prior to removal of the lymph node. Infrequently, a small portion of the node is removed for examination leaving the bulk of the node in place. The node or node section is sent fresh to the pathologist to allow frozen section. If lymphoma is present, the remaining fresh tissue can be used to assay for T cell markers. Portions of the fresh sterile lymph node are also submitted for bacterial and fungal cultures.

The incision is closed, often with absorbable sutures, and covered with a sterile dressing.

POSTPROCEDURE INFORMATION

Postoperatively there may be some incisional pain, usually controllable with mild analgesic agents. When the incision is large or deep, narcotic analgesia may be beneficial. Where there is a possibility of communicable disease, appropriate precautions should be taken.

COMPLICATIONS

Aside from incisional pain, aftereffects from lymph node biopsies are uncommon. There will be a small scar, the nature of which depends on the location of the biopsy. Patients who tend to form keloids should be aware of the possibility of keloid formation. As with all surgical procedures, the possibility of bleeding and infection exists. The presence of increasing incisional pain, erythema, induration, or purulent discharge should be reported to the physician. Lymphorrhea, (excessive drainage of lymphatic fluid from the incision) or lymphocoele (excessive collection of lymphatic fluid within the wound) are rare. Swelling of the affected extremity caused by lymphedema is extremely rare, and is more likely the result of underlying disease processes.

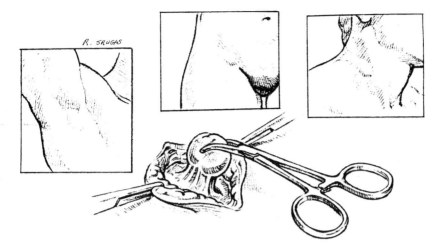

Figure 51–1. Lymph node biopsy.

PATIENT QUESTIONS

Will the procedure hurt?

The patient will feel only the injection of local anesthesia. The procedure itself should be painless although the patient may be aware of a pulling sensation as the biopsy is being performed. After the procedure, there may be some incisional pain similar to that following a simple laceration. This can be controlled with analgesics such as nonsteroidal antiinflammatory agents. Narcotics may be used in extreme cases.

Do I have cancer?

Unless there is a high index of suspicion of malignancy as a result of history, physical examination, and other findings, the patient can be reassured that most cases of lymphadenopathy result from nonmalignant causes. If malignancy is strongly suspected or if the patient reveals an obvious cancerphobia, the physician should reassure the patient that lymphatic malignancies such as Hodgkin's disease are always controllable and often curable.

When will the diagnosis be available?

If a frozen section is being performed, the patient will get a preliminary diagnosis within 1 hour following surgery. The patient should be cautioned, however, that a final diagnosis may require several days. Occasionally, lymph node biopsy is not diagnostic and further tests may be required in the future, including the possibility of a second lymph node biopsy.

How do I recognize abnormal lymph nodes?

Rounded, soft, usually freely moveable masses in the tissues just under the skin in the cervical, axillary, epitrochlear, or inguinal areas may be enlarged lymph nodes. Patients who are highly motivated can be taught to feel their own lymph nodes and make some evaluation about enlargement or other changes. In most cases, these will be attributable to localized infection such as cervical node enlargement occurring with pharyngitis or axillary node enlargement occurring with a superficial hand wound. In some cases, the cause of lymph node enlargement will not be obvious and will require a complete physical examination. In children, enlarged cervical and inguinal lymph nodes are common and usually of no clinical significance.

CONSENT

Fully informed consent is required.

SELECTED BIBLIOGRAPHY

Crowley KS: Lymph node biopsy. *Pathology* 1983;Apr:15:2:137.

Doberneck RC: The diagnostic yield of lymph node biopsy. *Arch Surg* 1983;Oct:118:10:1203.

Pandit AA, Candes FP, Khubchandani SR: Fine needle aspiration cytology of lymph nodes. *J Postgrad Med* 1987;Jul:33:3:134.

Slap GB, Brooks JS, Schwartz JS: When to perform biopsies of enlarged peripheral lymph nodes in young patients. *JAMA* 1984;Sept:14:252:10:1321.

52

Skin Testing for Allergy

RICHARD SADOVSKY

Direct skin testing is the most commonly used diagnostic test for allergy. A specific reproducible allergic reaction by a localized test is the most sensitive method for demonstrating immediate hypersensitivity. Allergenic extracts are manufactured by multiple companies and include hundreds of pollen, mold, food, animal dander, dust, or insect venom extracts.

Allergen expiration dates are usually 18 to 24 months after shipping date. Since suppliers may store the material for long periods, these dates may not correspond with actual biologic activity. The operator must be careful to ascertain the biologic activity of any allergen used.

INDICATIONS

The physician needs to recognize the large variety of symptoms and signs that hint at the possibility of allergy. Objective data suggestive of allergy include a large number of complaints dealing with the skin, eyes, nose, mouth, and ears. Generalized complaints of weight loss, wheezing, food intolerance, bowel movement changes, unusual drug reactions, and even behavioral and learning problems may be related to allergy.

A positive skin test can probably be caused in any person using a sufficiently concentrated allergen extract. With appropriate understanding of the legitimate levels of reaction to specific concentrations of the extract, the operator can make some evaluation of level of sensitivity to the allergens being tested. Interpretation should be correlated with the patient's history because of the incidence of false positive and false negative results.

Positive skin reactions do not always indicate clinical sensitivity. Adults with a history of hay fever during childhood may continue to exhibit reactions to weed pollens although they may have outgrown their rhinitis. It is generally thought that skin test reactivity is greatest during the third decade and declines significantly after age 50. Positive tests could be a predictor of future sensitivity to common allergens such as pollen rather than an indicator of current sensitivity.

Skin testing with mixes of allergens is less reliable than with specific allergens but is useful for screening purposes, especially in small children. Food allergy occurring as urticaria, or angioedema correlates well with positive skin tests.

ALTERNATIVES

Provocative testing using applications of allergenic extract material to mucosal areas such as the conjunctival sac, the nasal mucosa, and bronchial mucosa have been attempted. These tests are time consuming and imprecise.

The discovery that skin sensitizing antibody belongs to the immunoglobulin E class has allowed the development of radioimmunoassay and other assay techniques to measure this substance. Normal values have been determined, and can be influenced by age, genes, seasonal variations, and race. Although total IgE levels are elevated in most people with allergic (IgE-mediated) disease, this is not true for all patients. There are also many nonallergic diseases that may be associated with elevation of IgE including parasitic and immunologic problems. This nonspecificity has limited the usefulness of this test. Proper indications for IgE quantitation probably include (1) the prediction of development of allergic diseases in infants, (2) the need to evaluate immunodeficient patients, (3) the need to screen for infestation with tissue-invading parasites, and (4) the need to aid in the diagnosis and follow up of patients with allergic bronchopulmonary aspergillosis.

Procedures have been developed to measure allergenspecific IgE antibodies. These can be of use to the clinician, and the most commonly used procedure is the radioallergosorbent test (RAST). This test has been adapted to measure serum IgE antibodies to pollens, animal danders, house dust and house dust mites, foods, stinging insects, molds, and, recently, penicillin, although most physicians feel that the test is less sensitive than skin testing. RAST testing is indicated whenever skin testing is thought to be impossible, inappropriate, or potentially harmful. These would include patients who must remain on antihistamine medications, patients with widespread dermatitis, testing of an infant with minimal skin surface area, or patients with a history of extreme hypersensitivity to a specific allergen. RAST testing should be used in conjunction with a through history, skin tests, and provocative challenge tests to diagnose allergies. A positive RAST in a healthy, nonallergic individual is very rare.

Passive transfer skin testing (PK testing) involves the sensitization of skin sites in a nonallergic recipient by aseptically injecting serum from a sensitized donor. After 48 hours, the passively sensitized areas and the nonsensitized areas are tested with various test allergens. This procedure takes a lot of time and is not as sensitive as direct skin testing. This is mostly considered to be a research tool.

Leukocyte histamine release assays can measure both the quantity of cell-fixed IgE antibody and the capacity of the leukocytes to release histamine. This test appears to correlate well with skin testing in patients who are allergic to ragweed and insect venoms. The method of performing these assays limits their usefulness, and it is currently reserved for the research laboratory.

POSSIBILITY OF FAILURE

The lack of standardization between the extracts prepared by various manufacturers needs to be considered in evaluating patient reactions. Allergenic extracts are prepared and labeled according to weight:volume concentrations. This designation simply says how the extract was prepared. For example, 1:10 cat dander extract is prepared by extracting 1 g of dander in 10 ml buffer. There is no correlation with biologic activity. Therefore, the true biologic equivalents of two extracts that are identical in weight:volume may differ greatly. The problems associated with this can be avoided by the operators purchasing a large amount of the given extract so that the supply will be adequate for a long period. The operator must become accustomed to the biologic potency of each lot of extract purchased. This problem does not occur in some of the more common extracts that are standardized with respect to the content of major allergens such as ragweed, and insect venoms. Manufacturers are trying to standardize extracts in "allergy units" as determined by radioimmunoassay, but this is still in the early stages.

False-positive results can be caused by the presence of histamine-releasing agents in the extract, intradermal testing with an excessive volume or an extract that is too concentrated, or mechanical pressure from excessive trauma during the application of the allergen extract. False negatives can be caused by use of an inactive extract.

Care must be taken in the injection process when performing intradermal skin tests. The injection of air will reduce the precision of the test. In addition, intradermal injection of extracts containing large amounts of glycerine may cause nonspecific irritant-positive reactions.

CONTRAINDICATIONS

Recent history of an anaphylactic reaction may cause a false-negative reaction. Tests should be deferred for 2 to 4 weeks following such a reaction. The presence of an acute febrile illness may diminish skin test reactivity and requires the careful use of a histamine control.

Patients who have demonstrated extreme sensitivity to certain allergens should probably not have skin testing done for that allergen because of the increased possibility of a severe systemic reaction. Testing should be deferred during periods of symptomatic bronchospasms to prevent worsening of the clinical status.

The presence of chronic illnesses that affect T cell mediated immune reactions such as cancer, lymphoma, and sarcoidosis generally do not affect atopic skin test reactivity. Long-term immunotherapy, however, may cause a decline in circulating IgE and produce a negative skin test. Patients with acquired immunodeficiency syndrome (AIDS) often have decreasing IgE levels and may have markedly diminished ability to react to skin testing.

PREPROCEDURE PREPARATION

After a complete history and physical examination have been performed, a complete blood count and blood serology tests should be done. The blood count should include an absolute lymphocyte count and an eosinophil count. Cellular immunodeficiency is diagnosed if the lymphocyte count is abnormally low. The eosinophil count may be elevated in patients with hypersensitivity reactions involving IgE immunoglobulins.

PATIENT EDUCATION

Patients should understand that even with identification of the allergen and appropriate treatment, they will never be completely desensitized or allergy free. The interaction and importance of stress and environmental factors should be discussed so that the patient has realistic expectations of the results of allergy testing and treatment.

Patients should avoid the use of antihistamines, tricyclic antidepressants, or hydroxyzine for at least 1 week before to the test because these medications may suppress skin test reactivity. Patients should be warned that positive reactions to allergen skin testing may remain for 8 to 12 hours.

PROCEDURE

Skin testing is performed by either puncture or intradermal techniques. Puncture or scratch tests may be done on the back or the arm. When performed on the back, the upper or middle areas should be used because the skin here is more reactive. When performed on the arm, the ulnar side is used because it is more reactive than the radial. The patient's skin is cleaned with ethanol and allowed to dry. Sites for injection are marked with a pen and should be at least 7 cm apart to allow measurement of the resulting wheal and flare reaction. A drop of each extract is placed on the skin after which the skin is punctured by a sterile needle. The needle puncture should be deep enough to penetrate the epidermis, but not so deep as to draw blood. The diameters of the resulting wheal and flare reactions are measured 15 minutes later.

Intradermal tests are usually performed on the arm (figure 52–1). The sites are prepared and marked, and then a small quantity of extract, approximately 0.02 cc is injected intracutaneously raising a 3 to 4 mm diameter wheal. The resulting wheal and flare reaction is measured in 10 to 15 minutes. Depending on the type of allergen extracts being used, the skin areas used for testing may need to be observed up to 48 hours following the injections.

A less frequently used technique is the patch test where the allergen is applied to a small gauze square that is applied to the skin and taped in place. This technique is more often used to test potential allergens that come in contact with the skin such as perfumes, detergents, and other cosmetics. The operator should remain with the patient for the entire period regardless of which technique is used because of the possibility of anaphylactic reactions.

Allergy tests are graded on a semi-quantitative scale. Greater precision can be obtained by using skin test titrations where increasing concentrations of extract are used until a positive reaction is produced or until the most concentrated solution is tested. This latter titration system can be used for either puncture tests or intradermal tests.

POSTPROCEDURE INFORMATION

An adult patient can undergo skin testing without being accompanied by a friend or relative. It is a good idea, however, for someone to stay with the patient who has been exposed to concentrated allergen extracts for several days to observe and assist with discomfort or any delayed reactions.

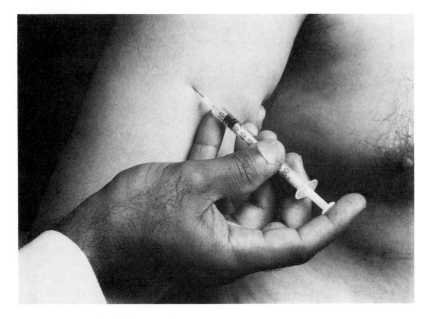

Figure 52–1. Skin testing by intradermal injection.

COMPLICATIONS

A positive reaction can occur for up to 12 hours or even longer. The skin can slough over a strongly positive reaction. This can be treated with a topical anti-inflammatory cream or mild steroid.

Generalized allergic reactions are rare after skin testing, but they can occur. Operators doing skin testing should have access to tourniquets, an oxygen supply, resuscitation equipment, and the appropriate medication for treatment of cardiovascular reactions. Appropriate doses of epinephrine and diphenhydramine should be available if needed.

PATIENT QUESTIONS

Should I have scratch tests or intradermal injection tests performed?

Scratch testing appears to be safer and faster, and it allows the performance of a larger number of tests at one time. It is probably more specific but less sensitive than intradermal testing. Therefore, important allergens may be missed if intradermal testing is not performed adjunctively. Intradermal tests may cause more discomfort to the patient. Careful evaluation of the patient's history and current status, and the skill and experience of the operator will help determine the relative usefulness of puncture or scratch tests and intradermal testing.

Should I stop my medications before the tests?

Antihistamines and tricyclic antidepressants should be stopped before skin testing is performed. Other medications such has theophyllines, corticosteroids, sympathomimetics, and beta-2 adrenergic agonists do not seem to suppress skin test reactivity.

Why should I go through skin testing when the RAST test simply requires a sample of blood?

Skin testing is clearly the best diagnostic tool in current allergy practice. In the opinion of most allergy specialists, skin testing is more sensitive than RAST testing in the vast majority of cases. Whether RAST testing will become more refined in the future will depend on further developments with the technique involved. In experienced hands, skin testing is safe and highly reproducible and can give immediate results. RAST testing is two to five times as expensive to perform.

Is skin testing painful?

Depending on the technique being used, skin testing can be completely painless. Even intradermal injections can be performed with a minimal amount of discomfort by an experienced operator. The most uncomfortable part of the examination may be the itching resulting from a positive skin test. No anesthesia is used for skin testing.

CONSENT

Informed consent should be obtained prior to performing skin testing for allergy.

SELECTED BIBLIOGRAPHY

Mangi RJ: Allergy skin tests. An overview. *Otolaryngol Clin North Am* 1985;Nov:18:4:719.

Nalebuff DJ: Allergen screening: using in vitro tests for initial diagnosis. Radioallergosorbent test (RAST). *Consultant* 1986;Aug:26:8:101.

Nelson HS: Diagnostic procedures in allergy. I. Allergy skin testing. *Ann Allergy* 1983;Oct:51:4:411.

Zeiger RS: Atopy in infancy and early childhood; natural history and role of skin testing. *J Allergy Clin Immunol* 1985;Jun:75:6:633.

XII
Orthopedic Procedures

53

Traction

RICHARD SADOVSKY AND RICHARD M. STILLMAN

Traction is a procedure in which a pulling force is applied to a portion of the body to stretch and separate soft tissue, bone fragments, and joint surfaces. The history of traction goes back to the earliest recorded medicine. Continuous isotonic traction became the preferred method in the early 1800s. To achieve separation of desired tissues, sufficient force with adequate duration must be applied. Traction can be applied using force on the skin or anchoring on pins inserted into bone.

INDICATIONS

The therapeutic use of traction should be limited to those conditions in which the mechanical effects of traction would be expected to cause improvement. These are generally conditions of pain caused by nerve root compression, deformity caused by disease or developmental problems, fracture caused by traumatic injury, and potentially deforming problems such as severe burns.

ALTERNATIVES

When possible, casting and splinting can be an alternative, as well as an adjunct, to traction. The oldest form of fracture treatment is immobilization, and splints have been used throughout history for this purpose. The advantages of casting and splinting include the nonoperative nature of the procedure precluding the possibility of wound infection and the avoidance of anesthesia. It is also less expensive than traction and, in most cases, can be done without hospitalization. Dynamic correction can also be established in certain cases by use of elastic pull straps, gradual wedging of the cast, and other techniques that are actually therapeutic.

Limitations of casting and splinting include incomplete immobilization, frequent inability to actually correct improper position, and the development of pressure points. An improperly applied cast can cause destruction of soft tissue and ulceration. These limitations can be decreased somewhat by careful technique and the judicious incorporation of pins to enhance the immobilization effect of casting.

The use of electrical stimulation therapy for management of traumatic bone injuries is discussed in a separate chapter.

POSSIBILITY OF FAILURE

Traction is only as good as its design and the cooperation of the patient. Well-performed traction yields good results if the underlying pathology is not excessively destructive.

CONTRAINDICATIONS

Contraindications to traction include malignancy, evidence of cord compression, active infectious disease, osteoporosis, severe hypertension or cardiac disease, rheumatoid arthritis, old age, and pregnancy. Depending more specifically on the location of the proposed traction, the procedure is contraindicated because of carotid or vertebral artery insufficiency, the presence of active peptic ulcers, aortic aneurysm, and gross hemorrhoids.

PREPROCEDURE PREPARATION

Traction should not be administered until a complete workup has been done, a definitive diagnosis has been made, and a specific indication for traction has been determined.

PATIENT EDUCATION

The patient should understand the reason for traction and its purpose. The effects of traction on activities of daily living should be discussed and all efforts made to help the patient cope with the new restrictions. Patients who are hospitalized for extended periods of time in traction often need supportive counselling.

PROCEDURE

Traction may be delivered by weights and a pulley system or by other devices. The direction of pulling forces may be vertical, horizontal, or angular. The patient may be sitting, standing, or lying in a supine or prone position.

The strength of the tractive force depends on the surface resistance to traction and the resistance to stretch of the soft tissue and muscle. Surface resistance to traction depends on the weight of the body or body segment, and the nature of the two surfaces in contact. Calculations can be made to determine the minimum effective force needed to accomplish the therapeutic goal but, in clinical practice, it is often the patient's tolerance that is the ultimate determinant in the therapeutic use of traction.

Types of traction depend on the utilization of various forces to obtain the desired result. Straight traction results in the application of some mechanism to create a pull on a portion of the body. The principal pull is in a straight line without additional support or without any additional traction in any other direction. Balanced traction is the most common type of traction used to treat traumatic bone injuries. The extremity is suspended in some form of frame that holds the entire extremity and establishes a single unit. This creation of a more or less weightless situation allows greater immobilization and eliminates movement at the fracture site. Vectored traction is used when it is not possible to provide traction in the direct line of pull needed to reduce a fracture or dislocation. The resulting "vectored force" occurs somewhere between the two lines of force being applied. This form of traction is used mainly in fractures of the long bones.

Traction may be continuous, sustained, intermittent, or intermittent-pulsed. Continuous traction uses the lowest tractive force in order to prevent patient discomfort. Sustained traction is usually applied for 20 minutes to 1 hours using somewhat larger forces. Intermittent and intermittent-pulsed traction (the latter using gradual increases and decreases of the tractive forces) permit the use of larger loads without significant patient discomfort. Many intractable pain cases appear to respond rapidly to application of adequate tractive load.

Attachment of traction to the body can be either skin or pin. Skin traction is easier to apply, and more commonly used in children, but has limitations in the amount of traction that can be tolerated. This limits the ability of skin traction to overcome strong muscle pull in areas such as adult extremities. Skin traction may include a cast or splint for some indications. Pin traction is more practical for long-term, higher-load traction. After a tiny hole is made in the skin, a pin is introduced by a drill through the bone, emerging on the opposite side. Recently, the relatively small-gauge Kirschner wire has begun to replace the solid pin for many indications.

In clinical practice, traction is frequently administered in conjunction with heat, massage, and immobilization. Exercises and manipulations may also be used.

POSTPROCEDURE INFORMATION

Traction should be used only under close supervision. Well-planned traction requires supervision to ascertain that the desired effect is being achieved. Traction may need to be altered slightly to assure proper alignment.

If a cast is included with traction, careful cast care should involve avoidance of cast dampness, management of appropriate skin care, and monitoring for cast softening or other deformities.

Exercise, as permitted by the treating clinician, is a good way to prevent weakness and improve patient morale. The patient should be encouraged to perform active range of motion exercises with any unaffected limbs.

Constipation can be relieved by use of a high fiber diet accompanied by large amounts of fluids.

Patients who are confined to bed for months in skeletal traction often feel helpless and angry. They should be encouraged to express their feelings and should be given as much control over their environment as possible. Multiple brief visits are helpful to decrease the feeling of isolation.

COMPLICATIONS

Complications of traction can be caused by several aspects of the procedure. The use of a pin for anchoring of traction can cause pin tract infections that may require removal of the pin itself. Ring necrosis of the bone can occur around the pin site. This may be caused by the heat of pin insertion, infection, or foreign-body reaction. In cases of the pins coming loose and slipping from side to side, thorough antiseptic cleansing is required along with an antibiotic ointment because of the increased possibility of infection.

There are few complications to well-supervised traction therapy. The possibility of malalignment and improperly applied traction is diminished by use of appropriate traction equipment and adequate monitoring. Occasionally, pressure sores develop and require conservative management. These may be difficult to heal, and every attempt should be made to avoid them in the first place. The patient may initially complain of a burning feeling in an area with excessive pressure. These complaints should be seriously considered by the clinician. When prolonged bedrest is required, the patient is at increased risk for all the complications of immobility including "compartment syndrome," which is edema in an area caused by trauma or fracture, excessive traction, or a constrictive bandage or cast. Edema causes vascular compression and muscle death, which may result in permanent paralysis and loss of sensation.

Anxiety in the patient in traction following trauma may be caused by emotional factors, but may also stem from a physiologic problem such as hypoxia caused by a fat embolism. This complication usually occurs early in the posttrauma period but has been reported as late as 2 weeks following injury.

Too much force can cause damage to nerves and tissues, while too little force can produce painful muscle spasms and delay healing.

PATIENT QUESTIONS

Is traction painful?

Pain associated with traction depends on a large variety of factors. These include the indication for traction, the type of traction used, and the emotional state of the patient. The patient will probably be aware of pain during the initial stages of traction therapy, but this discomfort should diminish with time. Different traction regimens as described above are associated with varying amounts of discomfort, and this may be a factor in determining the format of traction to be administered.

How can I get my child to comply with a traction program?

The child must view therapy in a nonpunitive manner and the use of a reward system might help to facilitate this.

Can my traction therapy be performed at home?

Certain kinds of intermittent traction can be administered at home (figure 53–1). The patient must be fully aware of the indications for the therapy and thoroughly familiar with how to apply the traction correctly. Frequent monitoring by an appropriate health professional is also a requirement. Strong motivation is required for home traction therapy.

How long will I require traction therapy?

Standards have been established for the more common indications for traction therapy that provide some guidelines concerning the length of treatment. This is

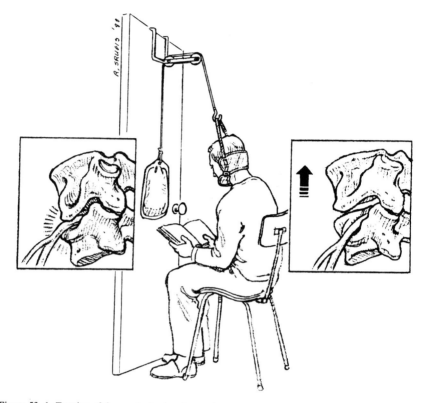

Figure 53–1. Traction of the cervical spine done at home.

dependent on the quality of traction planning and implementation, patient cooperation, and innate healing abilities. Close monitoring of patient progress and x-rays at appropriate intervals allow individualization of each course of traction therapy. The treating physician should be able to estimate the length of therapy needed.

CONSENT

Consent is required when traction involves an invasive procedure such as insertion of a pin or wire.

SELECTED BIBLIOGRAPHY

Fitz-Ritson D: Therapeutic traction: a review of neurological principles and clinical applications. *J Manipulative Physiol Ther* 1984;Mar:7:1:39.

Hickham JH: Directional forces revisited. *J Clin Orthod* 1986;Sep:20:9:626.

Simpson SA: Psychiatric problems on the orthopedic ward and the traction intolerance syndrome. *Nurs RSA* 1987;Aug:2:8:14.

XIII

Generalized Radiographic, Ultrasound, and Radionuclide Diagnostic Procedures

54

Computerized Tomography

DAVID H. GORDON

Computerized tomography, or CT scanning, involves the use of x-rays (ionizing radiation) that pass through the patient's area of interest and are attenuated by tissues that are in the path of the x-ray beam. The attenuated x-ray beam is then received by photomultiplier tubes that then transmit signals to a computer that synthesizes an image, viewing the body as though it were sectioned horizontally and viewing from below so as to put the liver on the right and the spleen on the left.

INDICATIONS FOR PROCEDURE

At this time a CT scan is used mostly for evaluation of tumor masses of various types in various locations in the body. In addition, information pertinent to abscess formation, stone formation, vascular diseases, bone and joint diseases, inflammatory processes, trauma, and follow up of tumors treated by radiation therapy and chemotherapy also are common indications. The CT scan is exquisitely sensitive to small differences in tissue densities, that is the four basic x-ray densities of air, fat, calcium, and water.

The information to be obtained from CT scan depends on the presenting clinical problem. This procedure is the examination of choice for evaluation of a number of intracranial abnormalities such as tumors or cerebrovascular accidents.

It is also the preferred modality for evaluating the mediastinum, retroperitoneum, and adrenals. It is useful in nearly every organ of the body and in the extremities as well. Most people who suffer various types of neurologic difficulties should receive a CT scan, either enhanced of nonenhanced, as part of their workup.

In the extremities, the CT scan is useful in assessing the presence of osteomyelitis, other bone pathology, and the extent of soft-tissue tumors. It has also proved to be of value, when combined with arthrography, in evaluating joints such as the shoulder, knee, wrist, ankle, and sacroiliac joints.

In the chest, the CT scan has been used for the assessment of pulmonary nodules, staging of lung tumors, and evaluation of the mediastinum for adenopathy and directing the surgeon in the mediastinoscopic biopsy of suspicious areas. CT can delineate only the presence of enlarged nodes or masses, but cannot usually diagnose the problem with histologic certainty. A specific diagnosis of hamartoma or granuloma may be possible if certain criteria are met. Other mediastinal tumors such as teratoma and lymphoma are well imaged. Aortic dissections and superior vena caval syndromes have been studied using this technique.

Below the diaphragm, the CT scan is an excellent modality for evaluating the liver, especially hemangiomas, where a near specific diagnosis can be made on an enhanced study. The presence of primary and metastatic liver tumors can be determined as can the presence of biliary dilatation, stones, or other biliary tract abnormalities.

The spleen can be viewed for abscesses, tumors, and granulomas, although lymphoma is imaged in the spleen in only approximately 30% of cases. Adrenal abnormalities can be well seen as can the retroperitoneum in the presence of lymphoma, metastatic tumors, and other abnormalities. The kidneys can be viewed for masses, stones, and even transitional cell carcinoma. Perinephric abscesses, hydronephrosis, and inflammatory changes can also be imaged. The pancreas can be well visualized morphologically, but, curiously, the advent of the CT scan has not impacted on the cure rate of carcinoma of the pancreas as was anticipated. Pancreatitis, as well as its complications of pseudocyst and stones, can be determined.

The bowel can be well imaged revealing inflammatory and ischemic bowel disease as well as the staging of tumors.

Scanning of gynecologic malignancies is a prime indication, both preoperatively and postoperatively.

The use of CT scans in the staging of prostate and bladder carcinoma is still under review.

Contrast material injected intravenously allows for vascular enhancement and the ability to distinguish vessels from a mass or a normal structure. Intravenous contrast may be administered as a bolus or as a slow infusion. General tissue enhancement is also seen following the vascular phase due to contrast in the vascular tree and diffusion into tissue parenchyma that has a vascular component. This technique is frequently helpful in liver and kidney evaluations.

The use of CT scans to guide biopsies is becoming more universal by offering a clear image of the needle tip in the desired area. Abscess drainage and ganglion block procedures can also be simplified using this technique.

ALTERNATIVES

The main advantage of the CT scan over other types of imaging techniques such as ultrasound and magnetic resonance imaging (MRI) is that a more panoramic view is more rapidly obtained than with either of the other techniques. In addition, linear attenuation of the x-rays is improved over conventional studies allowing better clarity in the distinction of tissues. With CT, contrast resolution—or the ability to distinguish adjacent areas of differing radio-density—is far superior to conventional radiology.

However, spatial resolution—the ability to distinguish between two structures a small distance apart—is somewhat inferior to conventional radiology. The size of the lesion that can be detected depends on the difference in the radiographic density of the lesion and the tissue surrounding it. This allows good resolution in the lung where contrasts are great and poorer resolution in areas of the abdomen or pelvis where contrasts are less. The disadvantage is that imaging can only be done in axial sections with reformatting into the sagittal and coronal planes, whereas ultrasound and MRI can general multiplanar images directly.

Intravenous contrast is often necessary when performing a CT scan to enhance vessels and to discriminate between tumors and other normal contiguous tissues that will have an enhancement that is different from masses or abscesses.

Often the information provided by CT scans can be provided by ultrasound and ultrasound is usually the initial procedure of choice prior to the CT scan in many situations involving children, women of child-bearing age, and very thin patients. This is because fat is a contrast material for CT scans, and peri-organ fat will enhance the chances of obtaining a satisfactory scan.

MRI is a newer technique and provides a similar type of information. It does not image calcium and cortical bone as well as CT and it depends on intrinsic tissue characteristic differences for its discriminatory ability.

Because loops of bowel can simulate masses in the abdomen, oral contrast nearly always has to be given for abdominal CT scans and rectal contrast may have to be given as well.

When properly focused on the clinical problem at hand, the CT scan will usually answer the posed question as long as the patient is able to cooperate with the procedure.

POSSIBILITY OF FAILURE

Limitations of the procedure include the presence of metal within the body, which tends to generate an artifact. This can be somewhat circumvented, but it does affect the quality of the information obtained. Inadequate renal function may contraindicate the administration of intravenous contrast material and, thereby, reduce the value of the CT scan.

The lack of tissue specificity is a major problem with the CT scan. A solid mass may be benign, malignant, or infected; cystic masses can be ascertained with some certainty. Another limitation is the inability to resolve lesions below a certain size. This varies depending on technique, the type of machine used, and the segment of the body being evaluated.

Organ movement affects the resolution possible by CT. The more sophisticated machines, which take images more rapidly, can eliminate some of the artifact caused by movement, but cardiac pulsations, for example, make cardiac imaging difficult.

CONTRAINDICATIONS

There are few contraindications to the procedure. The presence of metal or retained barium in the bowel works against optimal imaging. If the patient is extremely thin, the results of the CT scan are more likely to be inadequate because of the decrease in periorgan fat available to act as contrast for other tissues.

PREPROCEDURE PREPARATION

All retained barium from previous contrast studies should be removed. An intravenous line is usually started in anticipation of the possibility of administration of intravenous contrast. Renal function testing, including blood urea nitrogen (BUN) and creatinine levels should be obtained, especially in patients with diabetes.

The patient should not eat solid food prior to the procedure because of the likelihood of nausea or vomiting resulting from the intravenous contrast administration. The patient should be well hydrated, and this can be done by permitting a light liquid breakfast on the day of the examination. Some radiologists recommend a 4-hour fast prior to the examination.

PATIENT EDUCATION

Patients should' understand the procedure so that cooperation can be obtained, understanding that they may receive contrast material. Female patients are advised to wear a tampon to better delineate the vaginal vault in gynecologic evaluations.

PROCEDURE

The procedure involves placing the patient, head or feet first (depending on what part of the body is being scanned), on the examination table, which automatically enters the hardware, or "gantry" of the system (figure 54–1). A scout view or "topogram" is obtained, which is essentially a digital radiograph that delineates the body and allows the physician to prescribe various slices within the area of interest. The slices are usually done from 2- to 15-mm intervals depending on the size of the organ to be scanned and the size of the lesion anticipated. For example, an average abdominal survey for lymphoma would be done at 15 mm intervals with slice thicknesses of 10 mm.

Once the area of interest has been prescribed, scanning takes place. The patient is asked to hold his breath for chest and abdominal scans. It is not necessary to hold the breath for scans of the central nervous system, the pelvis, or the extremities. Modern CT scanners produce a slice in approximately 2 to 5 seconds so that breath holding is not a problem in all but extremely ill patients. Contrast material may be administered intravenously or through the mouth, rectum, or through a urethral catheter.

CT scanning can be performed on an outpatient basis if the patient is clinically able to come to, and leave, the procedure site unassisted.

POSTPROCEDURE INFORMATION

People living with the patient should not be affected by the CT scan and no special preparation is necessary. There are usually no aftereffects of the procedure although the patient may urinate an increased amount due to the administration of intravenous dye, which is eliminated from the body by the kidneys.

COMPLICATIONS

The procedure's morbidity and mortality is limited to the use of intravenous contrast material. In the absence of an allergic history, the frequency of death due to allergic reaction to the contrast is in the range of 1 in 30,000 to 35,000. If

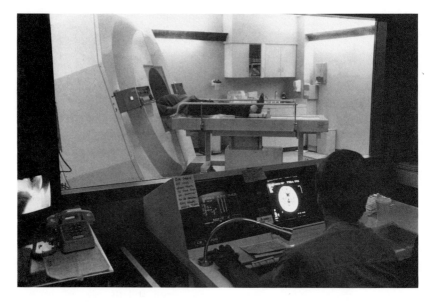

Figure 54–1. Computerized tomography (CT) unit.

an allergic history is present, prior preparation with a several-day course of steroids and the use of nonionic contrast material will reduce the risk substantially.

PATIENT QUESTIONS

Is there any pain involved in the procedure?

The procedure involves no pain unless a biopsy is combined with the CT scan procedure. The patient does have to lie in the gantry with the hands above the head for chest and abdominal scanning. The arms must be elevated in order to eliminate streak artifact created when the arms are lying close to the body. The arms can be left at the side during head scanning.

What is the dose of radiation involved in a CT scan?

The radiation dose received by the patient during the CT scan is within the range of other diagnostic x-ray procedures such as a barium enema or intravenous urography. The precise amount of radiation involved is determined by the slice thickness desired and the area of the body encompassed in the examination. Cardiac angiography requires a higher radiation dosage.

Will I have any after effects from the procedure?

The patient may urinate excessively for 12 hours because of the hypertonicity of the intravenous contrast material. There are no other after effects of CT scan.

CONSENT

Consent for the administration of intravenous contrast is routinely obtained.

SELECTED BIBLIOGRAPHY

Ghanem MH: CT scan in psychiatry. A review of the literature. *Encephale* 1986;Jan-Feb:12:1:3.

Lipton MJ: Cine computerized tomography. *Int J Card Imaging* 1987;2:4:209.

Lipton MJ, Brundage BH, Higgins CB, Boyd DP: Clinical applications of dynamic computed tomography. *Prog Cardiovasc Dis* 1986;Mar-Apr:28:5:349.

Murphy FB, Bernardino ME: Interventional computed tomography. *Curr Probl Diagn Radiol* 1988;Jul-Aug:17:4:121.

Noble PN: The changing face of computerized tomography. *Radiography* 1987;May-June:53:609:115.

55

Magnetic Resonance Imaging

DAVID H. GORDON

Nuclear magnetic resonance is a phenomenon that can be induced when nuclei are aligned in a strong magnetic field and then excited. Spinning nuclei develop a magnetic field around themselves with the orbits of rotation being randomly determined. When placed within a strong magnetic field, such as the magnetic resonance imaging (MRI) unit, the orbits align with the field. The nuclei (generally hydrogen, but sometimes carbon or phosphorus) give off energy and realign after excitation by pulsing with a radio frequency generated by the machine. Hydrogen nuclei are used because of the abundance of hydrogen in the human body and because it has a favorable characteristic called *gyromagnetic ratio*. The emitted energy is detected and translated into the magnetic resonance image. A specially designed wire coil that surrounds the patient both generates the pulsed radio frequency waves and detects the returning MR signal. The name *magnetic resonance imaging* was adopted by the American College of Radiology because of the concern that the previously used *nuclear magnetic resonance imaging* would be frightening to patients. MRI is a promising technique that is currently in its infancy in development and sophistication. The procedure is safe, noninvasive, and involves no exposure to ionizing radiation.

Tissues with the highest signal intensities are brightest (white), with those that emit no signal are black. Fat and bone marrow appear bright while cortical bone appears black. Tissues have specific characteristics termed T1 and T2 referring to relaxation times required to return from the excited to an equilibrium state. The radiologist often needs appropriate clinical information to determine the best imaging parameters and the appropriate pulse sequence for the specific patient. T1 weighted scans generally provide better anatomic information, T2 weighted images show bright signals in situations in which there is increased tissue water content such as tumors or inflammation.

Small surface coils can be used over specific areas or joints of the body in order to evaluate more specifically those areas.

INDICATIONS

Indications for MRI at this time are loosely defined, and, in many instances, MRI is a correlative imaging modality MRI allows better depiction of soft tissue than does any other modality and it makes cross-sectional pictures in any plane desired. It is the preferred modality for scanning the brain and spinal cord and the musculoskeletal system. The high signal intensity of normal bone marrow fat allows early detection of abnormal signals due to necrosis, tumor, or infection. The high soft tissue contrast in the images allows differentiation among soft tissue structures such as fat and bone marrow, muscle, synovium, joint fluid, ligaments, tendons, and cartilage. It is replacing computerized tomography (CT) scans to a large extent in these areas. In the body and the extremities, it has selected and limited applications although with the accrual of additional experience and increasing rapidity of scanning accompanied by enhanced resolution of images, it is clear that MRI will replace the CT scan for many clinical indications in the near future.

In the brain and the spinal cord, MRI is used to assess tumors, vascular malformations, stroke, hemorrhage, and infection. It is particularly applicable in the central nervous system because of the lack of motion of this area. Pulsations, however, of the cerebrospinal fluid may cause artifacts.

In the body, MRI is useful in the adrenal glands, liver, joints (knees, shoulders, ankles, tendons, and muscles) and in gynecologic and prostatic problems. It is also valuable in assessing vascular problems associated with the aorta, great vessels, and the heart. New developments in cineMRI promise to make this application in diagnosing cardiac problems very exciting in the near future.

The kidney can also be imaged by MRI although at this time it does not appear to be extremely helpful or to give information not obtainable by a CT scan. Within the adrenal gland, a mass discovered on a CT scan or sonography procedure can be characterized by the intensity of the mass on T2-weighted imaging. Adenomas are iso-intense with liver; metastases and primary tumors are somewhat hyperintense; a pheochromocytoma is markedly hyperintense; and cysts are extremely hyperintense, comparable to the gall bladder or a renal cyst. Therefore, it may be possible to define the nature of an incidentally discovered adrenal mass. However, there is overlap between these entities. MRI is the preferred diagnostic procedure when a pheochromocytoma is present because of the high signal intensity produced by this tumor. In the liver, MRI appears to be extremely sensitive in the diagnoses of metastases and primary tumors and is relatively specific in hemangiomas in which high signal intensity is noted on T2 weighted images. With the introduction of contrast agents (gadolinium, and iron oxides). MRI promises to become the imaging modality of choice for liver metastases and tumors.

MRI is not of great value in imaging the biliary tree or gall bladder. It is also limited in the evaluation of the spleen and pancreas. In evaluation of the kidneys, MRI is improving, but CT still has an edge at this time. The nature of a renal cyst (simple or complex) may be determined with MRI, but CT is preferable to evaluate this problem. Vascular abnormalities of the kidneys are also visible without injected contrast.

Evaluation of a dissection of the aorta and aortic aneurysms can be performed with MRI. The advantage here is that no intravenous iodinated contrast is necessary to delineate blood vessels because of the so-called *flow void* produced by moving blood. However, it may be difficult to distinguish slow flow from thrombus.

The retroperitoneum is seen well with MRI without intravenous contrast. Again, the same limitation as the CT scan exists, which is the inability to histologically evaluate, but only to note the size of the lesion. Preliminary results with the gynecologic organs reveal that MRI may be of value in delineating a tumor in the uterus and cervix with invasion of the vagina. Additional preliminary data hint at the value of MRI in the diagnoses of prostatic hyperplasia or carcinoma. Initial enthusiasm over staging of carcinoma of the bladder has not proved to be warranted to date. However, it is useful to do MRI in carcinoma of the bladder in searching for metastatic nodes and perivesicle fat invasion. MRI is not helpful in evaluating the gastrointestinal tract because of the nonavailability of suitable oral contrast agents. MRI is the preferred procedure for evaluation of the hips for avascular necrosis and has been shown to be more accurate and positive earlier than nuclear scanning techniques. It is also useful for the diagnosis of aseptic necrosis in other parts of the skeletal system. It may be of use in osteomyelitis in differentiating soft tissue from bony abnormalities. MRI is not useful in assessing bony cortical lesions, but it is very useful in assessing marrow abnormalities where the high intensity signals of fat may be replaced by metastatic disease, fibrosis, or other abnormalities. MRI provides a look at ligaments and tendons. The Achilles tendon and the fluid around tendons can be imaged providing diagnostic information. Magnetic resonance imaging of joints is the imaging modality of choice in assessing destruction of menisci and cruciate and collateral ligaments of the knee. Arthroscopic evaluations have proved the sensitivity of MRI in revealing these types of tissue damage in the knee. The shoulder joint has been well studied with reference to rotatory cuff injuries. The advantage of MRI over standard arthrography is that no contrast material needs to be injected and no invasive procedure performed.

Magnetic resonance imaging of the cardiovascular system remains a somewhat experimental technique. It can provide anatomic information as well as information about myocardial metabolism and blood flow.

The use of contrast-enhancing agents for MRI is being studied for the near future. These agents are considered to be much safer than those used in many radiologic studies.

ALTERNATIVES

MRI is not usually the definitive imaging modality at this time, but rather, with the exception of the knee, hips (for avascular necrosis), and the central nervous system, it is a correlative imaging method in most areas of the body. The information provided by MRI must often be confirmed by a CT scan or ultrasound. Ultrasound, however, is limited in its scope and CT uses ionizing radiation, often requiring the use of contrast materials. It is probable that MRI will replace the CT scan for many indications in the near future when faster imaging and improved resolution become available. The development of spectroscopic tissue analysis may make MRI a highly definitive, tissue-specific modality. At the present time, CT scans appear to be still preferable in the detection of meningiomas and acute intracranial hemorrhages although subacute hematomas 7 to 10 days old often show up better on MRI than on CT.

Arthrography for the evaluation of knee pathology is being replaced by MRI. Arthroscopy following screening MRI can confirm the findings and be therapeutic.

POSSIBILITY OF FAILURE

Because MRI is in its infancy, the chance of the necessary information not being obtained is substantial. In structures in which hydrogen is tightly bound or absent, such as in cortical bone, signal voids occur in the image. Motion and artifacts are frequent in MRI and, therefore, a CT scan or ultrasound is needed if the patient is unable to cooperate or if artifacts obscure the area being investigated.

There are little data on the potential for false positives with MRI, however there are probably fewer false positives in multiple sclerosis with CT. MRI tends to demonstrate an unacceptable level of false positives in the elderly population in evaluating dementia.

CONTRAINDICATIONS

Currently MRI is not recommended for use in pregnant women although no known biologic effects have been demonstrated to date. Contraindications to MRI are few, but include the presence of a pacemaker, certain types of heart values or inner ear prostheses, and cerebral aneurysm clips. Other types of metal in the body may produce artifacts, but, other than metal fragments in the eye, they are not contraindicative to the procedure. A relative contraindication is the presence of claustrophobia, as approximately 10% of patients will not be able to tolerate lying within the confines of the gantry for the long periods of time required.

PREPROCEDURE PREPARATION

Sedation may be given prior to the procedure to avoid motion and anxiety on the part of the patient.

PATIENT EDUCATION

Patients should be aware that the procedure may require a long time, usually an hour or more. They should be informed that there may be a claustrophobic feeling while within the machine, but that no other feelings or pain will occur. Communication with the technician and the physician performing the procedure will be by intercom. The patient must remain still during this period of time. They may be given an injection of glucagon to slow the peristaltic movement of the bowel. Women may be asked to insert a tampon into the vagina to help define the anatomic location of the vagina.

PROCEDURE

The procedure involves lying motionless on the table within the gantry for the time needed for the examination, which is generally around 1 hour (figure 55–1). Occasionally, EKG leads will be attached to the patient if cardiac gating techniques are employed. A surface coil is placed over the area of the body or the extremity to be scanned. The patient hears a knocking sound as the mechanism is being tuned. After that, little appears to happen and the patient can sleep for the duration of the study.

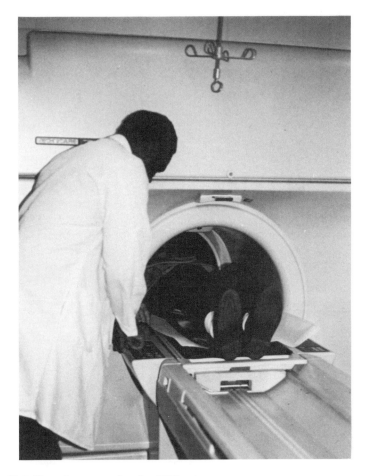

Figure 55–1. Magnetic resonance imaging (MRI) unit.

POSTPROCEDURE INFORMATION

There is nothing that the people who live with the patients need to know. There are no aftereffects of this procedure.

COMPLICATIONS

There are no known aftereffects of MRI, although the procedure is not recommended for pregnant women. There is some evidence that at high field strengths there may be some heating induced in the body, but this has not been a clinical problem to date.

PATIENT QUESTIONS

Will there be any pain or discomfort?

There is no pain, discomfort, or any other sensation involved with MRI. The patient may be distressed by the enclosed nature of the apparatus and the room in which the procedure is performed.

Is there any danger in having MRI performed?

The only danger known is the presence of movable metal in critical areas of the body such as metal within the eye, the presence of a pacemaker, or aneurysm clips. Conceptually, movement of small, unstable pieces of metal can occur, but no projectile injuries or harm to a patient due to torquing of metallic objects within the body have been reported in the literature. A large amount of metal such as a hip prosthesis or a plate can be safely imaged.

How long will the procedure take?

MRI usually requires about 1 hour to complete. During that time the patient will be asked to lie still without moving significantly.

Will I experience claustrophobia?

About 10% of patients will be claustrophobic while in the gantry, or body, of the MRI machinery and may not be able to tolerate the procedure.

Will there be any after effects of the procedure?

There are no known after effects to MRI.

CONSENT

Consent is not required at this time, although, when intravenous contrast materials become more available, it may be necessary to initiate this policy. Informed consent is obtained if pregnant women are to be scanned.

SELECTED BIBLIOGRAPHY

Bekllon EM, Keith MW, Coleman PE, Shah ZR: Magnetic resonance imaging of internal derangements of the knee. *RadioGraphics* 1988;Jan:8:1:95.

Glazer GM: MR imaging of the liver, kidneys, and adrenal glands. *Radiology* 1988;166:303.

Margulis AR, Crooks LE: Present and future status of MR imaging. *Am J Radio* 1988;March:150:487.

Merritt CR: Magnetic Resonance Imaging—A clinical perspective: Image quality, safety, and risk management. *RadioGraphics* 1987;Sept:7:5:1001.

Webb WR: MRI of the chest. *App Radio* 1986;Nov/Dec:69.

56

Positron Emission Tomography

ARNOLD M. STRASHUN

Positron emission tomography (PET) is a medical imaging technique that measures the location and concentration of physiologically active compounds in the human body. PET is a nuclear medicine technique that employs special radiopharmaceuticals produced by a cyclotron. The most commonly used medical positron materials include fluorine-18 (^{18}F) with a 110-minute half line, carbon-11 (^{11}C) with a 20-minute half-life, nitrogen-13 (^{13}N) with a 10-minute half-life, and oxygen-15 (^{15}O) with a 2-minute half-life. Work is being done to use the decay products of germanium-68 (^{68}Ge) and strontium-82 (^{82}Sr) because these have long half-lives and can be easily stored and shipped further distances. Early research in PET began in the 1970s, but the complexity and expense of the equipment at that time appeared to outweigh the clinical utility. Early PET centers began in academic settings with commercial development following later.

PET utilizes principles similar in certain respects to other computer tomographic methods such as computerized tomography (CT). In PET, radioactive elements (radioisotopes) that are injected into the patient are utilized emitting so-called "positrons" that decay rapidly, interacting with local electrons, in the process known as annihilation. At the point of each annihilation event, two high-energy photons are produced. These high-energy particles fly off in nearly opposite directions to be detected by the PET scanner, which surrounds the patient like a ring. This permits information to be gained on a line-by-line basis where these simultaneous annihilation events are detected 180 degrees apart, establishing the originating site of activity along that path (line). Image forming involves (1) the detection of the photon gamma rays emitted in the positron annihilation process, (2) the identification of the photon's direction of travel, and (3) the reconstruction of the distribution of the radiation into an accurate generic image. A circumferential array of detectors can establish the source of all coincident pairs of photon gamma rays.

As a result of substantial improvement in resolution, newer designs have provided images that are more familiar to the clinicians, no longer requiring color output to resolve distributional differences in the injected radiopharmaceutical, thereby providing better anatomic orientation. As of this writing, there are approximately 30 PET centers in the United States. It is anticipated that within the next 3 to 4 years, PET will make the transition from research to clinical practice.

INDICATIONS

Unlike traditional nuclear medicine, the ability to label the basic building blocks of biochemical structures (carbon, hydrogen, nitrogen, oxygen, and fluorine) without alteration of biologic behavior allows true physiologic evaluations of functional aspects of tissues. It is expected that PET will permit clinicians to assess the biochemical and physiological functioning of organs such as the brain and the heart and provide a quantitative method for monitoring a wide variety of common disorders. The range of PET application has been dramatically increasing with most attention being directed toward the neurologic system and, recently, in cardiovascular studies.

Neuropsychiatric applications of PET include the examination of the chemistry of the brain in living humans. The science of neurobiology is based on the electrical activation and transmission of impulses. This in turn causes release of chemical neurotransmitters. The total of all these neurotransmissions defines brain function, including behavior. A cyclotron-produced radioactive atom incorporated into a drug can bind to specific neuroreceptors allowing a view of actual functional activity. Diseases characterized by abnormal receptor function can be studied, such as Parkinson's disease, which is a true local deficiency of a neurotransmitter, dopamine, in the basal ganglia, and Huntington's Disease, in which an abnormally low number of receptors exist in the caudate nucleus. Many PET applications are being used to characterize other neurological disorders that are currently identifiable only with the full-blown clinical presentation. They can now be studied and diagnosed by neuroreceptor brain-labelling PET studies at earlier preclinical (and more treatable and potentially reversible) stages.

Untreated schizophrenics are noted to have approximately a 75% reduction in glucose metabolism of both frontal lobes as determined by PET studies. This, combined with the finding of increased uptake in the caudate nucleus, is helping to clarify the mechanisms involved in neuropsychiatric illness. Schizophrenia may, as a result of these studies, be reclassified as a neurological disease rather than a mental disorder.

Patients with dementia have demonstrated a decline of localized brain metabolism. Alzheimer's patients demonstrate with fair consistency decreased activity in temporal and parietal regions of the brain. Patients with multi-infarct dementia demonstrate scattered defects that parallel the small vessel intracerebral occlusive process. PET studies reveal defects often before the CT scan.

Increased activity has been found in primary brain tumors and at the site of epileptogenic foci with greater anatomic precision than with electroencephalogram (EEG).

The value of PET in monitoring treatment regimens for epilepsy, schizophrenia, and brain tumors is a rapidly expanding area.

Cardiac applications of PET involve the study of myocardial metabolism. Detection of small myocardial perfusion defects is becoming possible with resolution greater than that of Thallium scanning. The salvageability of at-risk myocardial tissue can be determined by metabolic activity and assist in the evaluation of patients for invasive clinical intervention such as angioplasty or emergency bypass grafting.

ALTERNATIVES

MRI and CT can also be used effectively in conjunction with PET to establish the morphological boundaries and spatial relationships of various disease states as well as defining the normal anatomy from which one can more accurately deduce the physiological and biochemical activities as well as tissue viability in the organ region of interest.

POSSIBILITY OF FAILURE

Standard PET machinery now permits a resolution of 5 mm. Due to the physics involved in the method, there is an inherent limit to the resolution that is theoretically possible with PET of approximately 2.5 mm. It is anticipated that improvement in detector position strategy will improve surface position detection and improve resolution to approach the lower number, which is comparable to that of CT and magnetic resonance imaging (MRI).

The sensitivity and specificity of PET techniques have yet to be proved in various clinical settings.

CONTRAINDICATIONS

The hallmark of the tracer principle is that radiopharmaceuticals represent picogram to nanogram chemical quantities that will have insignificant or undetectable physiological effects. There are not even any allergic effects because of the minuscule amounts involved. Therefore, there are no physiologic contraindications other than extreme physiologic instability.

PREPROCEDURE PREPARATION

Steady-state physiology must be present prior to the introduction of the positron-emitting radiopharmaceuticals. Thus, pretest clinical status must be sufficiently stable to allow placement of the patient within the remoteness of the detector gantry. The patient must also be prepared to remain stationary throughout the acquisition to eliminate resolution degradation by motion artifact.

PATIENT EDUCATION

In certain studies, a peripheral injection will be required to administer the radiopharmaceutical. In others, the patient will inhale the radiopharmaceutical through a mouthpiece. Patients will not be bombarded with radioactive beams externally but instead will be the source of the detectable radioactivity. The ultra-short half-life of the radioactive agent allows study results to be obtained without known side effects from the radiation. The patient is no longer a source of radiation on completion of the test. The results of the study will generally not be available at the conclusion of the study as the physicians and the technicians must process the acquired data through the computer. They will then inform the patient's referring doctor of the results. There will be no after effects of the study.

PROCEDURE

The patient will have a peripheral indwelling intravenous line placed to administer the radiopharmaceutical, unless it is being administered orally. The patient is then placed on a padded stretcher in a darkened room and aligned with laser beams within a doughnut-shaped radiation detector, the PET camera (figure 56–1). In an adjacent room, a cyclotron is bombarding accelerated, charged particles into a target material to allow the nuclear reaction required to produce the desired radionuclide. This radionuclide is then transferred via a vacuum tube into a chemical "hot" cell for further synthesis.

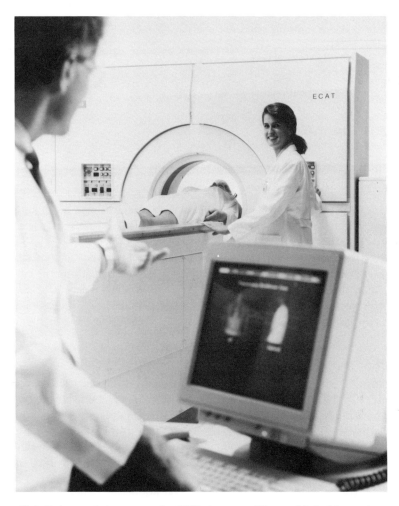

Figure 56–1. Positron emission tomography (PET). (courtesy of Siemens Medical Systems).

The final product is then tested to insure patient safety and sterility, that is, exact dosage to insure adequate radiation to provide the desired information yet not so much as to endanger the patient. This material is then injected via the intravenous line or inhaled into the lungs. While the patient remains motionless, the gantry stretcher is optimally positioned to collect data in the ideal patientcamera orientation for the organ of interest. The study generally requires 10 to 20 minutes.

POSTPROCEDURE INFORMATION

No postprocedure information is necessary.

COMPLICATIONS

There are no complications.

PATIENT QUESTIONS

Why is PET not offered at more locations?

Because the radiopharmaceuticals decay rapidly, it is necessary to produce them near the center where they will be used. This requires that a cyclotron be available in the institutions where the procedures are performed ar at least reasonably close to it.

Recent design modifications suggest that medical cyclotrons may be simpler, automated, and, therefore, easily operated in a conventional clinical environment, reducing installation costs and space requirements. These changes have also been associated with improvement in the design of the PET imaging units. These two factors may make PET more widely available in the near future.

Is there any danger from the radioactive material used?

The radiation dose absorbed by the patient during a PET study will depend on the energy of the emitted positrons and the distribution and effective half-life of the radionuclides in the body. For specific organs, the dose depends not only on the distribution within the organ itself, but on the distribution in the adjacent organs. Typical doses are 100 to 500 millirads to the target organ as well as the organ that receives the highest radiation dose, usually an excretory organ such as the lung for gas, or the kidneys and bladder for liquids. By comparison, the doses of an x-ray CT study are 1000 to 50000 millirads. Thus, these doses are far less than other noninvasive imaging studies. To date, these levels of radiation exposure have never been associated with any adverse effects.

Patient safety is insured by supervision of licensing agencies, although results useful in diagnosing and managing the referred patient's medical condition are not assured.

Is there any danger from the machinery?

There is no danger from the machinery.

Should I have PET performed for my "forgetfulness?"

Specific clinical questions concerning indications for PET scanning must be answered after consultation with the physician and, possibly, a consultation with a neurologist. In the premature or presenile dementia of the Alzheimer type (SDAT), the glucose metabolism of the brain is prematurely reduced, most prominently in the parietotemporal cortical regions (the posterior third of the brain surface neurons). Such findings may be determined years before the later stages reveal morphologic change of brain atrophy on CT and MRI. By that time, the SDAT is far advanced. Thus, the early warning signs of SDAT by cerebral glucose studies are valuable (although demoralizing) prognosticators of an insidious progressive decline in complex behavior related to memory.

CONSENT

Currently, certain studies of adults as well as children are approved for general use by the licensing agency that oversees all PET facilities for safety and reliability of their results. Thus, no consent is necessary. Other studies of a new and investigative nature to examine select medical conditions require the signing of a consent. This is the last step in a chain of checks and balances within the facility, its medical center, and the licensing agency to insure that the patient is aware of the investigative nature of the study.

SELECTED BIBLIOGRAPHY

Adam WE: A general comparison of functional imaging in nuclear medicine with other modalities. *Semin Nucl Med* 1987;Jan 17:1:3.

Anderson NC: Brain imaging: applications in psychiatry. *Science* 1988;239:1381.

Kessler RM, Partain CL, Price RR, James AE, Jr.: Positron emission tomography. Prospects for clinical utility. *Invest Radiol* 1987;Jul:22:7:529.

Positron emission tomography: Clinical status in the United States in 1987. ACNP/SNM Task Force on Clinical PET. *J Nuc Med* 1988;29:1136.

Wagner HN: Quantitative imaging of neuroreceptors in the living human brain. *Semin Nuc Med* 1986;16:51.

57

Radionuclide Techniques

DAVID H. GORDON AND RICHARD SADOVSKY

Radionuclide scanning involves the production of images of normal and diseased tissue by means of emissions from radiopharmaceutical preparations having specific distribution in the body. Various organ-specific compounds have been developed that are tagged with radionuclear isotopes that are then used to image the organ or body space in question. The current, most commonly used isotope is technetium-99m (^{99m}Tc), that has a suitable photon energy, a short half-life of 6 hours, and is easily produced by a technetium "cow" in a nuclear medicine department, which insures a constant supply of isotope. Additional isotopes used for specific scanning procedures include iodine (^{131}I, ^{125}I), xenon, gallium, and others.

The general principle of scanning is that a radioisotope is tagged to a carrier molecule (for example ^{99m}Tc is tagged to sulfur colloid for liver scanning). Most isotopes used in clinical nuclear medicine are injected intravenously although some are administered by aerosol inhalation when ventilation scanning is being performed or orally such as ^{131}I for thyroid uptake scanning.

A variety of detectors are used to display the pattern of dispersion of the radionuclide compound. The detector involves the use of a crystal to convert a gamma ray emitted from the organ into a flash of light. These flashes are translated into pinpoints on the oscilloscope screen forming an image that can be photographed, printed, or stored in a computer. Newer instruments involve a pinhole system or a rotating scintillation camera that allows three dimensional, tomographic imaging. The images obtained can be helpful in diagnosing, following the course of disease, and monitoring disease management. Scanning is a sensitive procedure but its specificity is low without the added information from other complementary examinations. To be most useful, scans must be interpreted in conjunction with other techniques. Interpretation is also enhanced by discussion of the clinical situation.

INDICATIONS

Nuclear scanning is helpful in patient care in many different ways. The indications vary depending on the organ or body space being evaluated. The discussion here will be limited to some of the more common uses of radionuclide imaging.

Indications for scanning the thyroid include anatomic and functional abnormalities. Thyroid scanning is based on the principle that normal thyroid tissue concentrates certain radionuclides while abnormal tissue does not. The major use of scanning here is to determine whether a thyroid nodule is likely to be malignant. Functioning nodules are usually benign while solitary, nonfunctioning nodules may be malignant. Anatomic abnormalities that can be revealed by scan include single or multiple masses, acute and chronic thyroiditis, various types of goiters, and carcinomas. Functional abnormalities of the thyroid can also be revealed by examinations involving both uptake and suppression. These tests involve the administration of various kinds of hormones or other chemicals along with compounds containing radioactive iodine or technetium. These procedures provide an anatomic and functional map of the gland.

Bone scans aid in detection and monitoring of bone and joint disease. Nuclide pickup depends on bone crystal surfaces, particularly where osteoblastic activity is occurring, as well as blood flow to the area. Indications for bone scan include elevation of alkaline phosphatase, presence of tumors known to metastasize to the bone, differentiation of single from multiple bone tumors, evaluation of skeletal pain, assessment of bone viability, detection of inflammatory diseases, evaluation for hip prosthesis, and serial followup of response of bone to treatments such as radiation or chemotherapy. Lytic lesions may not be visible if they are relatively static. In addition, evaluation of trauma, fractures, infarction, and mapping for biopsy sites can be done with bone scans. A survey whole body bone scan is generally performed. Bone scanning is sensitive but not highly specific and can frequently detect bone disease before radiographic changes are observed.

Isotope evaluation of the lung allows the detection of perfusion and ventilation defects. Perfusion scans illustrate the distribution of blood flow into the lungs and are most commonly used in the evaluation of pulmonary embolism. This study may also be valuable in assessing heart disease, pulmonary arteriovenous malformations, and other abnormalities. Ventilation studies illustrate the distribution of inhaled radioactive gas in the lung. Combined ventilation and perfusion studies are most accurate for evaluation of pulmonary embolism and for measurement of the degree of ventilation in a patient with obstructive pulmonary disease. Ventilation perfusion mismatches, in which the lung is ventilated but not perfused, can represent a pulmonary embolism with approximately 95% certainty when interpretation is not clouded by other pulmonary diseases such as chronic infiltrates or pleural effusions.

Brain scanning, which has been generally replaced by the computerized tomography (CT) scanning and magnetic resonance imaging (MRI), is performed to observe intracranial mass lesions and cerebrovascular disease. Isotopes can be used to measure cerebral blood flow and defects in the blood-brain barrier that can allow passage of the isotope and demonstrate a "hot" spot. Indications for brain scanning include all cerebrovascular abnormalities and the lack of availability of CT and MRI. Decreased flow patterns indicative of cerebrovascular accidents, subdural hematomas, space-occupying lesions, and meningitis can be determined. Radionuclide cisternography, in which the radioisotope is injected directly into the subarachnoid space, is used in evaluation of cerebrospinal fluid (CSF) dynamics and is useful in cases of CSF rhinorrhea, communication or noncommunicating hydrocephalus, and a dilated ventricular system. This technique may also be applicable for cysts in the brain to see if they communicate with the ventricular system. Brain scanning with the posistron emission tomography (PET) scanner is discussed in an separate chapter.

Tumor and inflammation scanning with gallium citrate is indicated when searching for neoplastic and inflammatory tissue throughout the body. This includes screening for neoplastic disease when other tests have been negative. It is particularly efficacious in bronchogenic carcinoma, various types of lymphoma, and hepatoma. Gallium may also be accumulated in other tumors, but with lower sensitivity and specificity. The presence of inflammatory collections, abscess formation, or osteomyelitis can also be defined since the inflammatory cells that migrate to the area will pick up gallium.

Gallium scanning is often correlated with a CT scan or MRI. Indium-labelled ^{111}In) leukocytes have recently been used to diagnose abscess formation. This is a sensitive and specific technique but is not readily available at all centers.

Kidney and urinary tract scanning permits evaluation of renal morphology, blood flow, tubular function, urinary excretion, and vesicoureteral reflux. Scans are most useful for discovering the location and degree of an obstruction, as well as determining the effect of the obstruction on renal function. Indications include evidence of renal enlargement or masses, nonvisualization of the kidneys by intravenous pyelogram, allergy to iodine-containing dyes, suspicion of renal vascular hypertension, the presence of obstructive uropathy, and renal transplant follow up. Specific radioisotopes are used since their excretion defines certain segments of renal function. Spatial resolution may be poor, but information about renal function is obtained.

Studies of the gastrointestinal system include scanning the liver, gall bladder, biliary tree, and bowel. Liver scanning is based on the uptake of radioactive colloid by functioning reticuloendothelial cells. Tumors, cysts, abscesses, and fibrous areas do not contain these functioning cells and will appear as areas of no uptake on the scan. Radionuclide study of the liver is a screening modality and is indicated in the evaluation of hepatomegaly and abdominal mass, diffuse liver disease, ascites of unknown origin, jaundice, inflammatory lesions or abscesses, and in screening for liver metastasis in patients with known primary tumors. The limit of resolution of a focal mass lesion is approximately 1 cm. Patchy uptake can be produced by diffuse disease such as cirrhosis, hepatitis, or fatty infiltration. Focal nodular hyperplasia is very accurately diagnosed by scanning techniques as hyperfunctioning or isointense areas. Labelled red-cell scanning is very specific for hemangiomas because of the large blood pool.

Gall bladder and biliary tree pathology can be imaged using radionuclide scanning. Nuclear cholecystography has become the diagnostic test preferred for the evaluation of acute cholecystitis with obstruction of the cystic duct and patency of the rest of the biliary tree. Nonvisualization of the gall bladder has a high predictability for ruling in acute cholecystitis with edema of the cystic duct or blockage with a stone. The common bile duct is also visualized as is its emptying into the duodenum. Indications for scanning of the gall bladder and biliary tree include evaluation of acute cholecystitis, gall bladder function, hepatitis versus biliary obstruction, postoperative biliary diversion procedures, biliary leakage or atresia, reflux into duodenum and stomach, and visualization of choledochal cysts. The pattern of hepatic uptake of the radioisotope is visualized as well as the gall bladder, the biliary tract, and the duodenum. Diagnostic liver and gall bladder examinations can be done with the bilirubin as high as 20 mg%.

Gastrointestinal scanning is useful in diagnosing the presence of abnormal gastric mucosa in a Meckel's diverticulum and this test is indicated in lower gastrointestinal bleeding in children or young adults. A negative study, however, does not rule out Meckel's diverticulum as only 60% of these anatomic abnormalities contain ectopic gastric mucosa that will concentrate the radioisotope.

Gastrointestinal bleeding, in general, may take place in sites from the stomach to the rectum, and includes vascular ectasia, ulcers, and tumors. Because bleeding may be intermittent, detection may be difficult unless active bleeding is present. The site of bleeding as well as the activity and quantity of bleeding can be determined. This procedure is 10 times as sensitive as angiography in the detection of active bleeding. Angiography is, however, more specific in terms of localization. Radioisotope-labelled red cells can be used in cases of intermittent bleeding to allow delayed scanning and increased sensitivity.

Radioisotope imaging of the spleen is indicated to obtain information concerning size, shape, and position of the organ, to evaluate left-upper-quadrant abdominal masses, to evaluate for infiltration due to lymphoma or metastatic disease, to evaluate splenomegaly, and to discern the result of abdominal trauma. Nuclear imaging of the spleen is a good screening test but specific disease often need to be characterized in other ways such as a CT scan or angiography.

Studies of the cardiovascular system, including the heart and the great vessels, allow evaluation of ventricular wall perfusion and motion. Indications are the evaluation of cardiac performance, delineation of cardiac perfusion, evaluation of cardiac viability and metabolism, quantitation of myocardial perfusion and damage, and assessment of cardiac function. Information that can be learned include ejection fraction, ejection rate, presence of intracardiac shunts, end diastolic volume, end systolic volume, pulmonary transit time, pulmonary blood volume, right and left ventricular volume and function, and the presence of myocardial ischemia or myocardial akinesis. In many centers, the information obtained by radionuclide imaging is comparable to that obtained by cardiac catheterization. Heart scanning can be used to identify coronary artery disease and to detect the extent of damage following myocardial infarction. Radioisotopic cardiac studies are expensive and require a skilled technical staff.

Assessment of venous function can be done by radionuclide venography. The major indication is the need for assessment of the deep venous system of the lower extremity with evidence of venous occlusion. The deep system in the lower extremity and the pelvis are imaged with this technique. This is a gross screening test and a negative result does not rule out obstruction in a patient with clinical evidence of venous blockage. This technique has also been used in the upper extremities.

Other radionuclide scanning techniques include voiding cystourethrography, testicular imaging, salivary gland imaging, and adrenal imaging.

ALTERNATIVES

Many other diagnostic procedures can offer information that will overlap with the information obtained by radionuclide scanning. A detailed description of all the procedures and their relative usefulness is beyond the scope of this text.

Anatomic information about organs and body spaces can be obtained using ultrasound. The image allows distinction between solid and cystic masses. Ultrasound is also the preferred modality for obstructive uropathy and the evaluation of gallstones, hepatic duct stones, and biliary stones. Intrahepatic biliary obstruction is best seen on ultrasound examination.

CT scan and MRI have also been applied to evaluate anatomic abnormalities. CT has good resolution for tumor diagnosis and greater sensitivity, especially in the brain and the central nervous system. MRI may be more sensitive than nuclide scanning in marrow evaluation, although cortical bone abnormalities are not well imaged. MRI is not useful in bowel examinations because of the inability to opacify the bowel. The rapidity and completeness of survey evaluations available using radionuclide techniques is still preferable to MRI studies. However, when emergency situations occur, the CT scan is more readily available than either radionuclide study or MRI. Dynamic CT scan and MRI are beginning to be used for functional organ studies in the heart and the kidneys, but more work is needed to standardize these results.

Plain radiographs may be used to evaluate the skeletal system, but are less sensitive than radionuclide techniques.

Angiography can be done to assess lung perfusion, the nature of a mass, quantitation of blood flow, and bleeding sites. Angiography does have a higher sensitivity and specificity than scanning for pulmonary embolism and it also permits evaluation of renal blood flow, whether intravenous digital study or direct study. This is an invasive procedure, however, and is accompanied by some morbidity and mortality.

Contrast studies using injections of contrast materials can be used to find leakage of cerebrospinal fluid (CSF) or to evaluate for hydrocephalus, but a larger leak is required than for radionuclide study. Intravenous pyelography can be used to define the renal parenchyma and qualitatively evaluate renal function. This cannot, however, be quantitated by computer as can renal function using radionuclide techniques. Endoscopy can be used to view sites of gastrointestinal bleeding, but this is an invasive procedure and carries some morbidity.

Venograms using direct injection of contrast material and, more recently, compression Doppler sonography and plethysmography are replacing radionuclide venography.

POSSIBILITY OF FAILURE

Radionuclide scanning as an anatomic test tells only whether an area is "hot" or "cold." It does not discern solid from cystic regions. Radionuclide studies should be considered a screening evaluation. The lack of specificity of radionuclide scanning techniques often makes additional tests necessary, although a higher degree of specificity can be obtained with some types of scanning such as lung evaluations. Additionally, no conclusion can be made about histologic changes. Fine needle biopsy is often helpful in this respect.

Gallium scanning is a sensitive method for detection of lymphoma in both the chest and the abdomen. The accuracy rate of gallium scans for lymphoma detection and abscess diagnoses is greater than 85%. The time constraints, however, often make gallium scans useless when rapid information is needed. In addition, gallium scanning is not specific. Operative scarring, acute inflammation, abscess formation, or tumor will all appear the same.

Because the resolution of radionuclide scanning is less than that of other noninvasive imaging modalities, it may be necessary to move on to other diagnostic procedures, If there is a high index of suspicion of disease and it is not discovered with radionuclide study.

If an organ is chronically diseased such as in chronic renal disease or chronic cholecystitis, poor concentration of the radioisotope will occur, reducing the diagnostic ability of the procedure. Intake of chemicals that compete with the organ radionuclide uptake, such as phenothiazine and steroids in thyroid scanning, can interfere with the procedure and affect its accuracy.

CONTRAINDICATIONS

There are no contraindications to radionuclide scanning although careful evaluation of the utility of scanning should be undertaken before testing patients during pregnancy and lactation. Certain scans such as ventilation studies require the patient's ability to cooperate with simple commands involving deep breathing and sitting up.

Radionuclide cisternography involves the injection of material into the CSF and, therefore, has the same contraindications as lumbar puncture. Specifically, this would be in the presence of increased intracranial pressure.

Poor hepatocellular function may decrease the uptake and concentration of the radioisotope making liver and gall bladder evaluation impossible.

PREPROCEDURE PREPARATION

The patient should be encouraged to drink large quantities of water since frequent voiding reduces the background uptake of the radioisotope. For ventilation lung scans, the patient must be able to sit up, take a deep breath, and generally cooperate with the technician in order to perform a successful study.

A careful review of patient medications is needed, and those that may affect the scan outcome should be tapered or discontinued.

Cathartics or cleansing enemas should be administered to the patient if the bowel has not been cleared of contrast medium following gastrointestinal contrast studies. Antihypertensives should be discontinued prior to renal scanning. If a scan using radioactive iodine is being performed on a pregnant woman or a young child, a potassium iodide solution (e.g., Lugol's solution) is often administered 1 to 3 hours before the test to block thyroid iodine uptake.

Fasting for 24 hours is required prior to gall bladder scanning to insure gall bladder filling. Parenteral nutrition or an intestinal bypass procedure may preclude gall bladder visualization. The use of meperidine or other medications that may cause spasm of the sphincter of Oddi should be avoided because they may diminish uptake.

Scanning for Meckel's diverticulum is generally preceded by administration of cimetidine, which enhances concentration of the radioisotope in the gastric mucosa without its being secreted or released.

Certain radionuclide scanning techniques may involve the insertion of needles or tubes into blood vessels, body cavities or body openings. For example, voiding cystourethrography requires bladder catheterization, evaluation of gastric reflux may require the placement of a nasogastric tube, shunt patency studies require injection of radioisotope into a body cavity, and venography necessitates needle insertion into the distal superficial venous system.

PATIENT EDUCATION

The patient should understand the procedure of radionuclide study and the purpose of the radioisotope injection. The possibility of the procedure requiring repeat scans up to 3 days following the injection should be made clear. If the radionuclide is being given intravenously, the patient may experience a slight tingling or burning sensation. Transient flushing or nausea which is (rare) may accompany the distribution of the radionuclide through the body.

PROCEDURE

The isotope is administered either intravenously, orally, or inhaled into the lungs. Varying amounts of time are required for the introduced radioisotope to reach the desired organ or body space. If radioactive iodine is used for scanning and the area of interest is not the thyroid gland, thyroid uptake of the ^{131}I is inhibited by administration of Lugol's solution. The scan is done at the standardized predetermined time required for uptake of the radioisotope to detect the deposition of the radioisotope at an appropriate interval (figure 57–1). Patients with chronic cholecystitis may have markedly delayed filling of the gall bladder. Gallium scanning is performed at intervals up to 72 hours following injection of the radioactive gallium.

POSTPROCEDURE INFORMATION

There are no side effects from radionuclide scan and the patient need not be accompanied to the procedure. Radiation poses no threat to anyone visiting the

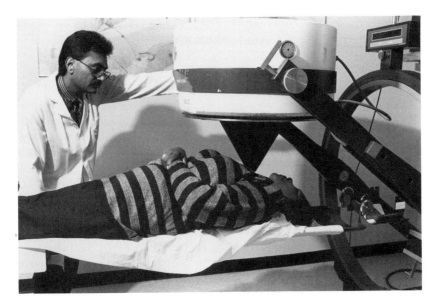

Figure 57–1. Radionuclear scan of the thyroid.

patient including pregnant females. Patients who have had renal isotope studies should flush the toilet immediately after each voiding for 24 hours as a radiation precaution. The possibility of needing delayed scans should be understood.

COMPLICATIONS

In general, nuclear scans are totally safe without significant complications. The material that is embolized to the pulmonary capillaries will compromise approximately 1 out of every 1,000 capillaries. This has not been demonstrated to stress the patient clinically.

PATIENT QUESTIONS

Is there any pain involved in having a scan?

There is no pain involved in radionuclide scanning. The only discomfort the patient may have is the in initial injection of the radioisotope.

Will the scan provide the information needed to resolve my clinical problem?

Radionuclide scanning provides a good anatomical map and often provides reliable functional information about the organ being studied. Scanning is generally used as a survey test and rarely can the diagnosis be made solely on the basis of the scan. Further testing is usually required to determine the actual pathologic process with greater precision.

Is the radioisotope dangerous?

Radiation from the diagnostic use of these agents is very small, and there have been no radiation effects reported. Certain studies may deliver several rads to a specific organ, but this is usually less than the radiation received during many standard radiologic procedures.

CONSENT

Consent is not needed for radionuclide studies unless the injection involves a lumbar puncture or some other procedure for the instillation of the radioisotope (e.g., catheterization for a voiding cystourethrography). Many centers, however, are beginning to obtain consents prior to routine intravenous injection of radionuclide material.

SELECTED BIBLIOGRAPHY

Acierno LJ, Worrell LT: Radionuclide imaging in coronary artery disease. *Radiol Technol* 1984;Mar-Apr:23:2:173.

Kogan BA, Hattner RS: Radionuclide imaging of the genitourinary tract. *Semin Urol* 1985;May 3:2:85.

Maid M: Radionuclide imaging in pediatrics. *Pediatr Clin North Am* 1985;Dec:32:6:1559.

Velchik MG: The clinical use of radionuclide bone imaging. *Semin Nucl Med* 1985;Jul:15:3:239.

58

Ultrasonography

RICHARD SADOVSKY AND DAVID H. GORDON

Ultrasonography involves the use of high-frequency sound waves to look at internal organs and body structures. A transducer that converts electricity to sound waves introduces the sound into the abdomen. The sound travels at different speeds in various tissues. It travels quickly in fluid tissues and is reflected by air. The sound that reflects back to the transducer is reconverted to electrical energy. The computers of the ultrasound equipment calculate the strength of the reflected sound and time intervals of travel, creating a grey scale image that reflects the examined areas.

INDICATIONS

Ultrasonography is a diagnostic tool that can reveal much about internal organs. It is used widely in the *abdomen* where, it is hoped, gaseous or bony medium will not interrupt the sound wave. The avoid this, liquids can be introduced into areas such as the stomach to allow sound wave transmission, although this does not obviate the obstacle of air in the large bowel. One of the greatest areas of utilization is the liver where not only solid or cystic masses can be recognized, but the ductal and vascular system can be seen quite accurately. The spleen may be evaluated for solid or cystic content as well as size, rupture, or perisplenic fluid. Ultrasound studies of the gall bladder have been found to reveal gallstones 3 to 5 mm in diameter and is the initial imaging modality for evaluation of stones. It is not clear what technique is best for diagnosing acute cholecystitis. Gall bladder wall anatomy is seen better by ultrasound while gall bladder physiology and acute cystic duct obstruction are seen better with nuclear medicine techniques. Practically speaking, the ability to obtain a scan quickly, the competence of the sonographer obtaining the radionuclide scan, and the expertise of the nuclear medicine specialist reading the images may influence one's choice of diagnostic method. In patients with chronic cholecystitis, gallstones are the hallmark of disease, and sonography has the clear edge. Evaluation of the common bile duct is possible in almost all patients. Determining the cause of obstruction may be difficult because the common bile duct passes posterior to the duodenum and may often be obscured by gas, preventing identification of the obstructing cause. Cholesterol stones may be hard to identify if they are not calcified so as to produce shadowing.

The pancreas is also accessible to this modality. Masses can be found and biopsy needles can be guided as they can for hepatic lesions. The abdominal aorta is readily recognized and aneurysms and branches of the aorta can be easily detected. The aorta can be measured as can the size of the aneurysm.

In the retroperitoneum, information can be gathered regarding renal size, content and location, renal mass evaluation, and guidance of biopsy needles. The urinary bladder can be evaluated if it is filled with fluid or water. The urinary collecting system can be evaluated and obstructions and stones may be found, especially if realtime imaging is performed. The adrenal glands are probably best seen by CT but they can be noted on ultrasound.

High-resolution sonography is ideal for evaluating the testes. A variety of scrotal lesions both solid and cystic can be detected. This feature may be particularly important in patients with overlying hydrocoeles or varicocoeles in whom testicular masses are not palpable. Doppler ultrasound can prove the vascular nature of a mass.

Ultrasonographic evaluation of the pelvis is helpful in identifying the urinary bladder, the uterus behind it, and the ovaries lateral to the uterus. If a pelvic mass is noted, the texture can be evaluated, especially in terms of solid versus cystic. Loculated fluid in the pelvis can be detected and aspirated by percutaneous needle biopsy.

In addition, the placenta and uterus are readily identified. The age of a fetus can be documented by measuring the biparietal diameter of the fetal skull and by other measurements such as the crown-rump and femur lengths. Fetal death can be diagnosed by the appearance of the fetal head, and the absence of fetal heart beat or movement with the M-mode evaluation.

The male pelvis is occasionally examined ultrasonically, such as for abscess, prostatic evaluation, or spread of neoplasm, but most pelvic sonography is performed in women. This may change as new research on using sonography for the early diagnosis of prostate carcinoma becomes more standardized utilizing intrarectal probes.

Evaluation of the *head* and *neck* are limited using ultrasound, but there are some specific areas of value. In the neonate and newborn infant, the presence of fontanelles allows passage of the sound waves. In adults, the adult brain is visible to the sonographer only in patients with bony defects or in the operating room when a craniotomy has created an acoustic window. This technique has been used effectively in locating deep-seated brain tumors.

As the frequency of a transducer increases and wavelength decreases, the resolution of the resultant image improves. Unfortunately, at present, the penetration of these higher-frequency transducers is limited to a few centimeters. The soft tissues of the neck are ideally located for scanning by high frequency transducers as are the eye, breast, testicle, and many parts of the neonate. The thyroid gland has been evaluated sonographically for years and studies have shown that simple cysts do not exist—that these lesions, when scanned with high-resolution technique are shown to contain septa, debris, or mural nodules. By definition, many of these should be classified as solid. So, does high-resolution scanning make sonography obsolete in thyroid diagnoses? This is not the case since ultrasound is capable of identifying nodules too small to be felt or identified by radioactive isotope scan. Therefore, the importance of sonography lies not in differentiating between specifically cystic or solid masses, but in classifying a thyroid nodule as single, with a high (approximately 15%) chance of malignancy, or multiple, with a low (approximately 4%) probability of cancer. These findings are controversial and require further elucidation.

Parathyroid adenomas can be localized by high-resolution real-time scanning and hyperplasia can be identified preoperatively. This is a tremendous aid and shortens the duration of surgery. The use of ultrasound in the evaluation of the carotid arteries is an evolving field. This will be covered more extensively in the section on Doppler techniques.

Ultrasound in the *thorax* has limitations because of the presence of air in the lungs surrounding the mediastinum producing an acoustic barrier. Locations of loculated pleural effusions can be done efficiently by ultrasound. Breast tissue is still best examined radiographically, which can better pick up microcalcifications and dense masses with surrounding fatty tissue. Sonography is of value in determining if a palpable mass is solid or cystic, with most solid masses being cancerous. Most classifications of criteria of solid masses for likelihood of carcinoma underestimate the number of malignant tumors. Therefore, most solid masses, even those with a benign sonographic appearance, should undergo biopsy.

Real-time, 2-dimensional echocardiographic scanning has dramatically changed imaging of the heart, where function and anatomic structure are so intimately related. This is discussed in the chapter on echocardiography.

Ultrasound technique can be used to determine blood flow by using the Doppler technique. This is discussed in the chapter on Doppler.

Ultrasonic needle guidance has been mentioned above. This technique has gained wide acceptance, but there is some difficulty in monitoring the needle tip constantly. Some researchers advocate ultrasonic guidance only for large masses, and CT is the preferred needle guidance technique in many institutions.

Contacting the sonographer directly to find out the areas with which he feels most comfortable is helpful in determining the likelihood that an examination will yield usable information since the modality is highly operator-dependent.

The use of ultrasound in pregnancy has been more clearly defined than in other circumstances. Where significant clinical questions exist, the resolution of which would alter the remainder of prenatal care, ultrasonography can be of benefit for a wide variety of problems around pregnancy including estimation of growth and fetal age, suspected multiple gestations, evaluation of pelvic masses, suspected ectopic pregnancy, fetal death, placental abnormalities, and uterine abnormalities.

There is no consensus that routine ultrasound evaluations for all pregnancies improve perinatal outcome or decrease morbidity or mortality. There is, however, evidence that there is a higher rate of detection of twins and congenital malformations as well as more accurate dating of the pregnancy, but without significant improvement in outcome.

ALTERNATIVES

Computerized tomography (CT) is the major competitor of ultrasound. In CT, structures are differentiated by variations in linear attenuation coefficients that are related to electron density of tissue. As a result, CT is most effective in distinguishing tissues with different atomic composition. The difference in attenuation coefficients is often small, as in the abdomen, and contrast material must be administered. Ultrasound reflects the acoustic properties of the medium on a macromolecular level and, therefore, echo-texture differences are noted between hepatic, renal, and pancreatic parenchyma, whereas CT attenuation values of these organs show minimal variation. CT is clearly more useful in situations in which the transmission and resolution of sound waves are difficult. This includes in the adult skull and brain, the soft tissue of the lung in most circumstances, the evaluation of the obese or fatty patient, and in specific organ evaluations such as the pancreas, especially when the patient has marked ileus in which the bowel is filled with gas and cannot accommodate the fluid needed to act as an acoustic window. The consensus appears to be that the retroperitoneal structures, lipomatous tissue, bone and soft tissue masses, the mediastinum, and tumor staging in the thorax are better evaluated with CT than with ultrasound. The presence of gas, abdominal sutures or dressings, and surgical wounds make ultrasound difficult.

A comparison of ultrasound with contrast radiography indicates many differences. Contrast studies outline hollow visci such as the bowel, bladder, or stomach and may reveal a mass by extrinsic compression. Ultrasound actually reveals the mass but the hollow viscus may cause shadowing unless filled with fluid. In some areas, the contrast studies are superior such as the mucosal detail in an air-contrast barium enema or the ureteral stricture seen on the urogram. In evaluating lesions and structures beyond the mucosa or lining, CT or ultrasound are superior.

Finally, patients who cannot properly adhere to the necessary preparation for ultrasound should be evaluated using different techniques. This would include patients who, for any reason, cannot fill their bladder or who have ileus or excessive bowel gas.

Ultrasound of the gall bladder may be adjunctive to oral cholecystography, which is a functional study as well, or even during cholecystography. Ultrasound should be done first since no radiation or chemicals are needed.

POSSIBILITY OF FAILURE

Ultrasound has specific limitations. The finding of common duct obstruction on sonography might require a transhepatic cholangiogram or an endoscopic retrograde cholangiopancreatogram (ERCP) to identify the cause of the obstruction.

Informed pattern recognition is the basis for all ultrasound interpretation. This procedure is the most operator-dependent of all the widely used techniques of imaging. Therefore, more than any other diagnostic procedure, ultrasonography requires a competent technician and physician working together to get high quality pictures and interpretations.

Some areas cannot be scanned using ultrasound. Bones and air cause problems for sound wave transmission, and scanning of obese patients is often difficult as fat is highly echogenic. Additionally, too great an acoustic mismatch between adjacent interfaces cause complete reflection of sound and do not permit scanning beyond these entities, as with gallstones and the frequent inability to see beyond them (shadowing). This also makes the adult brain impossible to scan unless a bone flap has been removed or the scanning takes place in the operating room during a craniotomy. In the chest, pleural based lesions may be visible, but an abscess within the lung is inaccessible to the scanner because it is surrounded by air. The normal lung sets up an impenetrable barrier and reflects all sound, whereas a dense pulmonary infiltrate fills the alveoli with fluid and allows sounds to pass. It is interesting that the consolidated lung has an ultrasonic appearance similar to that of the liver.

The imaging of fat is also a problem because it scrambles the beam and degrades the ultrasonic image. Organs of heavier patients are often better viewed by computed tomographic (CT) scanning. Intraabdominal fat that is not suspected by the clinician may cause the same problems. The sonographer must let the clinician know when the reliability of an exam might be compromised.

PREPROCEDURE PREPARATION

There is no specific preparation needed for ultrasound evaluation with the exception of tests done of the pelvic area. These require a full bladder, and the patient is requested to drink water for 2 to 3 hours prior to the examination and not to void.

Prior to sonography of the gall bladder, the patient should be instructed to eat a fat free meal in the evening and then to fast for 8 to 12 hours before the procedure. This promotes accumulation of bile in the gall bladder and enhances ultrasonic visualization. In addition, fasting will decrease the amount of gas in the bowel and improve visualization of abdominal structures. In patients who are dehydrated, ultrasonography may fail to reveal the borders between organ structures due to a lack of body fluids.

The patient should understand that this is a noninvasive exam that does not involve any injections, dyes, chemicals, or radiation. There are currently no known side effects or aftereffects of sonography. Following the sonographer's instructions is crucial and the patient should lie still and hold the breath when requested.

PATIENT EDUCATION

Prior to an ultrasound examination, patients should be informed of the clinical indication for ultrasonography, specific benefit, potential risk, and alternatives, if any. In addition, the patient should be supplied with information about the exposure time and intensity, if requested. A written form may expedite this process in some cases. Patient access to educational materials regarding ultrasonography is strongly encouraged. Patients should be told about the technique of ultrasound and should be assured that there is no risk of exposure to ionizing radiation. All settings in which these examinations are conducted should assure the patient's dignity and privacy.

PROCEDURE

Ultrasonography is the visualization of the deep structures of the body by recording the reflections of ultrasonic impulses directed into the tissue. Sound waves of approximately 20,000 cycles per second are employed (or 20 kilo-Hertz, where Hertz refers to the number of cycles per second). The skin of the patient is appropriately lubricated with mineral oil at the site of the sound introduction to produce acoustic coupling to the skin. The "transducer" is manually passed over the area to be imaged emitting sounds and recording the echoes.

The sound waves travel at a known speed until meeting a barrier from which they are reflected. The energy is transferred by spring-like forces binding adjacent molecules. The facility of energy transfer depends on the strength of these elastic forces and to the particle mass. The greater the "acoustic impedance" (product of the density of the material encountered and the speed of the sound wave) the greater is the amount of sound reflected from a boundary between these two substances toward the source of the production of the sound waves. The transducer is attached to a screen so that the distance between the source of sound and the returning interface is shown on the screen, producing the socalled "A-Mode" method of scanning. This is shown as peaks on the screen. Developments in ultrasonography have made A-mode imaging obsolete and B-mode imaging is currently being used.

In B-mode scanning, the brightness of the reflection (that is, its intensity) is recorded on the screen. These brightness spots are put together to produce a 2-dimensional representation known as a "compound scan."

In addition, there is a third form of ultrasonography called the M-mode. In this mode, one particular spot is watched over time. This is most helpful when the reflecting surface is moving in a regular manner such as does the mitral valve or other areas of the heart, including the myocardium. This can be helpful in distinguishing such abnormalities as pericardial effusion or hypertrophy of the myocardium.

Recent refinements of ultrasonography provide the ability to record a spectrum of echoes arising from within the substance of the organ displaying on the screen as varying shades of grey. A procedure producing an image similar to fluoroscopy called "real-time imaging" allow instantaneous images to be rapidly evaluated in sequence. This latter procedure utilizes either a linear array of sound-producing elements or a beam, swinging to produce a fan-like distribution of the sound waves.

The patient simply lies in a supine position as instructed by the sonographer. A small amount of lubricant is placed on the skin and the transducer is then positioned carefully and moved when appropriate (figure 58–1). The transducer does not cause any shock and the patient will feel only as though a microphone is being run along the skin. Occasional pressure may be needed to augment viewing of a specific organ or tissue area. The procedure generally requires less than 15 minutes although this can vary depending on complexity. Test results are usually available within 24 hours.

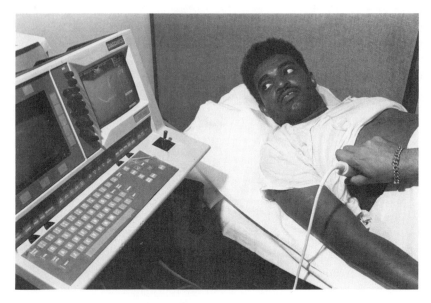

Figure 58–1. Ultrasound examination of the abdomen.

"High feedback" examinations, in which the fetal image is shown to the mother with appropriate explanation, are more anxiety-reducing to mothers and help encourage them to adhere to medically recommended regimens.

COMPLICATIONS

No harmful dose quantity has been identified for ultrasonography used in the diagnostic range. Variations in tissue properties between individuals as well as scanning conditions influence dose in an unpredictable way. For this reason, there is no information on the dose given to specific patients. Clearly, long-term prospective longitudinal studies are needed to determine what, if any, harmful effects occur to human tissue at diagnostic levels of ultrasound, but it is presumed that there are no after effects of the procedure and the patient should feel the same post-ultrasound examination as before.

POSTPROCEDURE INFORMATION

There are no special instructions for family members. The patient can come and go from ultrasonography without assistance.Outpatients can leave the test area immediately.

PATIENT QUESTIONS

Is ultrasonography safe?

Many studies have failed to show any damaging effects of pulsed ultrasound at diagnostic intensities when applied to intact mammals and human fetuses. These have included follow up studies of the growth and development of children who were ultrasounded as fetuses, with particular attention paid to the development of cataracts or hearing loss. All follow-up tests have been negative.

There have, however, been reports of biochemical changes to cells in suspension, including changes in DNA and in surface membrane behavior, clear at high intensities, but noticeable also at diagnostic levels. The significance of these changes is unclear, but the lowest level needed to obtain the diagnostic information required should be used.

Higher levels of ultrasound can clearly cause tissue damage. This has been demonstrated by the technique of renal stone destruction using an ultrasound probe. Local heat can be excessive at major boundaries. It is worth remembering that, with scanners, the pulses are transmitted for as long as the moving image is viewed. This means that it is likely that more energy will be used during a real-time examination than during a static scan. Doppler studies (see appropriate section) also use a higher dose because of the longer pulses or continuous nature of the pulses as in the case of continuous-wave examinations.

The entire subject of safety of ultrasound is under continuous review, but the procedure is felt currently to be totally safe when levels in the diagnostic range are used.

What are the risks to the fetus?

Some of the more than 35 published animal studies suggest that in utero ultrasound exposure can affect fetal growth. When teratogenic effects have been found, energies capable of causing significant hyperthermia have usually existed. In other experimental systems, results of ultrasound exposure have caused changes on the cellular level but (1) most of these studies employed energy levels greater than would be expected to exist in clinical situations, (2) in vitro exposure conditions to the ultrasound used in many of the experiments are hard to place in perspective for clinical use, and (3) some of the observations have not been reproducible. The existence of these studies, however, contributes to the decision that routine ultrasound screening cannot be recommended. However, when the clinical situation needs further clarification that might result in alteration of prenatal care, sonography is appropriate.

Can ultrasound be used to determine the sex of my baby?

Although the sex of the fetus can be determined with high accuracy, at this time, the performance of sonography solely to satisfy the family's desire to know the fetal sex, to view the fetus, or to obtain a picture of the fetus should be discouraged.

Should a scan be done simply to confirm the reality of the baby?

This confirmation of pregnancy prior to presence of the baby being realized by the mother has been shown in some studies to aid bonding between mother and baby and to reduce maternal anxiety. Although this may be considered an advantage by some experts and by mothers, this is not an appropriate indication for sonography at this time.

CONSENT

No informed consent is needed since the procedure is noninvasive and safe; however, most experts believe that informed consent should be obtained for all invasive procedures such as intrauterine transfusion and surgery, drainage of fluid collections and amniocentesis.

SELECTED BIBLIOGRAPHY

Goddard P: Indications for Ultrasound of the Chest. *J Thorac Imaging* 1985;Dec:1(1):89.

Holm HH, Kristenson JK: Indications for Ultrasonic Scanning in Abdominal Diagnostics. *JCU* 1974;Mar:2(1):5.

Neilson JP: Indications for Ultrasonography in Obstetrics. *Birth* 1986;Dec:3 Suppl:11.

XIV
Other Multisystem Procedures

59

Biopsy

RICHARD M. STILLMAN

The pathologic nature of skin and soft-tissue lesions is often suspected based upon history and physical examination by an experienced clinician. However, despite seemingly innocuous appearances, malignancy must always be considered. Initial mismanagement of potentially curable malignancies may compromise the definitive treatment. Common errors to be avoided include (1) wide disfiguring resection of benign lesions, (2) inadequate excision of malignant tumors, (3) electrodesiccation of malignant tumors without biopsy, and (4) dismissal of an early malignancy as benign (e.g., soft tissue sarcoma as lipoma, melanoma as nevus, epidermoid carcinoma as traumatic ulcer).

INDICATIONS FOR PROCEDURE

Although specifics of management vary widely with the suspected lesion (see table 59–1), the following basic principles should always be considered:

(1) Biopsy any lesion that fails to respond to appropriate therapy or if there is any uncertainty about its nature.

Table 59–1. Summary of the essential clinical features and the usual treatment of common benign lesions of the skin and soft tissues [Modified with permission from Stillman, RM: *General Surgery: Review and Assessment,* 3rd edition, Appleton & Lange, 1988.]

LESION	CLINICAL FINDINGS	TREATMENT
Lesions That Have Little or No Malignant Potential		
Cavernous hemangioma	Subcutaneous lesion present at birth; may ulcerate through the skin, and may involve deep structures; consists of mature vessels and arteriovenous malformations.	Excise surgically, but beware of bleeding from major arteriovenous fistulas; high-dose steroid therapy with prednisone 4 mg/kg po may induce regression in rapidly growing tumors in children.
Cavernous lymphangioma (cycstic hygroma)	Diffuse, deep, cavernous enlarged lymph-filled spaces usually located in the neck, axilla or mediastinum; appearing before age 2.	Usually regress during childhood. If there is functional impairment or infection, excision may be considered.
Condylomata accuminata (veneral wart)	Papillomatous lesions of perianal region, penis, or vulva of viral etiology.	Carefully apply 20% podophyllin resin in 70% alcohol or treat by electrodesiccation of cryotherapy using liquid nitrogen.
Dermoid cyst	Congenital lesion that manifests later in life; firm cystic lesion that does not dimple the skin but may be adherent to periosteum.	Excise surgically.

Table 59–1. **Continued**

LESION	CLINICAL FINDINGS	TREATMENT
Epidermal inclusion cyst	Unilocular, gradually enlarging, hard nodule that results from the growth of epithelial cells in the subcutaneous tissue as a result of trauma.	Excise surgically.
Fibroma	Pink to brown firm subcutaneous lesion, fixed to the skin.	Excise or biopsy to confirm the diagnosis.
Ganglion	Tense, subcutaneous cystic growth of the tendon sheath of wrist or ankle containing tenacious mucoid material.	Excise surgically.
Glomus tumor (angiomyoneuroma)	Severely painful or exquisitely tender, red, blue, or purple, small lesion, often occurring in nail beds.	Excise surgically.
Immature hemangioma (Strawberry mark)	Raised, irregular, flat lesion, present at birth; may enlarge during the first year, but regresses by age 7.	None needed; reassure the parents.
Intradermal nevus	Generally nodular in appearance, uniform in color and soft. Histologically, melanocytes are in the dermal layer.	Usually, no treatment needed.

Table 59–1.   Continued

LESION	*CLINICAL FINDINGS*	*TREATMENT*
Keloid	Raised, dense fibrous tissue accumulation replacing a surgical or traumatic scar.	No treatment required, but if removal is desired for cosmetic reasons, excise surgically and close wound. Avoid permanently buried sutures. Recurrence is common; therefore, adjuvant therapy with postoperative low-dose irradiation, corticosteroids or methotrexate has been used.
Lipoma	Multilobular, soft, fatty, subcutaneous lesions, freely movable in the subcutaneous tissue. Lipoma is the most common subcutaneous neoplasm.	Excise surgically.
Lymphangioma circumscriptum	Verrucose, opalescent patches with edema of the adjacent subcutaneous tissue.	Excise surgically.
Lymphangioma simplex	Grayish pink, soft lesion under 1 cm in diameter.	Excise surgically.
Neurilemmoma (schwannoma)	Encapsulated, firm solitary, small nodule of nerve sheath origin.	Excise surgically.
Port-wine hemangioma (nevus flammeus)	Dark red or purple, flat lesion consisting of dilated, abnormal capillaries.	Cover with opaque cosmetic cream, or use laser therapy.

Table 59–1.   Continued

LESION	CLINICAL FINDINGS	TREATMENT
Sebaceous cyst	Painless, unilocular, fixed to skin, often with visible punctum, contains cheesy material that may become infected.	*If infected,* drain, avulse cyst wall, allow to heal by second intention; *If not infected*, excise cyst and skin attachment using elliptical incision.
Seborrheic keratosis	Flat, yellowish-brown, hyperkeratotic lesion with a greasy surface, often multiple.	Usually, no treatment is required. If the problem is the cosmetic appearance, treat by electrodesiccation or cryotherapy with liquid nitrogen.
Verruca vulgaris (common wart)	Elevated or flat, well-demarcated lesion resulting from virus-induced hyperplasia of epidermal cells.	Treat by electrodesiccation under local anesthesia apply liquid nitrogen (cryotherapy), or apply caustic agent (40% salicylic acid plaster).
Xanthelasma	Elevated yellowish cholesterol deposits of the eyelids	Excise, if desired for cosmetic reasons.

Lesions That Have Malignant or Premalignant Potential

Compound nevus	Combination of junctional and intradermal nevi; *the junctional component is prone to malignant degeneration.*	Excise or biopsy for definitive diagnosis if there is any suspicion of melanoma.

Table 59–1. Continued

LESION	CLINICAL FINDINGS	TREATMENT
Junctional nevus	Flat, irregular in size and color, usually located in the genitalia, palms, soles, or mucous membrances. Histologically, melanocytes are at the junction of the epidermis and dermis. *Prone to degeneration to melanoma.*	Excise surgically for definitive diagnosis, and because of malignant potential.
Juvenile nevi	Rapidly growing nevi occurring in pre-pubertal children.	Excise surgically.
Keratoacanthoma	Rapidly-growing red papule that may ulcerate exposing a central keratin core, spontaneous regression usually occurs within 3 months; histologically, it appears to be a well-differentiated, squamous carcinoma that has regressed because of host resistance.	Treatment is surgical excision or biopsy to confirm the diagnosis.
Neurofibromatosis	Multiple, soft, globular, sometimes pedunculated cutaneous lesions that occur in patients with von Recklinghausen's disease; *malignant degeneration occurs in 10%.*	Excise those neurofibromas that interfere with function or show signs of change suggesting malignant degeneration.

Table 59–1.   Continued

LESION	CLINICAL FINDINGS	TREATMENT
Solar keratosis	Papular, firm, hyperkeratotic lesion usually in areas chronically exposed to the sun.	Treat with electrodesiccation under local anesthesia, or by liquid nitrogen cryotherapy.

(2) Perform a preliminary incisional biopsy before surgical excision of any large lesion that may be malignant.

(3) Send all biopsy specimens to the laboratory for pathologic examination.

The presence of an abnormal tissue mass is usually sufficient indication for biopsy. Biopsy will obtain tissue for microscopic examination by a pathologist in order to determine the exact nature of the lesion. In some cases, only a portion of the lesion will be removed by biopsy (incisional biopsy), while in other cases the entire lesion will be removed (excisional biopsy).

ALTERNATIVES

Tissue for pathologic examination can also be obtained by inserting a needle into the lesion (needle biopsy or aspiration biopsy). In some cases, this method is preferred. Nevertheless, needle biopsy specimens do not always provide adequate tissue for a definitive diagnosis, and subsequent surgical biopsy may be required anyway.

CONTRAINDICATIONS

There are no absolute contraindications to diagnostic biopsy. A history of allergy to local anesthetics will prompt the surgeon to consider the use of an alternative anesthetic technique. If the patient is known to have widespread metastatic disease, biopsy of what is likely to be yet another manifestation of the same malignant process is usually not warranted. If the patient has a transmissible disease such as human immunodeficiency virus (HIV), tuberculosis, or hepatitis, biopsy should be performed with great care to minimize risk to medical personnel.

PREPROCEDURE PREPARATION

In order to minimize the chance of postoperative infection, the patient should take a bath or shower before coming to the hospital. The patient must advise the surgeon about any history of allergy to local anesthetic agents. In some cases, the surgeon will ask the patient not to eat or drink anything for at least 8 hours prior to the procedure. In most cases, this precaution is not necessary.

PATIENT EDUCATION

The patient should be made aware of the reason for biopsy, and the possible diagnoses. The patient should be advised about when the result of the biopsy will be available, and should be reassured that whatever the result, the physician will be there to explain it and answer any questions.

PROCEDURE

Biopsy is usually performed under local anesthesia in the ambulatory (minor) operating room, or in a free-standing ambulatory surgery center. In some cases, biopsy may be performed in the physician's office or outpatient setting. For small cutaneous lesions, the incision encompasses the entire lesion, and the wound is closed with sutures or staples. The incision allows access to deep lesions by dissection within deep tissues, and the wound may require closure with several layers of sutures or staples. Rarely, a soft plastic drain will be left in place for 2 days to allow drainage of tissue fluids. Following incisional biopsy, the bulk of the mass will remain. After pathologic diagnosis is made, the proper approach to removing the remainder of the mass is determined. If infection is suspected, a portion or a swab of the tissue is sent for culture and sensitivity, including an examination for acid-fast bacillus and fungi when appropriate. The specimen is sent for pathologic examination, usually preserved in formalin for permanent (paraffin) sections. In some cases, the specimen should be sent fresh (not preserved in formalin) for a frozen section examination. In general, frozen section examination is indicated when an immediate diagnosis is required to determine the need for (1) continuation of the surgical procedure, or (2) performance of special tissue studies (e.g., breast cancer will require hormonal receptor assay; lymphoma requires cell typing).

COMPLICATIONS

Rarely, there may be postoperative bleeding, infection, poor wound healing, wound drainage, or hypertrophic scar or keloid formation. When a deep soft tissue lesion is removed, the resultant cavity may be the site of accumulation of tissue fluid. This fluid may cause noticeable deep swelling to the incision, and may drain spontaneously postoperatively. Postoperative pain following superficial biopsy is minimal, relieved usually with nonsteroidal antiinflammatory agents. Postoperative pain is greater following biopsy of deep soft tissue masses and may require narcotics for relief.

POSTPROCEDURE INFORMATION

In most cases, biopsy is performed as an outpatient procedure. The patient may leave the ambulatory operating room shortly after the operation. Depending on the depth, extent and site of biopsy, there may be short-term disability due to postoperative pain or limitation of motion of an extremity. The surgeon should be asked about prescribing required analgesics prior to the procedure so that a visit to the pharmacy will not be required in the postoperative period.

PATIENT QUESTIONS

Will there be any pain after the operation?

In most cases, the pain will be minimal, and will rapidly resolve over a period of 1 to 2 days. In some cases, a mild analgesic may be required. Usually, a nonsteroidal antiinflammatory agent is recommended, e.g., acetaminophen or ibuprofen. Occasionally, a more potent analgesic will be prescribed.

When will I know the diagnosis?

In most cases, pathologic examination requires that the specimen be embedded in paraffin and sectioned after the paraffin dries. Most skin and soft tissue lesions are examined using this relatively slow, but accurate, method. The patient will be advised of the diagnosis at the next visit to your physician for a postoperative wound check within about 1 week. For some lesions, earlier diagnosis is required to allow testing of the specimen for other features. A notable example is removal of a breast mass. If a breast mass is found to be malignant, it will be important to use a portion of fresh tissue for testing for hormonal receptors. Therefore, after removal of most breast masses, a portion the specimen will be frozen and examined immediately. In this case, the patient will know the diagnosis the day of the biopsy. When a lymph node (gland) is removed for biopsy, the potential need for special studies may also dictate the need for immediate pathological diagnosis.

If the mass is malignant, what will be done?

This is a complicated question because it depends upon the location and nature of the mass. Many skin lesions are treated only by excisional biopsy, requiring no further surgery. Some may require subsequent re-excision to achieve wider margins. Deep soft tissue lesions may require surgical removal of adjacent tissues to achieve tumor-free margins. In some cases, the nature of the malignancy may dictate treatment with chemotherapy or radiotherapy.

When will the stitches be removed?

Skin sutures or staples are removed anywhere from the third to the fourteenth postoperative day. Sutures on the face are removed earlier to improve the cosmetic result, while those on the extremities are removed later to allow more complete healing. Absorbable sutures do not need to be removed.

When may I take a shower or bath?

This varies depending upon the procedure and the surgeon's preference. Usually, the patient will be allowed to shower or bathe starting on the third postoperative day. An extremity that can be wrapped in a plastic bag to protect the wound from water may allow immediate showering. Despite the theoretical chance of contamination of the wound by the bacteria that thrive in our municipal water supplies, some surgeons advocate immediate bathing of the wound to minimize pain and speed healing.

How will I know if I develop an infection?

Wound infections tend to occur around the fifth postoperative day, but may occur somewhat earlier or later. A wound infection is signaled by redness around the wound, increasing wound pain, increased warmth in the tissues around the incision, drainage of pus, or fever. If any of these findings occur, contact your surgeon. In early cases, the physician may suggest only warm compresses and possibly antibiotics until the problem is better defined. If there is a clearcut abscess, he may reopen the wound to allow drainage until it heals spontaneously.

CONSENT

Because biopsy is a surgical procedure, signed informed consent is required.

SELECTED BIBLIOGRAPHY

Bart S, Kopf A: Techniques of biopsy of cutaneous neoplasms. *Dermatol Surg Oncol* 1979;Dec:5:979.

Brennan M: The management of soft tissue sarcomas. *Brit J Surg* 1984;Dec:71:964.

Cosimi A: Conservative surgical management of superficially invasive cutaneous melanoma. *Cancer* 1984;March:53:1256.

James, A: The extent of primary melanoma excision: A reevaluation. *Ann Surg* 1983;Nov:198:634.

60

Fine-Needle Diagnostic Aspiration and Biopsy

DAVID H. GORDON AND RICHARD SADOVSKY

In recent years, fine needle aspiration and biopsy cytology have been used increasingly in the diagnosis of many solid and cystic tumors inaccessible to exfoliative cytology techniques. This technique has been widely used in European countries for 30 years with great success. The actual technique involves needling both through the surface to palpable masses as well as under radiologic guidance to aspirate any organ within reach of the fine needle.

INDICATIONS

The fundamental indication for needle aspiration and biopsy involve the presence of an abnormal mass found clinically or radiologically in a location that can be reached by a needle and for which the relative number of diagnostic possibilities is limited. Aspiration is not suited for every vague swelling or for lesions that are inflamed, unless material is desired for culture. Superficial masses such as those in the breast, thyroid, head and neck area, or soft tissue, subtaneous regions and bone can be easily reached. Lymph node aspiration has been used frequently as a procedure for diagnosis of metastatic tumor. Deeper masses located in the prostate, lung, pancreas, liver, kidney, pelvis, and other structures in the retroperitoneal space can be biopsied. The pathologic finding of the aspiration may, depending on the clinical stage, type, and resectability of the tumor, be followed only by chemotherapy or radiotherapy.

Aspiration biopsy has been frequently used for breast masses. There are only rare false positives and fewer than 10% false negatives. Clinical correlation is essential. Aspiration of lymph node material is becoming more popular. Its greatest utility lies in the ability to diagnose metastatic carcinoma although the procedure has been helpful also in the diagnosis of lymphomas. Needle tissue sampling of the thyroid is becoming routine. Sensitivity and specificity have been greater than 90% at centers doing this procedure regularly.

Positive findings on needle aspiration assist the surgeon in determining the proper procedure. Positive lymph node aspirations may save the patient from disfiguring surgery such as radical neck dissections.

Specimens obtained by needle aspiration can also be tested for pathogens such as bacteria, fungi, and *Pneumocystis carinii*.

Future cell-analysis techniques such as electron microscopy, cytometric quantitation of DNA, computer-based image analysis of cells, measurement of DNA synthesis, and techniques to look for tumor markers will allow more precise identification of tumors and their biologic behavior by aspiration techniques.

ALTERNATIVES

Noninvasive diagnostic techniques, including radiologic procedures, physical examination, isotope scanning, and hormone measurements, can be used to assist in the diagnosis, but none of these will permit a tissue diagnosis of the mass in question.

Exfoliative cytology can be performed for areas such as the lung, cervix, and the genitourinary system. Comparisons between aspiration biopsy and conventional cytology have documented the superiority of the aspiration technique. This is true also when compared with brush cytology of the lung.

Some reports state that core needle biopsies requiring frozen section interpretation for immediate analysis have been shown, at some centers, to be less accurate than fine-needle biopsies. In addition, the procedure may be difficult in patients with small masses. The cost of core-needle biopsy is higher and there is a far greater potential for hematoma formation. The skill of the pathologists and the cytopathologists may determine the relative efficacy of the two biopsy procedures.

Open biopsy can be done using surgical techniques to obtain a sample of tissue from the mass. Fine-needle biopsy, when performed properly, is safer, faster, less expensive, and less stressful to the patient, than surgery. General anesthesia for this technique is unnecessary, and so needle biopsy is highly desirable. It can be performed on an outpatient basis on an individual with normal coagulation studies.

POSSIBILITY OF FAILURE

There is some concern that the diagnosis is based on limited amounts of material. As the experience of the operator and the pathologist increases, diagnostic accuracy also increases. Care must be taken that only those specimens that contain adequate material be described with certainty. In the presence of doubt, a specimen should be described as atypical or suspicious and further investigation should be recommended. False-positive results may be disastrous whereas false negatives rarely delay diagnosis or treatment if the surgeon and the pathologist are in close communication. Centers where needle aspirations are done frequently report sensitivities and specificities close to 90% when adequate material for evaluation is obtained. Accuracy, however, in fine-needle biopsy diagnoses in more recently evaluated areas such as the prostate, is lower and highly dependent on the experience of the operator and the pathologist.

The increasing combination of needle aspiration and biopsy with radiologic techniques such as computerized tomography (CT) and ultrasound are increasing the yields of this procedure.

CONTRAINDICATIONS

Fine-needle aspiration is contraindicated in patients with a tendency to bleed. Chest or upper abdominal aspirations are hazardous in patients with uncontrolled cough, severe pulmonary hypertension, or advanced emphysema.

Primary transitional cell carcinomas should not be biopsied by this technique because of the tendency to spread along the route of the needle insertion.

PREPROCEDURE PREPARATION

History of prior bleeding disorders should be obtained. Laboratory workup should include a bleeding and clotting evaluation and a platelet count. Some centers recommend prophylactic antibiotic use starting before the procedure when the needle is inserted through a potential source of infection as might occur with transrectal needle biopsies of the prostate.

PATIENT EDUCATION

The patient should understand the procedure and what information may be learned. It is helpful to describe the syringe pistol that may be used by the operator to manipulate the syringe with only one hand. The need for radiologic assistance in the placement of the needle for deep tissue biopsies should be discussed.

PROCEDURE

The technique of fine needle biopsy is ideally suited as an office procedure in a practice with a high volume of oncologic material. The actual procedure takes only a few minutes, and immediate results can be obtained within 20 minutes. Most needle aspirations are performed using a fine needle approximately 1 mm or smaller in diameter (less than 21 gauge). Larger needles have been used to obtain tissue fragments, but this is less common. Superficial masses such as breast masses and lymph nodes can be aspirated by an ordinary 20 cc syringe with a 22 gauge needle. The technique for biopsy of these types of subcutaneous masses involves cleansing the area with an appropriate antiseptic solution and infiltrating the biopsy site with a local anesthetic, although this is not needed in some cases. The mass is fixed by one of the operator's hands with the skin being pulled tightly over the tissue to be biopsied. The needle is advanced with the other hand, and, when the mass is reached, a vacuum is created in the syringe (figure 60–1). Special syringe pistols have been developed to allow insertion of the needle and aspiration using a single hand. With full suction on the syringe, the needle is moved from side to side and, when tissue material appears to reach the hub of the needle, air pressure is allowed to return to normal and the needle is withdrawn from the biopsy site.

Smear preparation involves careful expression of the sample onto the slide using air accumulated in the syringe. If the material is mostly liquid, a smear technique similar to that of peripheral blood is used. If solid particles are obtained, the specimen is crushed with another slide or a cover slip. The specimen should be fixed and delivered to the appropriate laboratory as quickly as possible. Close cooperation with the cytopathologist is of paramount importance.

POSTPROCEDURE INFORMATION

Any signs of bleeding, swelling, or infection should be reported to the physician. The patient can return to full activity almost immediately following a superficial aspiration. Following fine-needle biopsy of the deeper organs, several days of relatively little activity are advisable.

COMPLICATIONS

The complication of fine-needle aspiration and biopsy depend on the technique of the operator, the site being sampled, the general health of the patient, and the diameter of the needle used. Complications following thyroid aspiration are very

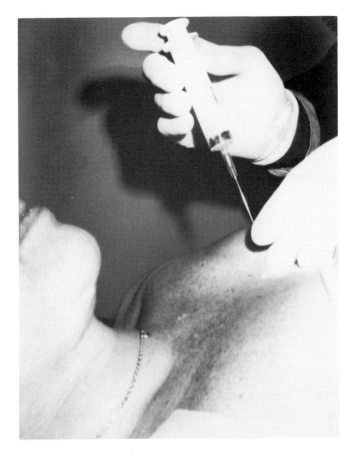

Figure 60–1. Fine-needle aspiration of a breast mass.

rare. Hematoma or ecchymosis formation has been reported, but these are generally not serious. The most common complication of chest and upper abdominal biopsies is pneumothorax, which has been found to occur in as many as 30% of patients in some studies. The incidence of these complications increases in the elderly and inoperable patients (although a minority of studies have a higher incidence of complications in younger patients, perhaps due to increased activity postbiopsy). About 10% of these patients will require a chest tube. Complications of needle biopsies of the kidney have also been studied and found to be (generally self-limiting) hematuria, perirenal hemorrhage, arteriovenous fistula formation, arteriolar aneurysms, infection, and inadvertent puncture of a different organ in the abdomen or the retroperitoneal space. Other serious complications that have been reported include gram-negative sepsis, acute peritonitis and shock, bile leakage, and broken needles.

It is apparent that tumor cells do leak out into the tissue and are deposited along the needle tract after needle aspiration and biopsy in many cases. However, there is rarely evidence of tract seeding and the tumor cells are probably destroyed by the host immune system or by some other mechanism.

PATIENT QUESTIONS

Is it possible that needling the mass might cause the spread of the tumor?

Although tumor implantation has been demonstrated, especially with needles larger than 21 gauge, it appears to have no clinical significance. Reports of cases of needle track implantation of tumor cells following biopsy of the lung have caused some objections to this technique. In most cases of seeding, a large bore needle was used in a patient who already had carcinomatosis and, in the few cases with seeding following fine-needle aspiration, the tumors present were already quite large and invasive. Clearly, however, approach to the lesion should be such that subsequent excision will encompass the needle tract. Transitional cell carcinoma does tend to spread along the tracts and, therefore, primary transitional cell carcinomas should not be biopsied by this technique.

If the aspiration is negative, does this mean that I definitely do not need a surgical procedure?

The sensitivity of needle aspiration depends on the experience of the operator and the pathologist. Assuming optimal experience, negative results of needle aspiration are accurate in approximately 90% of the procedures, and a lesion that is clinically suspicious should still be investigated further by the surgeon. In situ lesions are especially likely to be missed. The pathologic report must be correlated with the clinical picture.

Is the procedure painful?

If the patient is having a superficial biopsy, the procedure will probably not hurt any more than ordinary venepuncture. If a deeper aspiration and biopsy is being performed, the patient is given adequate local anesthesia to obviate any significant discomfort.

Can I rely on the accuracy of a positive result to make further therapeutic decisions?

Cytopathologists should and must be very conservative with positive reading of diagnostic needle aspirations and biopsies. This is generally well understood as a false-positive reading can have devastating results. The false-positive rate at most centers doing this procedure has been extremely low.

CONSENT

Informed consent is required for needle aspiration and biopsy.

SELECTED BIBLIOGRAPHY

Aretz HT, Silverman ML, Kolodziejski JL, Witherspoon BR: Fine-needle aspiration. *Postgrad Med* 1984;Feb:75:3:49.

Bottles K, Miller TR, Cohen MB, Ljung BM: Fine-needle aspiration biopsy. *Amer J Med* 1986;Sept:81:525.

Frable WJ: Fine-needle aspiration biopsy. *Human Pathol* 1984;Jan:14:1:9.

Smith EH: The hazards of fine-needle aspiration biopsy. *Ultrasound in Med* 1984;10:5:629.

61

Use of Lasers in Treatment

RICHARD SADOVSKY

The word *laser* is an acronym for light amplification by stimulated emission of radiation. The phenomenon occurs when a substance is excited to a higher energy state and stimulated to emit light when it returns to a lower energy state. Laser is a unique form of light with the special properties of monochromaticity, directionality, and coherence. These properties give laser a single wavelength, a single direction with a narrow convergence, and a fixed relationship between waves. The energy is used to stimulate the laser medium to form a beam of light. Mirrors at both ends of the medium allow trapping of the light energy and its reflection through the medium producing an intensely powerful light energy. The wavelengths determine the physical properties of the laser light.

The first medical use of lasers was by ophthalmologists in surgery for detached retina in the early 1960s. The more gentle, continuously working (as opposed to pulsating) laser brought about a renewed interest in this surgical tool in the early 1970s when the argon laser with its high absorption of blue-green light by red blood vessels was used in ophthalmology and dermatology. At around the same time, gastroenterologists began to use the near-infrared of the neodymium (Nd) YAG laser to cauterize bleeding ulcers.

Recently, red-emitting krypton lasers have been used to treat the eye, where the retina's low absorption of red wavelengths is important in reaching the subretinal choroid.

Advantages of the laser for surgical use include its high potential for accuracy, its intrinsic sterility, its hemostatic properties that make surgery relatively bloodless, and the lack of trauma to surrounding tissue that makes for less edema and faster postoperative recovery. Unlike radiation from a conventional source, all the power is easily collected and focused by a lens into a very small spot, the width of which depends on the focal length of the imaging lens.

Laser interaction with tissue can be separated into thermal and nonthermal actions. Thermal mechanisms account for the majority of applications and these can be divided into vaporization applications and photocoagulation applications. Nonthermal mechanisms imply short bursts causing micro-explosions that can disrupt tissue and produced small, desired perforations.

The types of lasers currently in use vary in the wavelength of the light. The **carbon dioxide** laser is used by surgeons as a high precision, "bloodless" scalpel because of its shallow penetration of superficial layers of tissue. Precision of dissection can be very accurate and the beam does not denature the tissues through which it passes. This minimal damage to normal tissue is one of the strong advantages of the CO_2 laser. Healing is rapid and remarkably free of pain. The **argon** laser has selective absorption by its complementary red color and has intermediate tissue penetration. This offers the surgeon the unique advantage of being able to treat lesions through clear, overlying structures. For example, lesions of the retina can be treated with no damage to the clear anterior parts of the eye, and abnormal capillary networks such as a port wine stain of the skin, without affecting the clear normal outer dermis. The **neodymium (Nd) YAG** laser, having the greatest depth of penetration, can be used to perform slow, but relatively bloodless tissue destruction and coagulation of bleeding tissue. Other lasers include the so-called "**cold beams**" used in beauty parlors that offer face lifts and f^cial toning.

INDICATIONS FOR USE

Clinical applications for lasers are increasing almost daily. Care must be taken to use them only when a clear and scientifically important advantage exists over established conventional techniques. General indications include control of bleeding, palliation of obstructing tumors, treatment of small malignant tumors, and cosmetic surgery (figure 61–1).

The use of lasers in **endobronchial surgery** has its greatest value in the palliative removal of inoperable and untreatable carcinoma of the bronchus espe-

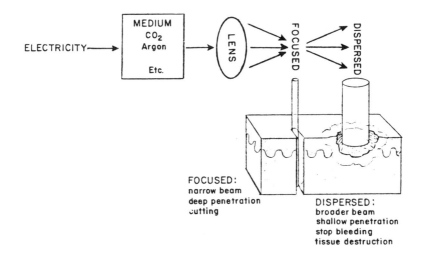

Figure 61–1. Production of laser beams and their function.

cially in patients regarded as highly at risk from anesthesia. This is done using the Nd–YAG laser through a rigid bronchoscope. Benign lesions of the endobronchial tree are rare, but also, can these, be treated in this manner. The CO_2 lasers can be used for the same purpose, and comparisons of the two types of lasers for this purpose are being done.

Dermatologic use of lasers include skin incisions, but there is probably no advantage over a scalpel incision except for patients with bleeding tendencies. Some advantages have been demonstrated in the sloughing of burns before skin grafting or of infected ulcers. In the removal of multiple lesions such as warts and condylomata, instant vaporization offers clear advantages over conventional methods, which are very time consuming.

Dermatologic practice takes advantage of the laser's ability to excise, vaporize, and coagulate. The argon laser has become the preferred treatment for port wine stains by causing thermal damage and thrombosis to the underlying capillaries that cause the discoloration. It has been shown that the thrombosed layer is eventually covered by a colorless layer of scar tissue causing a lightening in the color of the birth mark. Decorative tattoos can also be removed in this way, but some form of scar that may be a "negative" of the tattoo will remain.

Resolution of bleeding is the major indication for laser use in **gastroenterology**. Both argon and Nd-YAG lasers have been used to control acute bleeding and to prevent re-bleeding. Bleeding ulcers respond well to this treatment while esophageal varices are not as responsive. This is probably due to the fact that varices have thin walls, a large diameter lumen, and little surrounding supporting tissue making them unsuitable for laser therapy. Palliative tumor destruction is also an indication for use in the gastrointestinal system when the esophagus or stomach outflows are blocked. Tumor destruction is slow and several treatment sessions may be needed, but the benefits to the patient, although often short lived, are considerable. Almost every area of the gastrointestinal tract lends itself to use of lasers and they have been used successfully to treat duodenal, colon, and rectal lesions. Work is now going on to assess the feasibility of using lasers to fracture gallstones.

In the area of **gynecology**, CO_2 lasers have been used to treat cervical intraepithelial neoplasia, vaginal superficial lesions and carcinomas, endometriosis through the intraabdominal route, and vulvar lesions. This eliminates the need for anesthesia and the postoperative period is not complicated by heavy discharge as with cryotherapy.

Surgery of the brain requires working through a small bony window in the skull. In **neurosurgery**, lasers offer the potential of performing true no-touch surgery. Vascular tumors have been excised using lasers, as have aneurysms and arteriovenous malformations. This area is currently under study.

Regular use of lasers is being made in **ophthalmology**. Retinal photocoagulation is an established laser procedure. In addition, chorioretinal adhesions may be created by argon laser to prevent retinal detachment. Argon lasers are also used in glaucoma to relieve abnormal pressure.

In **otolaryngology**, the precision of the CO_2 laser in the removal of laryngeal lesions is well established, especially in children in whom much laryngeal pathology occurs. Tumors of the mouth and tongue can be removed bloodlessly often with analgesics postoperatively. The use of the argon laser in hemostasis during middle-ear surgery is also well established.

The use of lasers in **urology** is growing, performing excisional surgery on a number of conditions of the external genitalia and splitting the kidney for the removal of a stone. Bladder tumors can be destroyed with accuracy using the Nd–YAG laser with minimal damage to the bladder wall.

Lasers have been proposed in **cardiology** as effective instruments for surgical procedures of the intact cardiovascular system. The major problem at present in the use of lasers for ablation of lesions in the coronary arteries is that the operator cannot directly visualize the effect of the laser on the intravascular tissue. Prescribed energy doses coupled with fluoroscopic imaging are less precise ways of safely achieving desired effects. Vascular endoscopy might provide direct visualization in the future without compromising oxygen delivery.

Several applications of lasers in **cardiovascular surgery** are in the early stages. Laser-assisted microvascular anastomosis has been successfully done with a patency rate similar to conventional suturing. The tensile strength is slightly below that of a conventional repair but sufficient to prevent disruption at systemic blood pressures. Laser assisted myocardial revascularization is also being studied as is percutaneous transluminal laser angioplasty. All three biomedical lasers appear effective in dissolving atherosclerotic intravascular lesions. Laser appears to create a smooth-walled lumen that is less likely to undergo restenosis. Photosensitization of atheromata may be possible by staining techniques and sudan black is being experimentally introduced for this purpose. The problem of vascular perforation needs to be resolved.

ALTERNATIVES

With the circumstances in which lasers are being used encompassing so many parts of the body, a discussion of all the alternative therapies here would be difficult. Conventional therapies must, however, be evaluated before moving rapidly to laser treatment. For example, a variety of endoscopic treatments have been used to treat gastrointestinal bleeding. No one method is best in all situations, and in many instances nonendoscopic treatment (surgery, angiography, medication) is preferable. Nonlaser thermal devices such as the heater probe and electrocoagulation have been reported to be efficacious for gastrointestinal bleeding and, because of their much cheaper cost and portability, they may even be preferable. If the physician's hospital has a laser with a competent team to operate it, then the equation is slightly different. There is a trend in the United States to use thermal devices for nonvariceal bleeding but to use nonthermal methods such as medication, balloon tamponade, and sclerotherapy when variceal bleeding is present. Due to the lack of firm critical data it is difficult to evaluate clearly the efficacy of laser treatment.

Electrocoagulation is the use of high-frequency electrical current to generate heat. This is a new mode of therapy currently being evaluated. Early reports compare the efficacy of electrocoagulation to that of laser photocoagulation in randomized trials with active bleeding ulcers or nonbleeding visible vessels. The two modalities appear at present to be equally effective as assessed by initial or permanent hemostasis, and by the need for emergency surgery and the mortality rate.

The heater probe, which is a hollow aluminum cylinder with an inner coil, transfers heat from its end or sides to the tissue. Lesion washing is by an axial water spray. Preliminary results have been encouraging with good comparison to electrocoagulation. Advantages of these two procedures over the laser when used for hemostasis include less cost, portability of system, and the ease of use.

Comparisons of laser treatment to other conventional therapies such as balloon angioplasty have not yet been studied.

CONTRAINDICATIONS

There are no known contraindications to laser therapy besides the contraindications for performance of the procedure needed to maneuver the laser catheter into the appropriate position. Factors that predispose to poor results and complications with laser therapy include sepsis, myocardial infarction, polytraumas, and prior major surgery.

PREPROCEDURE PREPARATION

A review of medications and prior medical history should be done to identify patients with potential platelet problems since the failure of platelet function can delay laser coagulation markedly.

Premedication varies depending on the procedure. Generally, a sedative is given prior to the use of lasers in areas other than the skin. All patients wear special eye protection during laser treatment to prevent vision loss by accidental discharge of laser light into the eye.

PATIENT EDUCATION

The patient should understand the procedure and its risks.

PROCEDURE

The procedure for laser therapy varies depending on the treatment being done. Generally, a focal site is identified, the laser power is set to a predetermined wattage, the laser beam is carefully aimed, and multiple pulses are used to accomplish treatment. A continuous slow stream of gas or water is used to prevent secretions or other debris from creeping back into the tip and damaging the end of the fiber. The gas or fluid must be vented to avoid distention. In certain circumstances, water is instilled to clarify the surrounding tissue and to enhance the laser transmission.

A foot control is used to initiate the aiming beam and to operate the full power beam.

POSTPROCEDURE INFORMATION

All patients should receive written post-treatment instructions, individualized for their procedure, which include the telephone number of a knowledgeable staff member who can answer their questions.

COMPLICATIONS

The risk of complications from laser therapy increases with the amount of energy delivered and the length of the procedure. The benefit-to-risk ratio must be considered and alternate therapies must be reviewed.

Potential complications include bleeding, perforation, gas embolization, dissemination of viable cells, overdistention, fever, sepsis, pain, and danger of combustion and fire.

The greatest concern about percutaneous laser angioplasty is the possible danger of vessel perforation. The energy required for vessel perforation is no more than that required to penetrate fibrous plaque. In most cases, perforation energy is significantly less than that required to ablate calcific plaque. Several experiments have shown delayed damage to the elastic intima that could result in later aneurysms.

Rare perforations have been reported with either Nd–YAG or argon lasers. There is general agreement that lasers can paradoxically increase the severity of bleeding. If the laser beam causes vaporization of the vessel, increased hemorrhage is possible. This occurs in approximately 5% to 10% of cases reported in most studies. There are a few reports of patients who experience variceal bleeding or aspiration and death.

Thrombosis and atherogenesis are other concerns. Traumatic exposure of the arterial media to the bloodstream may cause thrombosis or new atheromatous formations. No long-term studies exist.

The fear of cerebral embolism following laser treatment of carotid artery plaque has slowed interest in this area. Although the problem of thromboembolic phenomena following laser plaque ablation has not been studied, several researchers have noted no evidence of limb-threatening ischemia following laser treatment of iliofemoral atherosclerotic plaque.

In an oxygen-enriched environment, combustible material must be carefully separated from an operating laser. Problems are most commonly seen with the CO_2 lasers. Occasionally, increased flaring can be noted at an operative site in the presence of increased oxygen concentrations. The probability of fire or burns can be reduced by ventilating patients with a nitrogen/oxygen mixture or by using only metal in the operating field when the laser is in use.

PATIENT QUESTIONS

Is laser therapy safe?

Studies that have been done so far show only rare complications when laser therapy is used in the hands of a capable clinician. The patient needs to understand, however, that the procedure is still in its early stages and that the therapeutic value must be compared with that of more conventional therapies.

Does laser use for skin lesions burn the skin?

The healing process for laser-induced burns may be different from that of thermal burns. There may be little or no pain and many patients may "forget" that they have had treatment and accidentally scratch or rub the treated skin surface. This can delay healing, and bleeding with scarring can result. In addition, laser treatment can affect pigment processes for a period following treatment, and the patient should be advised to avoid sunlight.

CONSENT

Consent is required for both the procedure allowing instrumentation to approach the lesion as well as to perform laser therapy on the affected area. Some lasers are considered investigational devices by the Federal Drug Administration (FDA) and require specific consent forms. In these investigational situations, the FDA requires that the consent form include all the potential complications applicable to the procedure, as well as a statement on the confidentiality of the records and the right of the FDA or the manufacturer to inspect the records.

SELECTED BIBLIOGRAPHY

Bailin PL, Ratz JL, Wheeland RG: Laser therapy of the skin. *Dermatol Clin* 1987;April:5:2:259.

Holloway RW, Barnes RW, Barter JF: The CO_2 laser: A guide to its use in lower genital tract disorders. *Female Patient* 1988;July:13:13.

Joffe SN, Schroder T: Lasers in general surgery. *Adv Surg* 1987;20:125.

Sanowski RA: Laser therapy in gastrointestinal practice. *J Clin Gastroenterol* 1987;9:1:83.

Stroh JA, Sanborn TA: Laser recanalization in atherosclerotic disease. *Med Times* 1988;Aug:116:8:55.

62

"Scopies" (Arthroscopy, Laparoscopy, Cystoscopy)

RICHARD SADOVSKY

The ability to use a scope to view the inside of the body has allowed physicians to directly view tissues not accessible during routine physical examination. Scoping can be done into a hollow viscus such as the urethra and the bladder, or directly into tissue through the skin as in arthroscopy or laparoscopy. Refinements of the scopes have allowed the development of instruments to do actual therapeutic procedures through the lumen of the scope. The development of fiberoptics boosted the instruments' usefulness and flexibility.

Arthroscopy, or endoscopy of the joints, is not a new procedure. In 1918 a scope was used in Japan to examine the knee; the technique was being used in the United States 5 years later. There was a lull in the use of the technique during World War II, but, in 1974, interest in the procedure resurfaced. At present, arthroscopy and arthroscopic surgery of the knee is the most frequently performed orthopedic operation. Joint evaluations are currently being performed with a rigid scope. The future of arthroscopy is being enhanced by advances in video equipment and light sources, and the use of holographic projections of the joint interior. The use of synthetic substances to replace ligaments is also under investigation.

Laparoscopy (also known as peritoneoscopy) was first performed in 1910, primarily for viewing the ovaries and the fallopian tubes. Seeing the living pathology through the laparoscope has given clinicians a new diagnostic dimension in the evaluation of abdominal and pelvic pathology.

Cystoscopy is the inspection of the urethra and the bladder wall by optical instrumentation. The instrument, called a cystoscope, uses a light source projected from its tip to permit visualization of the lower urinary tract. The quality of the equipment now enables the procedure to be performed even on newly born infants when needed.

INDICATIONS

Arthroscopy permits direct visualization of the interior joint structures of the knee, shoulder, elbow, ankle, wrist, and small joints of the hand. Although the knee is the most common joint for arthroscopic examination, the clinical value of the procedure in all these areas except the small joints of the hand has been established. The procedure permits photography, the performance of punch biopsies, and the accomplishment of small operations under direct visualization. Indications include the diagnosis of internal derangements, diseases, meniscus tears, loose bodies in the joint space, tumorous conditions of the joint, and arthritis. Arthroscopy of the knee is also being used to monitor progression of disease and the effectiveness of other therapies.

Therapeutic indications for arthroscopy include the need to wash out of debris or necrotic joint tissue, synovectomy, and other small surgical repairs.

Laparoscopy has been used to view the liver, gall bladder, peritoneum, spleen, stomach, small intestines, colon, and pelvic organs. Tissue diagnosis can be obtained and few lesions are missed. Clinical indications include liver disease, staging of carcinoma and lymphoma, peritoneal diseases, gall bladder diseases, infections, adhesions, hepatoma, fever of unknown origin, ascites of unknown origin, chronic jaundice of unknown origin, infertility, abnormalities of the female reproductive organs, and other symptoms localized in the lower abdomen. Gynecologic surgical indications for laparoscopy include resection of an ectopic pregnancy, aspiration of cysts or peritoneal fluid, coagulation of endometrial implants, tuboplasty, resection of adhesions, in vitro fertilization, ovarian biopsy, oophorectomy, myectomy, and sterilization.

Cystoscopy is used to evaluate symptoms of irritation, hematuria, voiding dysfunctions, recurrent infections, vesicoureteral reflux as well as for placement of uretheral catheters prior to percutaneous nephrolithotomy, extracorporeal shock-wave lithotripsy and retrograde pyelography. In pediatric patients, cystoscopy should be reserved for evaluation of urinary obstruction and severe congenital defects. It is probably not indicated in young patients for the evaluation of recurrent cystitis, primary enuresis, and most cases of hematuria.

ALTERNATIVES

The diagnostic accuracy of arthroscopy depends largely on the operator and the technique used. Double-contrast arthrography is an alternative to arthroscopy. The advantage of arthrography is that it can be performed as an outpatient procedure without anesthesia. There is, however, less accuracy of the diagnosis of most joint problems of the knee and there is no opportunity of treating the lesion during the same procedure. Use of the two procedures does, in select cases, increase preoperative diagnostic accuracy to almost 100%.

Arthrotomy is another alternative to arthroscopy, but the latter is preferred because of decreased patient morbidity, more rapid return to normal activities, decreased costs, and potentially better diagnostic accuracy.

Laparoscopy should be performed after appropriate diagnostic studies such as cytologic examination of peritoneal fluid, radionuclide scans, percutaneous trans-heptic cholangiogram, sonography, angiography, and CT scan have been performed. In patients with contraindications to laparoscopy, a small laparotomy incision may allow diagnostic evaluation. Laparotomy does require a longer hospital stay and a longer recuperation period. There is decreased morbidity with laparoscopy and there is a major reduction in expense. It is unclear at present whether operative laparoscopy is as effective as the more conventional laparotomy and whether there is any difference in the postoperative rate of adhesion formation and subsequent pregnancy success.

Culdoscopy has been done to aspirate peritoneal fluid. The advantage of laparoscopy is that it allows observation of peritoneal organs and permits direct biopsies. Postoperative pain has been described as less than that of culdoscopy.

Transabdominal ultrasonography has been compared with cystoscopy demonstrating good detection of bladder lesions. Intravesicular ultrasonography, however, is still an invasive procedure requiring instrumentation of the bladder and does not yield a specimen for analysis. Occasional false positives are noted on ultrasound because of large vesicular folds in a poorly filled bladder. Intravenous pyelography and cystourethrography can outline the bladder and the urethra when looking for larger lesions or anatomic abnormalities.

Urinary cytology can be performed but it has limitations and requires considerable skill on the part of the examiner. Normal cells may show marked variations in morphology. Both false positives and false negatives may be obtained. Cystoscopy is recommended in patients with any kind of atypia of voided cells.

POSSIBILITY OF FAILURE

The most common reason for an incomplete examination of the joint is failure to use the arthroscope properly. The combination of arthroscopy and arthrography can provide very accurate information about the status of the knee. Occasionally, a lesion is found that cannot be repaired through arthroscopic visualization. In this case, arthrotomy must be performed.

Laparoscopy is generally a highly effective diagnostic procedure and a route for minor surgical procedures. When laparoscopy does not allow an accurate diagnosis, or a desired procedure cannot be done through the scope, laparotomy is appropriate.

Cystoscopy is limited to viewing only the lower urinary tract. Problems occurring in the upper tract cannot be visualized, and an intravenous pyelogram and renal or uretheral ultrasound evaluation may be needed to view upper tract structures.

CONTRAINDICATIONS

There are few contraindications to **arthroscopy**. The presence of an infection anywhere in the body usually precludes arthroscopy. The evaluation of a grossly deformed joint is of unlikely value and joints demonstrating fibrosis or scarring may not permit adequate movement of the arthroscope.

Absolute contraindications to *laparoscopy* include bowel obstruction, ileus, abdominal hernia, peritonitis (although this is an indication for laparoscopy in a minority of centers), brisk intraperitoneal bleeding, and severe cardiorespiratory disease. Relative contraindications include extremes of body weight, inflammatory bowel disease, prior surgery, the presence of a large intraabdominal mass, and advanced intrauterine pregnancy.

Contraindications to rigid **cystoscopy** include conditions that do not permit the patient to tolerate the dorsal lithotomy position such as spinal cord injury and prosthetic hip devices. The ability to perform supine, bedside cystoscopic examination of these patients has eliminated this problem.

PREPROCEDURE PREPARATION

Laboratory tests that should be done prior to all scoping procedures include a hemoglobin or a hematocrit. The knowledge of prior history of allergy to anesthetics such as novocaine and xylocaine is important to the physician.

Arthroscopy should be used only as an adjunct to a complete history and physical examination as well as radiographic evaluation of the joint.

The patient should void prior to laparoscopy. Complete evaluation prior to use of general anesthesia should be performed. Premedication may be given to avoid anxiety the night before and 1 hour before the procedure.

The patient having cystoscopy should be fasting to permit full anesthesia and transurethral surgery if necessary.

PATIENT EDUCATION

The patient should understand these procedures and be aware of the associated risks and benefits. The use of anesthesia, the possibility of a hospital stay, and the postprocedure activities should also be discussed. The patient should be advised to fast from midnight prior to the procedure. The patient's history should be reviewed for hypersensitivity to anesthesia and a sedative may be given prior to the test.

PROCEDURE

The technique of **arthroscopy** is essentially the same for all joints with the exact positioning of the limb and the point of insertion of the arthroscope varying from one joint to another. Arthroscopy of the knee is, by far, the most common arthroscopic procedure. General anesthesia is commonly used, but local, spinal, or epidural anesthesia can also be administered. A tourniquet is often applied to decrease hemorrhage and enhance vision.

The procedure is done in the operating room with standard aseptic techniques. The skin is prepared with an appropriate antiseptic solution. The arthroscope is inserted through a skin incision into the joint in an angle that allows most convenience for the operator and best viewing of the internal structures (figure 62–1). Larger joints can be prepared for arthroscopy by distention with gas or saline. Manipulation of the intra-joint tissue can be done by use of a hook or a needle enhancing the visual field. If no treatable lesion is discovered, the arthroscope is withdrawn, the joint is irrigated, and the procedure is finished. Surgically treatable lesions can often be treated through the scope or through an arthrotomy.

Laparoscopy can be performed in an endoscopy room of a diagnostic unit, in the outpatient surgery unit, or in the operating room. Generally, regional anesthesia is used, although, under rare circumstances, general anesthesia may be necessary. Local anesthesia may be employed in the highly motivated patient. The patient is placed in a supine position on the table and the abdomen is prepared with an appropriate antiseptic solution. Using a large-gauge needle, a pneumoperitoneum is achieved by the injection of about 4 liters of air, oxygen, or carbon dioxide. Once this is done and the abdomen is tympanitic to percussion, a small incision is made to the right of the umbilicus and a trocar in a sheath is introduced. Placement of the scope through the sheath allows visualization of the peritoneal contents. The table can be manipulated for better visualization. Most laparoscopes have operating channels to allow passage and use of

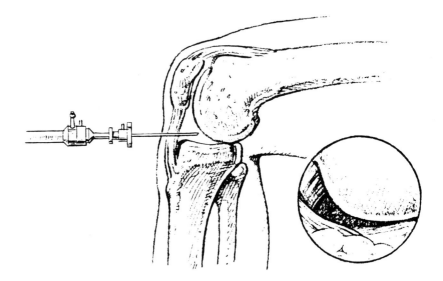

Figure 62–1. Arthroscopy of the knee.

probe, biopsy, and cautery instruments. Occasionally, a second incision or even multiple incisions are required for insertion of biopsy needles.

Operative laparoscopy usually requires general anesthesia, although sterilization under local anesthesia with sedation can be performed with little difficulty. Operative cases are usually longer and require adequate muscle relaxation. Various therapeutic techniques such as biopsy, electrocautery, thermocoagulation, suture, and laser permit surgical procedures through the scope.

After the examination is performed, the abdomen is deflated and all the equipment is withdrawn. A small dressing is applied to the incision site.

Cystoscopy usually requires general anesthesia when using rigid instrumentation and regional or local anesthesia when using flexible cystoscopy. Brief procedures performed through a rigid scope can sometimes be done under regional anesthesia. Generally, no skin shaving or other preparation is needed. The patient is asked to lie down flat in the cystoscopy room in a lithotomy position. Flexible cystoscopy has the advantage of being performed on a supine or prone patient. The actual procedure usually requires 20 minutes. The genital area is cleaned with an appropriate antiseptic solution and a local anesthetic is placed in the urethra. A cystoscope is then inserted and rotated permitting a view of the urethra and the bladder. Occasionally, the bladder is filled with an irrigating solution, and the sensation of emptying and filling may occur several times.

A tiny tube may be placed in the ureter in order to obtain a sample of urine, to take a radiograph, or to relieve a blockage. If a cause for the symptoms is discovered, the physician may decide to treat the findings at the time of the cystoscopy. If this is done, the patient is informed during the procedure.

POSTPROCEDURE INFORMATION

Following **arthroscopy** the patient should immediately be encouraged to move the joint and bear weight. The patient is usually discharged within 24 hours of the procedure, assuming complete recovery from the anesthesia. Exercise is encouraged and pain can be controlled with analgesics. The joint and limb involved should be observed for change in color, pulses, and sensation. Changes should be reported to the physician. The rehabilitation process is a little longer for patients who have undergone accompanying arthrotomy than for those who have had only arthroscopy.

Laparoscopy is a benign procedure leaving minimal scarring, minor discomfort, and little or no disability. Postoperative discomfort can be easily controlled with analgesics. The patient may shower or bathe, but should be careful not to rub the incision site.

Cystoscopy is frequently followed by some pain, and analgesics are recommended. If the pain becomes severe, the physician should be contacted. An antibiotic may be prescribed if an infection is found. The first urination following cystoscopy may burn slightly or contain a small amount of blood in the form of clots or pink urine. The urine should clear to normal color within 24 hours. The patient should drink large amounts of water and get plenty of rest. If normal urination does not resume following the procedure and several tries have been made, the patient may have to be catheterized for a short period so that urine can be emptied from the bladder. The patient should be able to return to work on the day following the procedure. The procedure should not affect sexual intercourse and normal relations can be resumed the day following the cystoscopy or as soon as the patient feels ready.

COMPLICATIONS

Complications following **arthroscopy** are clearly less than those following open surgery. The problem of infection has been rarely seen as have deep vein thrombosis and pulmonary embolism following arthroscopy of the knee. Other rare complications include persistent effusion, neurovascular damage, synovial adhesions, painful scars, bleeding from the puncture site, as well as sequelae of the anesthesia used or the position of the extremity examined.

Complications of **laparoscopy** include bleeding following trauma to major vessels or bleeding at the site of biopsy. Complications occurring during the induction of pneumoperitoneum and introduction of the laparoscope include subcutaneous emphysema, pneumothorax, introduction of gas into the lumen of the small bowel, perforation of the stomach, regurgitation of the stomach contents, direct trauma to major intraperitoneal structures, and cardiovascular collapse. Gas embolism is an extremely rare event. When operative laparoscopy is performed, damage can occur to any structure within the abdomen or the pelvis. The extent and type of complications depend on the technique of the operator and the surgical modality being used. Damage to the bowel is most serious and needs careful assessment. Frank perforation may require bowel resection and colostomy. Unrecognized damage will later present as acute peritonitis.

The few deaths that have occurred following laparoscopy for tubal sterilization were caused mainly by complications of anesthesia, followed by hemorrhage and sepsis.

The hazards of **cystoscopy** are minimal. Bacteremia, intravascular hemolysis, blood loss, and urethral strictures have all been reported in rare instances. The risk of infection is very small, and apart from the antibacterial substances within the lubricating gel, it is rarely necessary to supplement with systemic antibiotic prophylaxis or chemotherapy. However, chronically infected or at-risk patients should probably be appropriately medicated.

PATIENT QUESTIONS

What can I expect following arthroscopy?

Arthroscopy is considered a minor surgical procedure, but the patient may still have some pain following instrumentation. The patient should be reassured that normal activity will probably be possible within 24 hours of the procedure assuming that a therapeutic manipulation has not been performed. If a minor surgical procedure is done, the patient will still probably leave the hospital within 24 hours, but crutches or other limb support devices such as a sling may be needed for a brief time. There may be some swelling over the next few days accompanied by pain. The patient can generally return to work within 2 days. Those with highly athletic jobs may have to wait up to 4 weeks before resuming normal activity.

Is the procedure painful?

Generally, these procedures are all performed under local or general anesthetic and will involve little discomfort to the patient. Some unusual sensations may be noted when local anesthesia is used, such as pulling or tugging inside a joint, or a pressure-like sensation in the bladder. Any feeling that is stronger than mild discomfort should be reported to the physician.

Will laparoscopy affect my ability to conceive?

There is no evidence that laparoscopy will affect the fertility of a woman.

Will cystoscopy affect my sexual functioning or worsen urinary frequency?

There is no evidence that cystoscopy has a negative effect on sexual functioning or the flow of urine. If a urologic procedure such as dilation of the urethra is performed, the patient may note some increase in incontinence. Generally, problems following cystoscopy are related to functional causes rather that physiologic ones.

CONSENT

Informed consent is required for all the above scoping procedures.

SELECTED BIBLIOGRAPHY

Dandy DJ: Arthroscopy: the endoscopy of joints. *Br Med Bull* 1986;Jul:42:3:301.

Diehl JT, Eisenstat MS, Gillinov S, Rao D: The role of peritoneoscopy in the diagnosis of acute abdominal conditions. *Cleve Clin Q* 1981;Fall:48:3:325.

Ohlgisser M, Sorokin Y, Heifitz M: Gynecologic laparoscopy. A review article. *Obstet Gynecol Surv* 1985;Jul:40:7:385.

Siegler AM: Gynecologic endoscopy in infertility. *Obstet Gynecol Clin North Am* 1987;Dec:14:4:1015.

Snyder JA, Smith AD: Supine flexible cystoscopy. *J Urol* 1986;Feb:135:251.

Watson B, Gittes R, Walsh J: Instructions for patients for cystoscopy. *AUAA J* 1982;July–Sept:13.

SUMMARY CHART OF PROCEDURES

This chart is a reference for the majority of cases, but unique individual circumstances may require special management

Column 1. Absolute contraindications (+/-)
Column 2. Relative contraindications (+/-)
Column 3. Patient preparation required (Does the patient need to do anything before the test) (+/-)
Column 4. Consent required (+/-)
Column 5. Always done as inpatient (+/-)
Column 6. Always done as inpatient (x/-)
Column 7. Is sedation given? (+/-)
Column 8. Anesthesia (+/-)
Column 9. If yes, type of anesthesia (G = general, R = regional, L = local)
Column 10. Significant after effects patient will feel (+/-)
Column 11. Special instructions following procedures that are directly related to the procedure (+/-)
Column 12. Follow-up visit to physician recommended specifically as a result of having procedure (+/-)
Column 13. Do significant complications occur in more than remote instances (+/-)

Procedure (Chapter)	1	2	3	4	5	6	7	8	9	10	11	12	13
Acupuncture (15)	-	-	-	-	-	-	-	-		-	-	-	-
Ambulatory ECG Monitoring (1)	-	-	-	-	-	-	-	-	-	-	-	-	-
Amniocentesis (41)	-	-	+	+	-	+	-	+	L	+/-	-	+	-
Arteriography (2)	+	+	+	+	-	+	+/-	+	L	+/-	+	-	+
Arthroscopy (62)	-	+	-	+	-	+	-	+	LRG	+/-	+	-	-
Biopsy (59)	-	+	+	+	-	+	+/-	+	LRG	+/-	+	-	+
Biopsy, Lymph Node (51)	-	-	+	+	-	+	+/-	+	L	+/-	-	-	-
Bone Marrow Aspiration and Biopsy (13)	-	+	-	+	-	+	-	+	L	+/-	-	-	-
Bone Marrow Transplantation (13)	-	-	+	+	+	-	-	-		+	+	+	+
Bronchoscopy (20)	-	+	+	+	-	+	-	+	LG	+/-	+	-	-

Procedure											
Cardiac Catheterization and Coronary Angiography (3)	+	+	+	L	+/−	+	−	+	+	+	−
Cardiac Electrophysiologic Studies (4)	+	+	+	L	+/−	+	−	+	+	+	−
Cardiac Pacing (5)	+	−	+	LG	+/−	+	+	+	−	+	−
Chest Tube Insertion (21)	−	−	+	L	+/−	+	+	−	+	+	+
Colonoscopy (25)	+	+	+		−	+	−	+	+	+	+
Colposcopy and Colpocentesis (42)	−	−	+		+	+	−	+	+	+	−
Computerized Tomography (54)	−	−	+		+	−	−	+	+	+	−
Cone Biopsy and Conization (43)	+	+	+	LRG	+/−	+	−	+	+	+	−
Culdoscopy and Culdocentesis (44)	+	+	+	L	+/−	+	−	+	+	+	−
Cystoscopy (62)	+	−	+	LRG	+/−	+	+	+	+	+	+
Dermabrasion (48)	+	−	+	L	+/−	+	−	+	+	+	+
Dialysis (38)	+	−	+	L	+/−	−	−	−	+	+	+
Digital Subtraction Angiography (2)	+	−	+	L	−	+/−	−	+	+	−	−
Doppler and Plethysmography (6)	−	−	−		−	−	−	−	−	−	−
Echocardiography (7)	−	−	−		−	−	−	−	−	−	−
Electrical Stimulation Therapy (16)	−	−	−		−	−	−	−	−	−	−
Electroencephalography (28)	−	−	−		−	−	−	−	−	−	−
Electromyography (29)	−	+	−		−	−	−	−	−	−	−
Endoscopic Retrograde Cannulation of the Pancreas (24)	+	+	+	L	+/−	+	−	+	+	+	−
Enzymatic Thrombolysis (8)	+	+	+		+/−	−	−	+	+	−	+

Procedure (Chapter)	1	2	3	4	5	6	7	8	9	10	11	12	13
Esophagogastroduodenoscopy (25)	–	+	+	+	–	+	+	+	L	+/–	–	–	–
Evoked Potentials (30)	–	–	–	–	–	–	–	–		–	–	–	–
Fine – Needle Diagnostic Aspiration and Biopsy (60)	+	+	–	+	–	+	+	+	LG	+/–	+/–	+	+
Fluorescein Angiography of the Eye (33)	+	+	–	+	–	+	–	–		+	–	–	–
Gastrointestinal Motility Studies (26)	–	–	+	+	–	+	–	–		+/–	–	–	–
Gastrointestinal Radiographic Dye Contrast Studies (27)	+	+	+	–	–	+	–	–		+/–	+/–	–	–
General Anesthesia (17)	–	+	+	+	+		+	+	G	+/–	+	–	+
Intraocular Foreign Body Removal (33)	–	–	–	+	–	+	+/–	+	LG	+/–	+	–	+
Laparoscopic Tubal Ligation (45)	–	+	+	+	+		+	+	LRG	+/–	–	–	–
Laparoscopy (62)	+	+	+	+	+	+	+	+	LRG	+/–	–	–	+
Laryngoscopy (34)	–	+	–	+	–	+	+/–	+/–	LG	–	+/–	–	–
Lasers (61)	–	–	–	+	–	+	+/–	+/–	LG	+/–	+	+	+
Lithotripsy (39)	+	+	–	+	–	+	+/–	–	LRG	–	–	–	–
Lumbar Puncture (31)	+	+	–	+	–	+	–	+	L	+/–	+	–	–
Magnetic Resonance Imaging (55)	–	+	–	–	–	–	–	–		–	–	–	–
Mammography (46)	–	–	–	–	–	–	–	–		–	–	–	–
Mediastinoscopy (22)	+	+	+	+	+		+	+	G	+/–	+	+	+

Procedure	1	2	3	4	5	6	7	8	9	10	11	12
Myringotomy (35)	−	−	−	+	−	+	+	+	LG	+/−	+	+
Nasal Packing for Epistaxis (36)	−	+	−	+	−	+	+/−	+/−	L	+	+	+
Percutaneous Transluminal Angioplasty (9)	+	+	+	+	+	−	+	+	L	+	−	−
Phototherapy (49)	+	+	−	+	−	−	−	+		+	+	+
Positron Emission Tomography (56)	−	−	−	+	−	−	+/−	−		−	−	−
Postoperative Pain Management (18)	+	+	−	+	−	−	+/−	−		−	−	−
Proctosigmoidoscopy (25)	−	+	+	−	+	−	−	−		−	−	−
Pulmonary Function Testing (23)	−	+	−	−	−	−	−	−		−	−	−
Radionuclide Diagnostic Procedures (57)	−			+/−		−	−	−		−	−	−
Regional Anesthesia (19)	+	+	−	+/−	−	+	+/−	+	R	−	−	−
Skin Grafting (50)	−	+	−	+	−	+	+/−	+	LRG	+	+	+
Skin Testing (52)	+	+	−	+	−	−	−	−		−	−	−
Stress (Exercise) Testing (10)	+	+	−	+/−	−	−	−	−		−	−	−
Traction (53)	+	+	+	+	−	+	+	−		−	−	−
Transfusion (14)	−	−	−	−	−	−	−	−		−	−	−
Ultrasonography (58)	−	−	−	−	−	−	−	−		−	−	−
Urethral Catheterization (40)	+	+	−	−	+	−	−	−		−	−	−
Vasectomy (47)	−	+	−	+	−	−	+/−	+	L	−	−	−
Vestibular Function Testing (37)	−	−	−	−	−	+	−	−		−	−	−
Vein Stripping and Ligation (11)	+	+	+	+	+	+	+	+	G	+	+	+
Venography (12)	+	+	−	+	−	+	+/−	−		−	−	+

Index

RELATED TITLES OF INTEREST

PATIENT CARE PROCEDURES FOR YOUR PRACTICE
edited by Charles E. Driscoll, M.D. & Robert E. Rakel, M.D.
ISBN: 0-87489-444-1   1988   280 pp. $32.95

PATIENT CARE FLOWCHART MANUAL, 4th Ed.
edited by Steven R. Alexander, M.D.
ISBN: 0-87489-430-1   1988   672 pp. $59.95

CARDIOLOGY: PROBLEMS IN PRIMARY CARE
Thomas H. Lee, Jr., M.D. & Richard T. Lee, M.D.
ISBN: 0-87489-463-8   late 1989   320 pp. (tent.) $39.95 (t)

PULMONARY MEDICINE: PROBLEMS IN PRIMARY CARE
Robert D. Brandstetter, M.D.
ISBN: 0-87489-468-9   1989   768 pp. $52.95

OTOLARYNGOLOGY: PROBLEMS IN PRIMARY CARE
edited by D. Thomas Upchurch, M.D.
ISBN: 0-87489-442-5   1988   325 pp. $42.95

UROLOGY: PROBLEMS IN PRIMARY CARE
edited by Elroy D. Kursh, M.D. & Martin I. Resnick, M.D.
ISBN: 0-87489-419-0   1987   344 pp. $43.95

NEUROLOGY: PROBLEMS IN PRIMARY CARE
James L. Bernat, M.D. & Frederick M. Vincent, M.D.
ISBN: 0-87489-407-7   1987   656 pp. $46.95

Send me the following Medical Economics Books on 30-day approval.

Quantity   *ISBN*   *Title*

_____

_____

_____

☐ *Check enclosed, including $3.00 handling.*
  Publisher pays postage. NJ, NY, and CA residents add sales tax.
☐ *Bill me, including postage and $3.00 handling.*
☐ *Bill my credit card + postage and $3.00 handling.*

Name _____

Signature _____

Address _____

City/State/Zip _____
        P.O. Box not acceptable

Prices subject to change without notice.

Mail completed coupon to:
Medical Economics Books
Box C-779 Pratt Station
Brooklyn, NY 11205-9066
Or call: 1-800-666-6525

NBA9